URBAN, SOCIAL, AND EDUCATIONAL ISSUES

Third Edition

Edited by

LEONARD H. GOLUBCHICK, Ph.D.
BARRY PERSKY, Ph.D.

A Doctorate Association of New York Educators Series

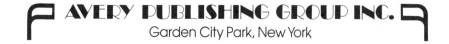

AVERY PUBLISHING GROUP INC.
Garden City Park, New York

Library of Congress Cataloging-in-Publication Data

Urban, social, and educational issues / edited by Leonard H.
   Golubchick, Barry Persky. – 3rd ed.
      p.   cm. – (A Doctorate Association of New York Educators
series)
      Includes bibliographies.
      ISBN 0-89529-377-3
      1. Education–United States.   2. Educational sociology–United
States.   3. United States–Social conditions–1945-   I. Golubchick,
Leonard H.   II. Persky, Barry.   III. Series.
LA217.U73 1988
370'.973–dc19

87-30649
CIP

LA
217
U73
1988

Preface

These are interesting times for those involved in urban development. In virtually every MSA (Metropolitan Statistical Area) one finds a declining core city in terms of residents and jobs, while the surrounding area is growing with both. (The *city* of Miami is about 400,000, while the Miami *Metro* Area is 2 million people). As our economy becomes even more dominated by service jobs and income, we can see a new American Dream—to live in one suburb and work in another. Among other things, this totally defeats our mass transit systems, which are "Hub–Spoke" systems designed to get you from your suburban house to your downtown job. These new "Suburban Growth Corridors" are expanding all over America, moving out along freeways, with new housing on one side of the freeway and new clean, quiet service jobs on the other.

As a result, the "middle" of the core city's population will decline even more, as bright black and hispanic workers are now moving to the suburbs in very large numbers, along with whites. (In the past, barriers to middle class access for talented minorities meant that there was a talent pool *within* the core city which today has been successful and has moved to the Suburban Growth Corridors, leaving less talented minorities behind in the core.)

If one looks at the school reform movement in 1987, one is struck by the over-emphasis on *picking* winners through education, and the lack of emphasis on *creating* winners. In the 40 states that have passed some legislation requiring higher standards for the high school diploma, only 4 have passed *money* bills that will allow each child an equitable chance at meeting these higher standards. At the moment, most states resemble a track coach with an athlete who can't clear the high jump bar at five feet. Rather than providing additional coaching, the coach suggests that the bar be set up to six feet, just as an experiment. The experiment isn't needed—if you can't clear five feet, you certainly won't make six feet without some increased coaching and help.

There has been limitless talk about the *nation* being at risk, and no talk about *youth* being at risk. Yet, today in America, 40% of the poor are children (13 million) while only 10% of the poor are over 65 (3 million), the highest figures on childhood poverty in four decades. If we add physically and emotionally handicapped, as well as children who don't speak English, the numbers begin to leap out at you, even though the Reagan administration has consistently ignored the issue.

The burden of these and other social problems has been heaped on America's cities, which are *clearly* more "at risk" than they have been for years. The papers in this volume have been carefully selected to indicate the enormous *range* of issues that impinge on urban education as we move inexorably toward the year 2000, only 14 years away as this is written. Although the problems of urban education are immense, it is clear from this book that we have learned many things about successful urban schools, that we can face the future with a modicum of hope. And, indeed we must, in that the demography shows a decline in youth populations for at least a decade. There is no youth surplus—*everyone* must succeed. Particularly the 37% of our public school students who are minority, and who are concentrated in urban schools. If minority children fail in school, the future of *whites* will be diminished as well.

This volume presents the range of urban school issues as a series of challenges and opportunities. The problems are severe, but we know enough about urban school successes to be optimistic. It is hoped that the reader will come away from this volume with the same view.

Harold L. Hodgkinson
American Council on Education

Contents

the creation of connections or links throughout our culture. The schools can build such links.

Teachers and parents need to regain some of their lost authority and help youth contribute to society—not just borrow from it.

Violence and school discipline are separate problems, insists Dr. Wayson. Confounding them only reduces the likelihood of solving either.

School desegregation is not just another school reform; it also reforms the socialization function of schools. The authors present evidence that school desegregation leads to desegregation in several areas of adult life.

Magnet schools offer a strategy for low-cost, highly visible, incremental change, say the authors. Though magnet schools are not a panacea, they are certainly a powerful tool for educational change.

The authors describe a collaborative effort between the New York City Board of Education and the Board of Higher Education. The program is designed to curb the high dropout rate in secondary schools.

With the exception of desegregation, no other subject has aroused as much passion as that over schools educating students with limited English proficiency. A pro-con look at bilingual education is presented.

A discussion of the current ''child abuse'' crisis, its presumed causes and putative cures, from a critical perspective.

Dr. Holman describes recent research in the area of ''latchkey children'' and programs designed to meet their needs.

The author discusses the scope of the teenage suicide problem and how we can develop programs to prevent teenage suicide.

The area of school finances has been influenced by court decisions, legislation, and public interest in the last few decades. Aspects of these changes are discussed.

This article examines the merits of proposals to increase the length of the school term.

The author outlines why peer review works in Toledo and why he established an intern/intervention program for his union and its members.

State-required testing of teachers is spreading to nearly every state. The author discusses the pros and cons of these tests.

Recent research on teaching effectiveness is reviewed and the arguments for its practical usefulness are summarized.

The preservice teacher should have exposure to existing theory and programs for gifted and talented students. Such a program is discussed by the article.

In light of the present-day focus on educational reform, a review of current practice in preservice education is offered together with a rationale for extended field services.

Drawing on his extensive research on teacher incompetence, the author discusses the nature, origins, and detection of incompetence and describes how administrators deal with this problem.

The author explores the nature of the educational work setting and the characteristics of teachers themselves in order to understand teacher job satisfaction.

Field research discloses that the work of classroom teachers is pervaded with many philosophic elements. Suggestions are offered by the author as to how the quality of such philosophizing can be improved.

An industrial quality circle technique is making its way into service organizations, including schools. The author outlines the quality circle technique in accordance with John Dewey's educational philosophy.

The author discusses the status of literacy today—from what it is and whether it is getting better or worse to how and why we got here. Current research is looked at, including dyslexia and learning disabilities.

The author contends in his article that there are various models of the learner and that the appreciation of that variety is what makes the practice of education something more than a scripted exercise in cultural rigidity.

This article reviews the literature on characteristics of effective schools, classrooms, and instructional processes.

The "SMRT-STEPS" Project (pronounced "smart steps") is described by the authors. This project can provide a school-level diagnostic-prescriptive "school mastery of reading test" system to enhance the progress in schools.

Under the auspices of the National Academy of Education's Commission on Reading, the country's leading experts on reading and language development addressed the question "Which approach to phonics works better?" The result: "Becoming a Nation of Readers," a 147-page booklet giving a systematic account of what we know about learning to read. This article is a synopsis of that report.

The author discusses the "adultification" of childhood in the media, especially television.

The author discusses the research as well as programmatic consideration in the area of mainstreaming.

The author discusses the scope of learning disabilities in terms of what is a learning disability, identifying learning disabilities, and the interaction between left and right hemisphere processes.

The authors discuss the implementation of the all-day kindergarten programs as well as developing the most effective program possible.

The author discusses our needs in meeting the demands for trained personnel in science and math.

The presence and influence of computers in education continue to grow, yet the uses to which computers are being put are often disquieting. The author sketches two possible but very different futures for education, in the hope that educators will learn to use computers effectively for learning.

The school-home partnership is a growing phenomenon and needs to be recognized. We need to learn how to deal with this relationship and render it useful to serve the best interests of educators, students, and parents.

This article examines the forces which lead to the adoption of a curricular innovation in the middle school of an urban community.

The current crisis in urban education is symptomatic of a general crisis in urban life. The crisis is in part reflected by the population patterns and projections impacting upon urban America. These have policy implications for American Educators.

This article surveys the latest waves of immigrants to our shores and their problems in terms of acculturation.

By the end of the century, approximately two-thirds of all work will be information work. If information is now our "crucial resource," what does this portend for citizenship and the education of citizens? This article attempts to answer this question.

This article discusses different conceptualizations of intelligence and focuses on family factors that influence children's intellectual development; research on trends in national SAT scores is highlighted.

Day care fulfills a tremendous need. Young children growing up in families in which both parents work, or who are brought up by parents who are struggling with the financial and emotional demands of single parenthood, need the nurturance and care that good day care programs can provide.

The traditional family—with mother in place—remains the best setting to nurture self-confident and well-adjusted children.

The way we care for children and other dependent family members has not changed nearly as much as we have thought, but there is concern that the personal element of caring not be lost.

In certain aspects of development, peer relationships play a key role. Indeed, chronically poor peer interaction is one of the most potent indices of trouble ahead.

The author explores the extent of the drug problem in our society and the implications for educators in designing drug prevention programs.

Foreword

Urban, Social and Educational Issues must be treated jointly if our public schools are to remain viable centers for the transmission of our culture and heritage. Education is facing a great reform movement; if the schools are to meet their mission there must be a concerted effort by the entire community to ensure that the schools are to educate our youth. The bulwark of our democratic way of life is an educated populace.

The editors can remember sitting in university courses dealing with social problems such as gangs, drugs, and school busing. Many of the students from the suburbs strenuously objected to the emphasis on these issues which they felt were strictly related to the inner-city and had no relevance to their communities. We have seen that these issues make no distinction regarding social class or distance from the core of the city. What is unfortunate is that efforts to combat these social problems by government agencies are only fully mobilized when the influential middle and upper citizenry are affected and can make their feelings known. Such can be viewed in the drug dilemma. No mass efforts were made to combat it until it affected the middle class and the suburban communities. In the same light, educational reform movements are a response to illiteracy and high dropout rates and the ability by our educational system to meet the demands of a high-tech society.

In putting together a book of readings, the selection of what to include and what to exclude is of primary concern. In this case, the editors were indeed fortunate to have a great resource of talented authors to draw upon. Therefore, editors were very fortunate in being able to be highly selective about what to include. The negative aspect of this is that many excellent articles had to be ex-

cluded. We hope to use these articles in a future publication. The use of all materials would have produced a book of unwieldy proportions and too diverse a scope for students of the social sciences and education.

The articles are written by professionally trained educators and social scientists who are active in the field of education. Thus, the contributions are of a relevant nature and offer insights into the science of education. Most of the articles were written specifically for this sourcebook.

The text is divided into six sections: Section I: Overview of Critical Issues; Section II: School Climate and Behavior; Section III: National issues; Section IV: Teaching as a Profession; Section V: Curriculum Issues; Section VI: Urban Issues.

The editors feel that we have compiled a book of readings on educational and social issues which is as pragmatic and meaningful to the beginning student as it is to the graduate student and the experienced professional in the field of education or the social sciences.

We wish to extend our thanks to our friends, colleagues, and members of the Doctorate Association of New York Educators. We also wish to thank our editorial board who had the difficult task of selecting the articles which appear in this book from a great source of talented authors. We wish to extend special thanks to Eleanor Cook, Rebecca Edwards, and Elaine Morenberg who have helped us assemble this text, as well as to our wives Judy and Regina and to our children Jeffrey, Craig, and Sherry.

Dr. Leonard H. Golubchick
Dr. Barry Persky

Editors

Section I
Overview of Critical Issues
Introduction by James P. Dixon*

This section is about social change and the common school. In a broad sense it is about dissatisfaction with the performance of public schools and what can or should be done to improve the situation. It is about reform rather than radical social change. Although for differing reasons, none of the contributing authors consider abandonment of the common school to be an appropriate course of action. This failure to support radical action places the discussion in the context of social change commonly called reform. Reform is incremental social change. It often occurs in systems and organizations in which goals are expressed in terms of value preferences and which provide services in a publicly sanctioned monopoly to a demographically diverse clientele.

The common school is such an organization. It is a social institution of professional teachers. Traditionally, professionals in human services fields, be they teachers, physicians, psychologists, or ministers, have viewed the application of their particular expertise as means to the larger end of maintaining the integrity of individuals who are seen as the smallest indivisible component of civilized society. Despite their monopoly status, they have defended against complaints of elitism by offering services to all comers regardless of race, creed, national origin, type of employment or economic status. This traditional behavior is under a severe challenge in post-modern society from those who claim that learning, health and salvation are not human rights but marketable commodities. Such a challenge is a powerful stimulus for counter offensive organizational reform. The outcomes are far from clear. While it is not yet apparent that the challenge will affect all human service organizations in similar fashion, it can be said that the notion of service as commodity is gaining currency in the health field. As this occurs it appears that social class distinctions are accentuated.

For reforms to succeed requires agreement about issues, consensus upon values, and information to de-

fine interventions. While these authors have different views about the underlying causes of dissatisfaction and the appropriate actions to be taken, they show a consensus on the nature of the dissatisfactions and the constraints on change. While he intends to speak only for himself, Erdberg describes key issues in much the same terms as the others.

Goodlad, employing a typology of academic/intellectual, social/citizenship, vocational, and personal goals, found that students, parents, and teachers agreed about goals in general but were unable to agree on a top priority. He interprets this finding as supportive of the existence of a consensus on goals and aspirations. He believes that there is a working consensus on both the kind and amount of formal education which children should have and on the organization and conduct of schooling. Simply put, this is that all students require education that is at least equivalent in function to what the common elementary school provided at the end of the century. In other words, secondary education is now included in the definition of the common school. It is the high school which now controls direct entry to the workforce and indirect entry to the workforce through control of entry to the university. The new common school is at the epicenter of the definition of work and workers in an emergent, information-dependent, entrepreneurial and service-oriented society. The impact of reform in the common school influences social change in all human service institutions.

Reform is a process. Its viability depends upon consensus, information, and intervention. The establishment and maintenance of consensus for reform in an open society enthralled by a dream of hope and the possibility of abjuring violence as agent of change is problematical. Success requires not only an agreement about values, constraints, outcomes, and issues. It requires also the support of a majority of the citizenry.

*Dr. James P. Dixon is Professor, University of North Carolina, Chapel Hill.

In a systemic view, consensus involves agreement about the nature of a complex of variables interacting dynamically within external constraints. One of the important constraints acting on the common school is the Constitution. MacMurtrie and Zirkel remind us that there is not a constitutional guarantee of education. Education is a matter for the states. The common school is subject to constitutional provision separating church and state. It must operate under law. Laws can and do prescribe eligibility for service to students as well as terms of employment of teachers.

There are other constraints to reform in the schools. Bureaucracy and hierarchy are common characteristics of social order in advanced industrial countries. Both severely limit intrinsic institutional innovation and change. In the United States, meritocracy seems to be a distinctive quality of public employment and as such is viewed as an impediment to both the preparation and the employment of teachers. An equally important constraint, which may weigh in most heavily in large cities, is the phenomenon of local control, which appears to some to block the development of special schools for the gifted. These constraints notwithstanding, the authors of this chapter seem to prefer to base reform on the continuation rather than the abandonment of the common school.

There is little disagreement about the presence of a profound dissatisfaction with schooling. In the aggregate, the schools have generated a reasonably adequate workforce, perhaps because mandated attendance at present population levels produces a significant oversupply. But illiteracy persists, and many high school graduates are unemployable. These apparent failures undermine the American dream. It may be that this is because of an excess of hope. It could be that attitudes, behaviors, and experiences crucial to the support of learning for many individuals lie outside the purview of the school, just as most of the effective supports of health lie outside the purview of the hospital.

Argument by analogy is useful in examining the potential of reforms. Shanker makes effective use of analogy in his proposal to support increasing the professionalization of teaching by comparing it to the reform of medicine which commenced in the first quarter of the twentieth century. At the general level of the transfer of knowledge this analogy is apt. The role of teachers in support of learning is rather like the role of doctors in support of health. Physicians, however, devote their major attention to intervention in disease. Their orientation is fueled by a national preoccupation to defeat death which is vastly more obsessive than the national preoccupation to defeat ignorance.

This difference aside, Shanker seems correct in his perception of the potential power of higher education to create and defend professional monopolies. The power to make this happen is concentrated in the elite research universities. Presently, the attention paid to teaching as contrasted to the attention paid to medicine in these institutions is minor indeed, and resistance to reform is as strong as in the common schools.

While it may be true, as Goodlad hopes, that democratic values and aspirations are constant and ubiquitous forces guiding the natural experiment of the common school, the statistical evidence reported by Passow and the informed opinion of Erdberg make clear that the outcomes of the experiment are far short of ideal for the growing concentration of the disadvantaged, the poor, and the racial and ethnic minorities who occupy central cities. Passow argues that reform of urban education is contingent upon understanding urban change and underscores the role of demographic and cultural research in contributing to that understanding.

The essence of institutional reform is the belief that social change is best served not in abandonment, but in continued improvement of existing institutions, when this belief in reform can be supported by plausible hypotheses that can be tested without reckless risk to institutional survival. These authors seem to agree that while it is reckless to view the common schools in isolation from the institutions of the community, the state and the nation, within a systemic view of social structure, reform is possible.

Chapter 1
Our Profession, Our Schools: The Case for Fundamental Reform
Albert Shanker*

Once in a great while, and usually spurred by crisis, a combination of forces and ideas come together in a way that makes real change possible. In the field of education and in the lives of teachers and students, I believe that now is such a time. I would like to recount for you some of the events of the past few years, and particularly of the last few months, that have brought us to this point of both crisis and opportunity.

This year marks the three-year anniversary of the beginning of the education reform movement in this country. In the spring of 1983, the National Commission on Excellence in Education released its report, *A Nation at Risk,* which was soon followed by well over a dozen others. This union supported the basic thrust of those reports even while we had serious disagreement with some of their specifics. We did that for two reasons. First, we saw that the reports did not represent an attack by the enemies of public education. These were friends and potential allies talking, and they were powerful ones. Not a single report recommended tuition tax credits or vouchers. On the contrary, they accepted public education as the delivery system and said that what is needed is not to provide an alternative or destroy what we have, but rather to make it a high quality institution.

Second, many of the criticisms in the reports were accurate. While the schools had made admirable progress in some areas—particularly in reaching out to new populations that had been previously ignored, such as the handicapped—the overall picture was not encouraging. Standards had fallen. SAT scores had declined rapidly over two decades. Although there were isolated gains, significant numbers of our children were growing up without basic literacy and numeracy skills, and even larger numbers could not craft a well-structured sentence, explain basic concepts of science, or advance a logical argument. Discipline problems, particularly in urban settings, were draining and demoralizing teachers. High schools had too many electives, and too

many of those were frivolous. In many places, student grades, promotions, and graduation certificates were becoming devalued currency.

The Gallup polls reflected the public's concern. Each year, a higher and higher percentage of the American people gave low or mediocre marks to the schools. Meanwhile, demographic changes—people having fewer kids, people living longer—meant that a smaller and smaller percentage of the adult population felt they had a direct stake in the public schools.

So, when the reform reports came, we welcomed them, both because we were deeply concerned about the problems they described and because they were authored by people who cared about public education and were in a position to do something about it. Throughout the period that followed, the AFT, its local affiliates, and its members engaged the debate fully. We led the fight for some of the changes that followed; we were strong supporters of others; equally important, we were able to beat back many of the dangerous and simple-minded proposals masquerading as education reform. Indeed, our receptivity to the reports enhanced our ability to be critical.

I don't think I have to tell all of you how successful our approach has been. Our open and welcome attitude toward school reform has evoked a tremendously positive response from governors, state legislatures, and the business community. People who once wanted to unilaterally impose their views on us now respect the positions that we have taken; generally, they no longer do what they once did as a matter of course, which is to act without talking to us first.

More often than not, we are now called in at the very beginning, and we are told, "You people took a

*Albert Shanker is president of the American Federation of Teachers. This article is based on a series of speeches. Reprinted with permission from *The American Educator,* the quarterly magazine of the American Federation of Teachers, Fall, 1986.

responsible and courageous position three years ago. Without you, this entire reform effort would have been destroyed or seriously hampered. From now on we don't want to make any moves without bringing you in as partners."

What we did over these three years has been a tremendous success, and I think we should enjoy a round of self-congratulations for a good strategy.

In these first years of the reform movement, not only has the voice of teachers been firmly established, but also, progress has been made in the schools. Course requirements have been stiffened. Teacher salary has gone up, in some cases significantly. Education budgets have gotten healthy new infusions of money—in South Carolina a 32 percent increase in just one year, teacher pay up 33 percent in Texas in a year, education spending up 12 percent in California in a year. In addition, important new alliances have been cemented. The business community, keenly aware that its own competitiveness rests on an educated workforce, has moved beyond token gestures to serious, long-term support for public education.

Yet, while the early reform reports were needed to get things started, they didn't go far enough. Not by a long shot. Their recommendations were compromised by a central flaw: They told us where to go but not how to get there. It is fine to call for three years of math and science. We're for that. But simply sounding the alarm will not produce the thousands and thousands of math and science teachers without whom those classes can't be taught. We don't have nearly enough math and science teachers to teach the classes now required. The National Science Teachers Association estimates that 30 percent of the teachers now assigned to teach science are doing so without the appropriate academic background.

The same is true of the other recommendations. The reports called for children to write more—a paragraph a day, a paper a week, two papers a week, three papers a week, more writing all across the curriculum. We're for that. We know that writing is important not only as the development of a craft in its own right, but also because it is probably the best way to teach children to think clearly, cogently, critically. But for a teacher with five classes a day and thirty kids per class, where is the time going to come to really help a child learn to write? The marking and critiquing of a paper and the coaching of children—how to organize their thoughts, how to build an argument or create an image, how to know when to end—takes time. As Ted Sizer pointed out in his book *Horace's Compromise,* if a teacher with one hundred fifty students takes ten minutes for a marking and coaching session, each set of papers will take

twenty-five hours to complete. Two sets would take fifty hours. Whom are we kidding? So we agreed with the reform reports on the necessity of more writing, but the much harder question of how to structure our schools to make that possible went unanswered, indeed, unasked.

Many of the other reform proposals were also only half-measures. They described the symptoms. They could even tell you what a healthy patient would look like: He would have so many years of English and math and science and history and foreign language. He would do his homework and listen attentively. His teachers would all be from the top of their class. They would engage him in Socratic discussion and he would develop his critical thinking abilities and be ready to take on the twenty-first century.

It is easy to agree on the final outcome. But how do we get there? How do we attract and retain the talented teachers? How do we create such a community of learning?

If we are serious about reform—and we are—we must be unmercifully honest about the problems we face. Otherwise, we are dealing only with slogans and wishes.

The first problem is that, given the way schools are currently organized, there is no conceivable way we can get the enormous numbers of talented teachers we need. The nation's talent pool isn't that big. There simply will not be enough high-caliber college graduates available to us. No single sector of the economy—not medicine, not industry, not transportation, not law and the judiciary, not the military—can successfully bid for 25 percent of the country's college graduates, which is what we need. The numbers just do not add up.

Secondly, even assuming we could capture one-quarter of the country's educated workforce, if we simply placed them into the existing structure of our schools and told them to do their best, their best would not be good enough. That structure, and the rigid, confining approach to teaching and learning that it imposes, never did work well for more than a minority of our students.

Let me first take up the problem of the limited talent pool.

The reality that casts its shadow over any discussion of education reform is the massive teacher shortage that we are now facing. I want you to walk through this with me, to add up the numbers, consider the alternatives, and grapple with the dilemma. After all, it is *our* profession; we are the ones who care most about what happens to it.

Over the next few years and at exactly the time that the public will be expecting results from the new monies they have voted for education, we will lose one-half of all current teachers. Just think of it. Within the next six years, through normal retirement and attrition, over 50 percent of all of you and of all your colleagues will no longer be teaching.

Who will replace you? The prospects are not good. Let me rephrase that, for some of you may have read reports saying that there will be no shortage. The prospects are fine if we don't care about quality. One can always fill a shortage by lowering standards. Shortages are always relative to standards, and if you have no standards, there is never a shortage.

Consider what happened last year in Baltimore, Maryland. The school district there instituted a new examination for all its prospective teachers. Although it was elementary, we should keep in mind that thousands of other districts don't even bother to test their applicants. The Baltimore exam was a simple writing test. But some of those who took it couldn't compose a simple note to a parent without making errors in grammar, spelling, and punctuation. Since they failed the test, they were not supposed to be hired. But on the opening day of school, they were given the jobs anyway because there were no better candidates available.

So that is one way to solve a shortage problem, but it spells disaster for our students, our profession, and the future of public education.

Teacher supply and demand are not within striking distance of each other because of an unfortunate confluence of demographics—a baby boomlet generation entering school while a baby bust generation graduates from college and an earlier baby boom generation retires from teaching. Let's look at the potential supply of teachers now moving through our colleges. Keep in mind that even with no reduction in class size or work load, we will need 1.1 million new teachers in the next seven years. That means 23 percent of each college graduating class must enter teaching if the demand is to be met—23 percent this year, 23 percent next year, and so on into the 1990s. However, in 1983, only 4.5 percent of college students said they were planning to become teachers. Last year, things got a little better, and now 6 percent say they will join our ranks. Even if more students eventually become teachers than say they will, the gap remains enormous. There will still be hundreds of thousands of missing teachers.

The gap becomes even more insurmountable if we want to recruit only from the top half of the college graduating class. Not an unreasonable standard, but it means we would need to take 46 percent of that group. To add to the discouraging picture is the fact that—as we've all seen reported in the papers for a number of

years now—a majority of those who say they are going into teaching are in the bottom quartile of all college students in the country.

There have been reports recently of former teachers re-entering the teaching force, but that surge is likely to be short-lived and certainly won't make much of a dent in the situation.

The second problem that any serious education reform effort must deal with is the limitations imposed by the current structure of our schools. Even at its best, that structure produces good schools for some of our children but not for all of them. It is hard to face up to this one, because it requires that we give up some of our nostalgia about the past. I know it took me awhile to do so.

Let's suppose that there were plenty of outstanding teachers available and that all of the commonly proposed reforms of the last few years were put into effect.

If this were the case, what would schools look like? Students would be required to learn reading, writing, and arithmetic in the early grades or they would not be promoted. Later they would learn science, math, literature, history. They would be tested on their knowledge before being passed on. Teachers would be tested in their subject areas before they were employed, and they would teach the mandated curriculum. There would be pressure on both students and teachers for greater achievement.

Does anyone recognize these schools? I do. They are very much like the schools I attended as a child in New York City and, I suspect, like many public schools across the country in the 1930s and 1940s. Is this what we want again? Weren't these schools good? They were certainly good for me and for many, many others. We were pushed and pressured; we were forced to learn things whether we liked them or not. There were many oustanding teachers. Some of them waited over five years to get their jobs during the Depression. The schools had their pick of the best and the brightest. And as students we did learn and later came to love and enjoy subjects that we hated at first.

Is this what the current reform movement is all about? Should we go back to the good old schools we used to have? That is exactly what we will do if we follow most of the reform reports. But, if we do, the results may be disastrous. According to statistics in the Spring 1986 issue of the *Teachers College Record,* in 1940 the high school dropout rate was 76 percent; it was not until the 1950s that the dropout rate fell below 50 percent! A traditional, tough academic program, even with outstanding teachers, did not benefit the majority of students. Therefore, if we simply return to the schools we once had, we can expect a huge dropout rate in the 1980s and 1990s, particularly among disadvantaged students, at a time when students will not have the benefit of the same family support system they had in 1940.

Furthermore, a dropout in 1986 is considerably worse off than he would have been forty years ago. In earlier periods, it was much more possible than it is today for a person to succeed on the basis of hard work even if he was not well educated. In contrast, our high-tech society will continue to demand an extremely sophisticated labor force; a person without basic skills will be defeated before he has begun.

These two problems—the demographic wall that we have now bumped up against and the limitations of the current structure even under the best of circumstances—must serve as the take-off point for any consideration of education reform proposals. If we don't come to grips with these problems or if we just make incremental change, we had better be prepared for the issuance of hundreds of thousands of emergency credentials to people who are not qualified to enter our profession. We will also have to live with the tragedy of millions of children ill equipped to take up a full life. We can't just sit this period out. If we do, we not only place in jeopardy an entire generation, but, in my opinion, we will irrevocably undermine the public's faith in our schools. This system that has played such a unique and noble role in this nation of immigrants could disappear or become unrecognizable.

What do we do? In 1986, two groups of people have been grappling with that question. AFT leaders from around the country spent long days gathering the statistics, taking testimony from the experts, and, most importantly, reflecting upon the problems our members face in the classroom. Simultaneously, another group was taking up approximately the same agenda. This one was convened by the Carnegie Forum on Education and the Economy and was composed of governors, corporate executives, state legislative and university leaders, myself, and Mary Futrell, president of the NEA.

In the spring of 1986, the Carnegie report, *A Nation Prepared: Teachers for the 21st Century,* was issued; in July 1986, AFT delegates meeting in convention in Chicago endorsed the basic thrust of the Carnegie report and adopted one of their own: *The Revolution that Is Overdue: A Report of the AFT Task Force on the Future of Education.*

While the reports differ in some respects, they are kindred spirits. They both say that the time is past for marginal reforms that uphold the status quo. They both refuse to accept defeat, and they both dare to

think of new ways of doing things. At their core are two ideas: First, we must seek the full professionalization of teaching. Second, and interwoven with the first, we must redesign our schools and rethink the way we approach teaching and learning. It is to these two interlocking ideas that I would now like to turn.

Professionalizing teaching means all the things this union has long stood for and worked for: higher salaries; smaller class size, a manageable work load, and relief from nonteaching chores. It means working conditions that other professions so take for granted that they often go unmentioned: an office, a desk, a telephone, a quiet place. It means enough textbooks to go around, equipment that doesn't fall apart, school buildings that are clean and safe. It also means time for preparation and new learning and for discussion and work with one's colleagues.

But true professionalism requires an even more basic prerogative than these, and it is the recognition of this that distinguishes the AFT report and the Carnegie report from those that preceded them. The central recommendation of the new reports is to *empower* teachers, to give teachers control over the standards of their profession and the conduct of their work.

If there is one principle on which all the studies of effective schools—and effective businesses—agree, it is this: Top-down management does not work. Neither does top-down reform. We cannot help Johnny overcome his reading problem by turning to page 234 of a state regulation. The people who wrote those regulations are not qualified teachers, nor have they spent six months in the classroom observing Johnny and trying out and discarding four different approaches to solving his particular difficulty. The fifth approach—the one that may work—is not to be found in a state law or a school district's administrative directive. It can only come from the mind and hands of a creative and sensitive teacher.

Teaching, like medicine, cannot operate by remote control. There is no formula that fits all children. The only treatment that works is one that is constantly adjusted and fitted and fine-tuned by the people on the scene. Intelligent change has its best hope in teachers because nobody knows better than teachers what is going on in schools.

This concept is not only honored in all the other professions, it is increasingly becoming the operating principle in blue-collar industries.

I had the privilege a couple of months ago (Summer, 1986) of being at a conference where a group of labor leaders met with a group of university presidents under the sponsorship of the Labor/Higher Education Council. I was especially pleased to be present when the international secretary of the United Steelworkers of America, Edgar L. Ball, described some of the new work arrangements that are being tried in the steel industry. His remarks have now been published, and I would like to read one section from them, because it will show how far behind public education is compared to the innovations in private industry with blue-collar workers.

Earlier this year we finished a two-year plan to redesign labor/management relationships in an ALCOA plant in Arkansas. For forty-five years, a very strong, militant, adversarial relationship existed. The union faced the problem of changing the adversarial relationship and redesigning jobs and methods of doing work.

After two years, autonomous work crews went into effect in every department, almost eliminating the need for the shop floor management in the plant. Instead of eighteen job classifications, there are no more than three in any department. The crew in every department designed its own jobs based on what they felt would work and what they were willing to try to make work. The craftsmen also agreed to do away with pure crafts and go to multicrafts. They decided what the groupings would be and what the new jobs would be.

I talked to a group of employees in the first department that tried the new system. The first three months the plan was in effect, down-time was reduced by half, and within the next three months decreased by half again. I asked them, "Why? How did you do it?" and this is what they said: "What we used to do was come to work, punch time cards, go to our work station, and stand there until the foreman came by and told us what to do. If he didn't tell us to do something that needed to be done, we didn't do it. If he wasn't there enough, that was his fault, he was the boss. If he told us to do it wrong, we did it wrong even if we knew it was wrong, because we were subject to discharge if we didn't do what he told us to do.

"If something went wrong, after we knew it was going wrong with the equipment or process, we didn't say anything to anyone about it. If the foreman happened to come by and catch it, fine. If he didn't, we let it go. If equipment broke down, we shut the power off. We didn't call anybody. We stood there until someone from management came by and looked at it, and they had to decide to call maintenance. When maintenance got there, we didn't tell them what was going wrong with it and we didn't help them. If they knew how to fix it, fine, and if they fixed it wrong, too bad, that wasn't our concern. We weren't being paid to do those things. We were being paid to do the few little things that were in our job description and that's all we did."

I asked, "What are you doing now?" Their reply: "We know how to run the plant. We come to work; we start operating it. We are running maintenance even though it's not in our job description. We help each other. If one is having trouble, we help. If we think something is going to go wrong, we plan around that and we alert maintenance in advance and we have them there and we tell them what's wrong, and we show them and we help them fix it."

I have heard similar descriptions of auto plants, steel plants, and other companies all across the country that are starting to turn decisions over to the people who are closest to the work. These are companies that were going to close down or decide to take their operations overseas.

I would like to know why, if blue-collar workers can be trusted to run their own plants and organize their own jobs, why can't teachers be trusted to do exactly the same thing?

Putting teachers in charge of instructional decisions will lead to experimentation with new kinds of management in schools. Different models will emerge, but they will all be marked by a movement away from authoritarian, hierarchical structures. School management may look more like the professional partnerships of law firms. In some cases, teachers will want to hire administrators to carry out many of the noninstructional chores now assumed by the principal, much as a hospital hires a business manager. Whatever the particulars, the relationship between administrative functions and professional functions will be different from what it is now. Those not expert in the teaching field will not oversee those who are.

In discussing the empowerment of teachers, I want to be very clear on two points: First, we do not suggest that teachers should be the instructional leaders because we are a well-organized, powerful group that can commandeer that position. We are that, but that is not where the legitimacy for teacher authority lies. Doctors, too, are well organized and powerful, but their authority lies elsewhere: in their knowledge and expertise. It was not always so. Not until medicine had a substantial knowledge and clinical base underlying it, not until medical education was transformed from its once-scandalous state into a rigorous program, and not until the profession acted to establish high entry standards did authority, autonomy, and respect follow. And so it must be with our profession. The call for teachers to be the instructional leaders must rest on the demonstration of our expertise.

It must also rest upon our professional integrity. Let me return for a moment to the situation I described earlier where the school district in Baltimore, Maryland, hired clearly unqualified teacher applicants because, according to school officials, there were no better candidates available. The message that such a decision sends is that the school's custodial role takes precedence over its intellectual mission. If teachers were in charge of professional standards and instructional issues, we could not allow such a decision. We would have to make some hard choices and fashion some creative solutions. In doing so, we would make it clear that the overriding consideration is the protection of our professional standards and the safeguarding of the education of the children who are placed in our care.

Other professions frequently have shortages, but they find ways to serve their clients without sacrificing their standards. There often aren't enough doctors in rural areas or in certain specialities. Would anyone even consider issuing emergency or temporary medical credentials to ill-prepared "doctors"? Or accepting to the bar candidates who had flunked their law exams? To do so would be a betrayal of those professions, and to do so in our schools is a betrayal of the meaning of education.

As a profession, we would have to grapple with alternative solutions, none of them easy. For example, in the Baltimore situation, qualified teachers might be asked to volunteer to teach an additional period after school for extra pay, just as some now volunteer to coach. This would permit class-size limits to be maintained, but students would be divided in classes over a longer day. Or, teachers might be asked whether they would agree to an increase in class size for the year by one student per teacher, with the money saved on the salaries given to the teachers now in the system. Increasing class size or lengthening the school day are certainly not good, but is it more desirable to risk the education of hundreds of students? Spending a year with an unqualified teacher is not just a question of losing that year, as serious as that is. It could also permanently damage a child's desire to learn, undermining his confidence in himself and discoloring his whole outlook on school.

Another way to avoid hiring unqualified teachers would be to try to entice back former teachers who left the system five, seven, or ten years ago for jobs in industry by offering to place them at a step on the salary schedule that would give them credit for their outside experience. Likewise, appeals could be made to the thousands of people in the vicinity who were once licensed and qualified teachers in other states, offering to give them full salary credit for their work elsewhere.

None of these solutions is perfect, but they are better than letting our professional standards erode or jeopardizing a child's future. Making these difficult

choices—some of which would involve real sacrifice on the part of teachers—would make it clear that our professional code of ethics has as its center a concern for what is best for our students. Once the resolve is made never to lower our standards, the discussion can then turn to how we can best deal with dilemmas like the one in Baltimore and the many others that we face on a daily basis.

What I'm saying, in effect, is that we cannot assume the prerogatives of a profession without also assuming the responsibilities. This brings me to one of the key recommendations of both the AFT and Carnegie reports: the creation of a national board of professional teaching standards. This will be a national, non-governmental board composed of a majority of outstanding teachers. It will set standards for what teachers ought to know and be able to do. Based on those, it will develop and administer a national certifying examination for teachers comparable to the bar and other professional exams.

The assessment process developed by the national board of teaching standards will stand in sharp contrast to the trivial, paper-and-pencil, multiple-choice, context-free questions that are all too typical of existing teacher tests.

The exam for basic certification would consist of three parts. First, there would be a stringent test of subject matter knowledge. The second part of the exam, which probably would be given on a different day, would test knowledge of pedagogy, educational issues, and the ability to apply educational principles to many different student needs and learning styles. Video presentations of actual classroom problems might be used, much as the medical boards are now utilizing computer simulations of real-life medical problems. Whatever the format, the tests would not be looking for a single "right" answer (there usually isn't one) so much as they would be assessing the candidate's thought processes and decision-making skills, based on known principles of effective practice. Finally, the third part of the assessment would be a clinical induction program of from one to three years in which teachers would be evaluated on the basis of how well they work with students and their colleagues. Rather than a sink-or-swim approach, staged induction would give novice teachers the time and opportunity to learn from and reflect on their practice with experienced teachers.

The certification process will be a voluntary one. In addition to basic certification, those teachers who choose to do so will also have the option of pursuing advanced board certification, much as a doctor can become board certified in his specialty. Advanced certification will be a mark of superior quality. It will mean that teachers will finally have available to them a way of advancing in their profession without leaving it. No more phony merit pay schemes. No arbitrary limits on the number of teachers allowed to prove themselves. The standards will be visible and verifiable. Anyone who examines them will agree that anyone who meets them is an exemplar of the profession's highest reach.

A national board certification process would be a major leap toward the professional standards and status teachers have sought. Indeed, if the history of other professions, such as medicine and law, is a guide, such certification is one of the prerequisites of professionalization. Its potential is also great for breaking the grip of the present array of low-quality, low-cost, ill-conceived teacher tests and securing for teachers more rigorous and helpful training. Moreover, a fair assessment that candidates could prepare for and that minimizes the importance of test-taking skills would remove some of the obstacles that now stand in the way of our ability to replenish the ranks of minority teachers and thereby perpetuate their tradition of service to the nation's schools. As a powerful quality-assurance signal to the public, professional board certification also could spell an end to demeaning and bogus schemes to "improve" the teaching force.

The creation of such a national board would put teaching standards in the hands of the profession. After all, isn't that where they belong? Should commercial testing services—the developers of current teacher tests—determine our standards? Are state legislators or district administrators the appropriate people to say who is fit to enter and advance in our profession? The lay members of school boards? Do they know the research and practice base that underlies good teaching? Shouldn't it be to the best of our own ranks that we look? We will set our standards. They will be high ones and they will be fair ones.

Monumental as these proposed changes are, they will not be enough unless they go hand in hand with a rethinking of the way we now approach teaching and learning. I go back to the basic dilemmas I raised before—the limited talent pool available to us and the need to design an approach to teaching and learning that can do a better job of reaching all our students.

Suppose medical care were structured so that everyone involved in patient testing, diagnosis, treatment, and care had to be a doctor? No nurses, no nurses' aides, no lab technicians, no operating room assistants, no pharmacists, no interns, no residents. What if everyone who operated a CAT scan, drew blood, took temperatures, handed out medication, made the early morning and middle of the night rounds, bathed pa-

tients, and kept their charts—that is, everyone who had anything to do with patient evaluation and care, from the most basic maintenance to the most sophisticated diagnosis—had to be a doctor? If that were the case, instead of having 520,000 doctors, as we now do, we would need 4.8 million.

They, of course, wouldn't be "doctors" as we now understand that term. If medicine were structured like education, with undifferentiated staffing—and it is hard to even imagine—each "doctor" would be assigned the near-total care of a certain number of patients.

In evaluating such a structure, one question outweighs all other considerations: Would medical care be improved? The answer is, it would be worse. Where would we find 4.8 million people capable of doing the broad range of work called for? Some patients would have very good "doctors," although they would be so busy running the X-ray machine and dispensing medication at the appropriate intervals, they would have very little time for what we now consider doctoring. Many of them would not want to stay in a "profession" where they were not able to make the best use of their talents and where they were constantly frustrated by not having the support staff required to free them to concentrate their efforts on the more demanding aspects of their art and science.

The great majority of patients would not have "doctors" drawn from the top 10 percent or the top quartile or the top half of college graduates. Medicine would have to dip deeper and deeper into the talent pool. Salaries would be commensurately low, perhaps at about the average level of teacher salary, since the country—even one that values good medical care—could not afford to pay 4.8 million people $100,000 each. There would be calls for closer supervision of the less capable people; state legislatures would adopt rules and regulations governing the treatment of each disease. Talented young people would not be drawn to such a restricted, nonprofessional field, thus the downward spiral would continue.

Well, there are of course differences, but there is much food for thought in this analogy. We can't get 46 percent of the talented college graduates; no other profession and indeed no single sector of the economy can either. But we can get our fair share. And we can begin to think of new ways of organizing the way education services are delivered. The Carnegie report calls for teaching to be structured closer to the way other professions are:

Professionals are a valuable resource in our society. It takes a lot of education and training to produce them and costs a lot of money to pay them. For that reason, most employers work hard at making the most of these professionals.

That is why professionals are typically supported by many other people who do the work they would otherwise have to do. The services of these other people come at lower cost, so it is more efficient to use them to perform such tasks than to have them performed by the professionals. For the same reasons, professionals also have available to them a host of machines and services that improve their efficiency in countless ways, from computers and copying machines to telephones and adequate work space. These services are not perquisites for professionals. They are regarded by employers as necessary investments, enabling the professionals on their staffs to reach the highest possible levels of accomplishment.

Not only do professionals typically have a range of support staff and services available, but they are usually organized so that the most able among them influence in many ways the work that others do, from broad policy direction to the development of staff members who might some day take on major responsibilities. This, too, is a matter of simple efficiency, making sure that the experience and skill embodied in these valuable people makes itself felt throughout the enterprise. . . .

America's schools can, without doubt, greatly improve their performance. They will not do so unless they prove to be an attractive employment opportunity to some of the most able college graduates in the country. But the schools cannot realistically expect that all 2.3 million teachers will be the best and brightest the country has to offer. Education, like other professions, will have to structure itself so that it can make the very best use of a distribution of talent. That means reorganization, because the current "eggcrate" organization does not permit efficient shared use of highly skilled people, support services, and equipment.

The Carnegie Task Force points out in its report that teacher salaries are not only extremely low but also extremely compressed compared to other occupations demanding a college degree. After ten to twelve years, most teachers have reached the top of the scale. The Carnegie report estimates that if teaching were restructured to be more like other professions, with different levels of teachers and corresponding levels of responsibility, starting salaries would be about what they are today, average teacher salary would be significantly higher, and a substantial number of people—those holding advanced certification—would be making $60,000 to $100,000, with local and regional variations determined by the same kinds of factors as they are today.

In a restructured teaching profession, certified teachers could be assisted by interns and instructors and computer lab technicians, by paraprofessionals and clericals and administrative staff, by tutors and volunteers, and by an increasingly sophisticated and accessible selection of computer and video technology. Interns will be finishing their final stages of teacher preparation. Some instructors will be on loan from businesses for a year or two; others will be recent college graduates who have chosen to work in the schools as part of a tuition loan plan; still others may be drawn from the rapidly growing ranks of college-educated retirees who still have much to offer.

The professional teaching staff will be freed up to practice their profession. They will have more time to spend with their students—not setting up machinery, conducting routine drill sessions, or filling out forms, but teaching. They will have time to do what the earlier reform reports called for: to teach writing; to help children sort out fact from opinion; to lead discussions that take students beyond scattered names, dates, and places to real knowledge and understanding. They will have the time to develop new ways and new materials for conveying difficult concepts; and they will have time to work with the child whom no one else can reach.

With the aid of new technology and a diverse complement of teaching staff, new options of time, teaching method, and class arrangement will open up. While some students are analyzing ideas in a small seminar, others will be gathered around a computer station. While some are receiving intense assistance through one-on-one tutoring, others will be viewing historical footage in the video screening room. The effectiveness of our teaching will no longer be compromised by having to fit it into fifty-minute time slots. Nor will teachers be forced by an inflexible class schedule "to teach to the average."

Teachers will no longer be isolated all day long in a self-contained classroom. Like other professionals, they will have time during the school day to consult with their colleagues, to share ideas, and to brainstorm solutions to stubborn educational problems. Some teachers will want to divide their time between teaching and other professional responsibilities, such as the development of discipline policy and grading standards, the assignment of students, the allocation of their school's budget, the design of a staffing structure into which various categories of support staff would fit, and the evaluation of a mushrooming array of new software. Certified teachers will not only be on top of the latest research but will themselves be identifying the questions for which we do not yet have answers and will join with their colleagues at local universities in the development of classroom-based studies. In addition, they will do what every doctor in a teaching hospital does: perpetuate their profession by passing on the best of their science and art to the young interns who will eventually replace them.

Other instructional staff and support personnel, under the direction of certified teachers, will be available to conduct drill-and-practice sessions, lead small-section review classes much as teaching assistants do in graduate school, mark multiple-choice tests, coach multiplication tables, prepare a hands-on science lesson, read a story aloud, organize field trips, check a book review report, run the video equipment and monitor the viewing room, tinker with the mechanical problems that arise at computer work stations, persuade parents of the importance of providing time and space for homework, and so on.

The central function of the professional teaching staff will be to shape the climate and the structure of their school and its curriculum and to develop the best learning program for each individual child and see that it is executed.

I've been talking about how a new structure would enable teachers to do their best teaching. Let me turn once again to our students, for the same system that has confined teachers has also confined children. As I mentioned earlier, even under the best of circumstances—when the supply of talented teachers was plentiful, when family structure was stronger than it now is, when homework time didn't have to compete with TV—even then, one-half to three-quarters of our young people did not complete high school. And is it any wonder? To again use a medical analogy, suppose that a doctor had to try to diagnose and treat patients in groups of thirty instead of individually. Ridiculous? Of course. But are the needs, the problems, the strengths, the achievement levels, the attention spans, or the learning styles of students any less diverse than the history and symptoms presented by patients?

How do children best learn? Is there any one of us who really thinks that it is by putting them together in groups of thirty, sitting at their desks for five or six hours a day? Do any of us believe that the lecture format—which numerous studies show constitutes approximately 85 percent of classroom time—is the desirable method for all subjects and all children? Is it any wonder that teachers, who on a daily basis are required to get thirty fidgety youngsters to master the same topic at the same pace and with the same instructional approach, are suffering from job stress?

Many critics have attacked teachers for the problems in our schools. But it is not teachers' fault, anymore than the problems of the auto industry are the auto workers' fault. Our auto workers are as good as

the Japanese, but they are working in a defeating structure. What if you are a junior high school teacher and you get a student in your class who can't read? What do you do? You can't really help him. He needs a different setting. He needed a different setting six years earlier. He didn't get one because schools aren't structured to give him one.

But they could be. The new approaches to the staffing and design of schools that we have been discussing will do much more than enable us to cope with a teacher shortage, as important as that is. They will also allow us—finally—to begin to move in the direction of more individualized learning, fitting the structure to the child rather than the other way around.

Students learn at different paces and in different ways. Most students need more time in some subjects than in others, and most learn better through one method than through another. Some students learn best by reading a chapter in a book, others by watching a videotape, or by using programmed instruction on a computer. Some children can best master new material by teaching it to younger students, by reviewing it in a structured coaching session, or by analyzing it in a teacher-led seminar. Some students can master a concept the first time around. Others need two tries, or three, or more. Some students shine in large groups; others are too shy to participate. Some students can pace their efforts over a five-month semester; others need the sharper incentive of shorter time spans. The rigidity of the current structure forces us to try to fit these very different children into the same mold. The fit often isn't a good one.

Teachers know this better than anyone, but we've never had the flexibility or the personnel or the technology necessary to plan and oversee more individualized learning programs. We now have the possibility of bringing all those elements together for the first time. Teaching would be broadly defined as connecting students with the materials, experiences, and resources that will best help them learn. The teacher's job would be more like the doctor's: to diagnose and then to develop and execute a plan of educational action—like writing an educational prescription for each child. Sometimes that program would be carried out by the certified teachers and sometimes by other instructional staff. And if the first prescription doesn't work, we will be able to try a second, or a third, or a fourth.

In thinking about the way things could be and should be, there is no blueprint before us. Our only sure principles are to hold to our standards and to give teachers the leeway to exercise their judgment and to start thinking about how to restructure and reshape our schools and our profession so that teaching and learning can flourish. We of course do not abandon what we have. We experiment; we refine; we try again. It will take time.

If we sit by and do nothing, or if we just make marginal repairs, we will see the quality of our teaching force rapidly decline. Emergency credentials will be issued in the hundreds of thousands. The country has built up great expectations. If things get only slightly better—or if they get worse—all the powers we can exercise at the bargaining table or in the legislative arena will not be enough to stop an angry public from getting even with the public school system.

But even if we could fool the public, we cannot fool ourselves. Nor would we want to. In the end, it is we who must serve as the protectors of our students and our profession. We wouldn't want it any other way.

We have before us the great possibility of forever transforming the lives of teachers and students in America. Many good people are on our side.

For students—especially those to whom life has not been so kind—it will be a new chance. And for teachers, it will mean the opportunity to give them that chance. It will mean a real profession and a real community of learning.

In closing, I want to acknowledge that many of the ideas I have been discussing will mean change, and change is always hard. Over the past couple of years,

as these ideas have begun to take form, we have experienced two feelings in tension with each other. On the one hand, there are many things about our schools and our profession and our jobs that we do not like, so we project an image of hope, and hope gives us a picture of how things might be.

But at the same time, there is the fear of change. Is the change going to be in the direction we want it to be? Will things really get better, or will they get worse? So in the middle of our hopes, our fears take hold and we experience a kind of paralysis. Maybe, we say, it is better to hold onto things the way they are now; the terrain is familiar, and we have adjusted our dreams to fit the landscape.

I would hope that in this battle between hope and fear, we would be instructed by our experience over the past few years and indeed over the last seventy years. This union and its members have always been good for taking risks. We stood for unionism when no one else believed in it. With only a handful of members, and when others said it would be suicidal, we called for collective bargaining elections because we believed that when teachers had sketched before them a vision of what could be if they joined together, they would go with their hopes and not their fears. They did then, and I believe they will now.

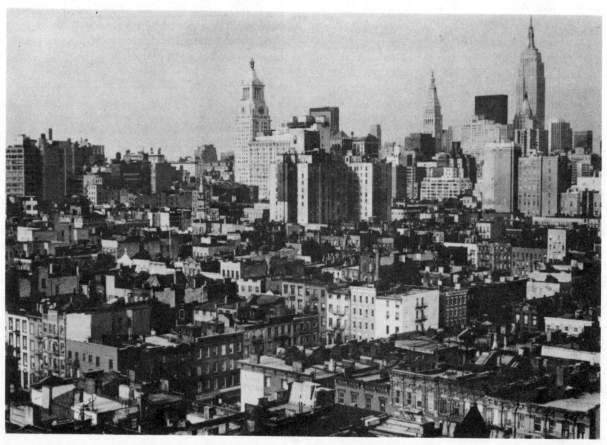

Ken Robinson

Chapter 2
Major Issues in Education
Carl B. Erdberg*

This article represents the thinking of an educator with fifty years of experience in the profession. It is hoped that the thoughts herein will lead to discussions, pro and con.

Here are fifteen major issues in education in the mid-eighties. There is hesitation to go beyond the mid-eighties because change is so rapid in modern times. For example, it was not very long ago when colleges and universities were shutting down their departments of education. Yet, now, we are facing intense shortages of teachers throughout the land, with special shortages in inner-city schools.

The presentation of these major issues will not be given in order of importance. In fact, major issues may vary according to the author who perceived them. Here, then, are fifteen, as they come to the mind of one educator who has spent fifty years in the field; as a teacher, chairperson of a social studies and an English department in high schools, elementary school principal, high school principal, district superintendent, and chairperson of a department of educational administration at a university. At present, he is still active in education as a consultant to a system which prepares examinations to test future school supervisors.

Issue I—Accountability

When students demonstrate weakness in educational achievement, who should be faulted? There are an appreciable number of educators who place the blame completely on the shoulders of teachers and principals.

There are others who feel that the sociological conditions under which these failing students live develop in them a lack of receptivity to learn which the school basically cannot overcome.

A third group are of the opinion that there are out of school factors (e.g., child abuse, wife beating, drugs, poor housing, poor health, poor nutrition, wide-spread teen-age pregnancy, drug addiction, etc.); and, in-school factors (large class size, low teacher expectancy of stu-

dent achievement, poor teachers, lazy teachers, poorly-trained supervisors who are not skilled in upgrading instruction, poor school administration, lack of adequate materials of instruction, poor school plants, etc).

Those who feel that the major cause of student failure lies in the hands of teachers and supervisors point to inner city schools which they deem to be successful. They ask why other inner city schools cannot emulate what is being done in these schools considered to be successful by these school critics.

There are others who are concerned that every effort must be made to improve the sociological conditions under which the students live, simultaneously with the upgrading of school programs. With this in mind, some schools are organizing medical clinics to be housed on school grounds to work hand in hand with school staffs in a combined thrust to advance student progress.

At any rate, it must be noted that the idea of holding teachers accountable for the educational retardation of pupils is a distinct phenomenon of the latter half of the twentieth century.

Issue II—The School Dropout

A major issue, quite related to that of accountability, is the fact that so many students fail to complete high school. Especially is this true of students of minority background.

Therefore, those who are so angry with public schools state that these are not dropouts but pushouts; that they are harassed, neglected, or both by high school faculties who hope to rid themselves of these students considered by them to be troublesome.

There are others who are of the opinion that everybody attends high school these days; that, in the first quarter of the twentieth century such students would have never reached high school. Thus, not having at-

*Dr. Carl B. Erdberg is Professor Emeritus, Department of Educational Administration, Pace University.

tended, they could very well not be considered high school dropouts. They would have dropped out before leaving high school. When it became impossible to drop out of school before age 16 rather than age 14, the dropout problem became a glaring one.

Some school superintendents of large inner-city school systems have lost their positions recently, mainly because of the large percentage of dropouts in the school areas over which they had jurisdiction.

Hence, school supervisors, and, indeed, state commissioners of education, and entire state legislatures are giving their attention to slowing down the rate of school drop out. Principals of high schools are replaced, special assistant superintendents are assigned to give their attention completely to the drop-out problem, cooperative education is flourishing, partnerships with industry are being established, the universities are lending their skills, and appreciable amounts of money are voted earmarked for stemming the tide of dropouts.

However, a curious contradiction has developed; namely, the very state legislatures which are voting funds hoping that such actions will result in fewer dropouts, are demanding higher academic standards (verified by the outcomes of standardized tests) of those who are graduated from high school. Many are asking, therefore, whether such an increase in standards will actually not increase the number of dropouts.

Another line of thought suggests itself in regard to the dropout problem; namely, the out-of-school factors mentioned above. And, tied to this, steps which might be taken in school from kindergarten to the twelfth year to plan an end-to-end school program to combat the tendency to drop out before completing high school.

Issue III—Family Living

There are many citizens who are of the opinion that such topics as sex education, planned parenthood, abortion, and pre-natal care do not belong in the school curriculum; that these matters are best left for instruction and discussion in the home.

There are others who feel that the subject of family living including such matters as child rearing, proper nutrition, birth control, pre-natal care, avoidance of wife beating, etc. is the most important offering that should be offered in the curriculum today. This argument is bolstered by the huge increase in teen-age pregnancy in recent times. They point out that along with teen-age pregnancy there are a host of other problems which develop. These problems then find themselves impacting adversely on school performance.

For example, it is argued that if secondary school students, both male and female, were to be taught to rear children with tender, loving care rather than to abuse

them, children would be less angry and hostile when attending school. Many teachers will speak of children who angrily strike out at others physically because these children themselves have been the victims of extremely harsh child rearing. Hence, the psychology of positive child rearing would be taught in school to all students in the hope that fewer cases of child abuse would ensue because of this greater understanding which has been taught in school.

Again, the matter of the effective nutrition of children is considered by many educators to relate to receptivity to learning; for example, the ingestion of excessive amounts of sugar which could lead to hyperactivity in the classroom. What is commonly known as junk food may well be a factor in the matter of a child's receptivity to learning.

There is also the "Right to Life" movement which is sensitive to school involvement in such areas as the teaching about abortion, birth control, sex practices, the AIDS disease, and other sensitive situations.

Issue IV—School Discipline

The item which is rated by parents regularly as the most serious problem in the annual Gallup poll on education, is poor discipline in schools.

Educators frequently express a relationship between poor discipline on the part of individual students with the out-of-school factors which prey upon children. In short, the children bring their problems with them.

The Kozals, Kohls, Leonards, Friedenbergs, Levins, and Holts, on the other hand, state that teachers, principals, and school curricula "turn off" the students, as a result of which they misbehave.

In the past decade the use of drugs by students, even in the elementary school, has increased tremendously. Basically, there is little debate about this extremely serious problem. Almost everyone agrees that the schools must do their utmost to educate students to the harmfulness of drug use and abuse. In addition, there is no doubt that drugs are a major source of poor discipline in schools, both public and private.

One answer which is developing is the joining of community resources with the schools in a unified effort to fight the drug problem.

One other issue has some relationship to poor discipline. Namely, it is the matter of class size. Teachers are almost unanimous in requesting smaller class sizes not only to improve discipline, but also to reach the reluctant learner who needs so much individual help and encouragement.

Also related to discipline is the matter of school safety. There are a growing number of parents who have stated that they have opted for private school because they fear for the safety of their children in public schools. This option on the part of parents is especially true in the inner city.

Issue V—Drug and Alcohol Addiction

Closely related to poor discipline and lack of safety is the matter of the use of drugs, starting as low as the upper grades of K-6 schools. The use of alcohol is more frequently found in the high schools.

The majority of students may not be considered to be addicts, but recent studies have found that an appreciable number have experimented with drugs.

Governments, federal, state and local, have infused large sums of money in varied programs to combat addiction. Yet, drug sales continue in and near schools. Young people who sell drugs can earn a great deal of money although they themselves may be users. It is a vicious cycle with governmental leaders currently stating with increasing frequency that it is a losing battle unless the United States can successfully negotiate with countries which are the source of the drug crops to eliminate this nefarious product, because law enforcement agencies, and anti-drug education programs have had a measure of success, but hardly enough to really meet this problem.

Issue VI—Vouchers

There has been a move on the part of federal governmental authorities to ask Congress to pass a law granting a specific number of dollars to parents who have chosen parochial or private schools for their children. This would probably be distributed in the form of a chit which would be submitted by the parent to the non-public school, upon enrollment.

Opponents of this plan point out that the amount would probably cover tuition at most parochial schools, but would be far from adequate to cover the tuition of those wishing to attend a secular private school. In addition, opponents claim that if poor parents in the inner city wished to switch from the public schools they would be limited to the inner city parochial schools.

Proponents state that poor parents, for the first time, would have the option as consumers of making a choice between the public and non-public school. They also claim that the competition between public and non-public school would have a salutary influence on the public school, which might be faced with a severe drop in enrollment, thereby necessarily having to strive harder to provide quality education.

A third approach to voucherism in education limits itself to competition among public schools. It would remove current limits of school enrollment to the school in the immediate neighborhood with a student allowed to attend any one of an appreciable number of public schools. This, it is felt, would mean that individual public schools would have to demonstrate quality or face a drastic cut in enrollment as parents scamper to the public schools with outstanding reputations.

Issue VII—Tuition Aid

Highly related to the issue of vouchers is that of tuition aid. Powerful figures in government have been campaigning for governmental tuition aid to families with children in non-public schools. The argument given in favor of this move is that these families are taxed in their communities to support public schools, yet they do not send their children to the schools for which they are taxed.

Opponents state that the public schools are open to their children and that free public education is basic to a modern, democratic form of government.

And in the case of parochial education, support of such schools by the government through tuition aid would seriously threaten the separation of church and state, the opponents of tuition aid aver.

Issue VIII—Censorship of Textbooks and of Other Materials of Instruction

The recent debate between Creationists and Darwinites is an illustration of pressures which are brought to bear on educators, especially in the public schools. As the United States moves toward greater conservatism in politics, there appear to be greater demands that materials of instruction reflect this trend to the right.

Another great issue, related to the debate over the origin of the species, calls for prayer in the schools. President Reagan has been a strong supporter of this movement for prayer in the schools with the current Supreme Court standing in his way.

Issue IX—The Quality of the Teaching Staff

State after state is adopting examinations both for experienced teachers as well as for those coming into the profession.

There has developed great alarm in regard to the academic capabilities of public school teaching staffs. Hence, a move toward recertification has taken place with teachers with years of experience concerned that they may lose their positions. The two major national teachers organizations are opposed to this. They differ, however, on the testing of incoming teachers.

On the whole, there is concern that teachers of minority background will not do as well in paper and pencil tests as teachers of middle class background. The problem is compounded by the desire to recruit more minority teachers when, at the same time, a good percentage fail the statewide and national examinations.

Some leading educators are recommending that more teachers of minority background will be successful in the examinations if they receive a solid undergraduate college education and, second, if they are given special training in how to pass the examinations.

Issue X—School Integration

Allied with the trend toward conservatism in politics is the move away from busing, and the reorientation toward the neighborhood school.

The magnet school appears to have become more popular as a way of attracting a mixing of races in school rather than moving school populations by various other means. Certain schools are designated to specialize in a specific type of curriculum so that students of all colors, nationalities, and creeds who wish to avail themselves of this specialization, will seek to enroll.

The idea of busing, however, is not dead, being revived from time to time by federal district judges.

Reverse busing has taken place, also, in a few instances. This calls for busing students from the suburbs into the inner city as well as from the inner city to the suburbs.

Issue XI—Bilingual Education

Bilingual education may be looked upon in one of three optional ways:

1. Transitional: When a child learns to use his native language as a bridge to move into the use of English.
2. Maintenance: Where, even though a child has made a transition, he continues to learn in two languages in order to maintain a proper respect for the culture from which he has come.
3. Planned Immersion: Where the child is immersed in English, but his native language is called upon from time to time, to illustrate English words, sentences, and general concepts. This method is accompanied by textbooks and workbooks which specialize in moving the child from foreign language structures to English.

Recently there has been movement by the federal government, which funds bilingual programs, to allow each local educational community to make a determination by itself as to which way it would like to go in teaching the language-handicapped child. Prior to this, federal bilingual educational laws had called specifically for the transitional philosophy and methodology.

Issue XII—Special Education

Public Law 194-42 is a federal law which mandates that the states provide the handicapped child with an education. There are various handicapping conditions, going from the physical to the mental, and emotional. This type of education, and corollary mandates such as the provision of proper physical equipment, is very costly. Indeed, some local governmental leaders have stated that the cost of special education will make "the tail wag the dog," in the sense that special education will outspend the cost of educating children in regular classes.

Another problem is that of mainstreaming so that special education children will join regular classes to provide them with a situation which is "the least handicapping."

Curricular problems within special education classes have also arisen, with differences cropping up between state education authorities and local education specialists.

Issue XIII—The Basics

Reading, Mathematics, Writing—concern over these areas by the lay public has been with us over the last thirty years. Methodology comes to the fore here—e.g., phonics versus the "look say" method, or should it be a combination of both? Developmental mathematics through the process of experiencing, representational materials, thinking through, and the final use of the algorithm, or the use of the algorithm first backed up by a memorization of the tables. Writing—should we learn how to read through writing, or should we follow the learning sequence of listening, speaking, reading and writing with writing as the last step in the process?

Concern over the basics has led many local educational administrators to end what is called "social promotion" or 100% promotion. It calls for holding over in a grade students who are weak in the basics, notably reading, until they can demonstrate some degree of mastery.

The debate still goes on as to whether academic progress is actually made by holding children over for another year or longer.

Another curricular area which is beginning to loom large today is that of pre-kindergarten education. Assessment of the Headstart Program points to positive development, especially of disadvantaged children.

The issue is, however, that once such public education of pre-kindergarten children is accepted more widely, how will it be presented? There are already arguments pro and con as to whether we should begin to teach the basics formally to children as young as those who are in pre-kindergarten classes.

Issue XIV—The Use of Computers in Education

Accompanying the hardware represented by the computer itself is the necessary software. Will this software replace the presentation of the curriculum by the teacher? Or will it be, at most, a supplement to the teacher's instructional program?

One thought is definite. The vast majority of students will have had to have contact and some understanding of the operation and potential of the computer in order to be considered a well-trained, educated individual. Computers have become basic to modern existence. The issue is—Will they replace the human instructor?

Issue XV—Quality Circles in Education

The Japanese are known to involve workers in the operation of their industrial plants. This appears to be a major reason for that nation's vast industrial growth. In the United States, labor and management, in the main, have had an adversarial relationship.

An appreciable number of educators are now calling for quality circles in which school supervisors and teachers will have a joint role in decision making. Some teachers say that their input in helping to "steer the ship" in their schools is even more important to them than an increase in salary. Peer supervision appears to be gaining ground because the rank and file classroom teacher is of the opinion that students will benefit from teachers who have an enhanced self-image. And such image development can only come about if the school supervisor sheds his paternalistic mannerisms and comes to consider the teacher as a partner in the educational process.

Final Commentary

No doubt there are other issues which were not presented among the above fifteen. On the other hand, frank discussions around each of the fifteen presented herein, may lead toward thinking-through advances in the educational programs of our nation.

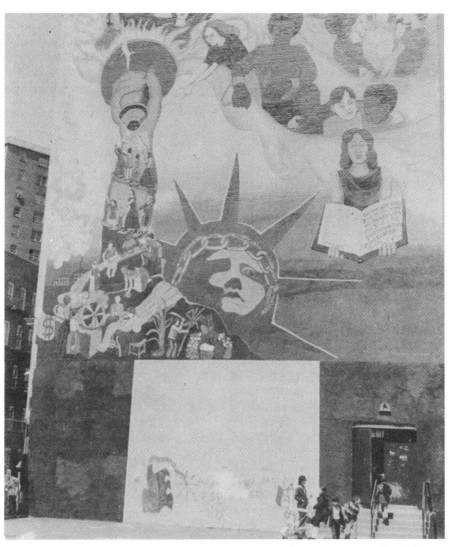

Ken Robinson

Chapter 3
Supreme Court Decisions Affecting Education
Perry A. Zirkel and Faith L. MacMurtrie*

Although the United States Supreme Court has been less active in recent years with regard to education issues (La-Morte & McCollum, 1986), its decisions continue to be a significant source of legal activity affecting the operation of the public schools (Reutter, 1984; Zirkel, 1978a, 1982). Various empirical studies, summarized in Zirkel (1985; see also Arbegglen, 1985), have found that preservice and inservice educators are not particularly knowledgeable about the education-related decisions of the Supreme Court and other such sources of law.

A useful technique for ascertaining and improving one's level of knowledge concerning the Court's education-related decisions is a checklist-type test with brief explanations accompanying the answers. An updated version of such a test, on which a national sample of educators scored approximately 50% (Zirkel, 1978b), appears on the next page. You may wish to quiz yourself and then compare your results to the answers and explanations that follow. This material is also useful for preservice and inservice training.

Quiz on the Supreme Court's
Education-Related Decisions

Circle one of the first three answers below each item to indicate whether the U.S. Supreme Court has held that practice or procedure to be mandatory (''Must''), permissible (''May''), or prohibited (''Must Not''). Circle the fourth answer if you don't know what the Court has ruled for that item. *Note:* These decisions were based on federal law; the answers may differ depending on legislation or regulations in your state that may exceed the minimum legal requirements established at the federal level.

1. A school district . . . have a statutory funding system that relies largely on the local property tax and

that offers at least a minimum education to its pupils.

MUST   MAY   MUST NOT   DON'T KNOW

2. A school district . . . have a program permitting religious instruction within its facilities during ''released time.''

MUST   MAY   MUST NOT   DON'T KNOW

3. A school district . . . require, in accordance with a state statute, the posting in each classroom of a copy of the Ten Commandments which has been obtained via private contributions and which is expressly labeled as nonreligious material.

MUST   MAY   MUST NOT   DON'T KNOW

4. A school district . . . provide classes to nonpublic school students in classrooms located in nonpublic schools.

MUST   MAY   MUST NOT   DON'T KNOW

5. A school district . . . allow an exemption from compulsory high school attendance for students affiliated with a religious sect that has a long history of informal vocational training during the adolescent ages.

MUST   MAY   MUST NOT   DON'T KNOW

6. A school district . . . have maternity leave rules that require a pregnant teacher to stop work at a fixed point 4 to 5 months before the expected date of giving birth.

MUST   MAY   MUST NOT   DON'T KNOW

7. A school district . . . provide a hearing prior to the nonrenewal of a nontenured teacher if: (a) under

*Dr. Zirkel is University Professor of Education and Law at Lehigh University, where Faith MacMurtrie is a graduate student in the M.P.A. program.

state law that teacher had a reasonable expectation of continued employment, or (b) s/he can show that the nonrenewal would severely harm his/her reputation in the community or foreclose employment opportunities elsewhere.

MUST   MAY   MUST NOT   DON'T KNOW

8. A school district . . . require, under the authority of a state statute, that teachers or other school employees take a broad or vague loyalty oath as a requisite of employment.

MUST   MAY   MUST NOT   DON'T KNOW

9. A school district . . . dismiss a teacher for expressing criticism of school policies or practices that are not of public interest.

MUST   MAY   MUST NOT   DON'T KNOW

10. A school district . . . dismiss teachers who are engaged in an illegal strike where the teachers do not show that the board's decision was based on personal, pecuniary, or antiunion bias.

MUST   MAY   MUST NOT   DON'T KNOW

11. A school district . . . allow teachers who are not members of the teachers' organization that is the exclusive bargaining agent to speak at a public board meeting about matters subject to collective bargaining.

MUST   MAY   MUST NOT   DON'T KNOW

12. A school district . . . have regulations that prohibit deliberately making disturbing noise close to classroom facilities while school is in session.

MUST   MAY   MUST NOT   DON'T KNOW

13. A school district . . . provide special language-based instruction for national origin children who have limited English proficiency.

MUST   MAY   MUST NOT   DON'T KNOW

14. A school district . . . provide oral or written notice and an informal hearing prior to suspensions of up to 10 days for students whose presence does not pose an immediate threat to persons, property, or the academic process.

MUST   MAY   MUST NOT   DON'T KNOW

15. A school district . . . permit nonexcessive corporal punishment of students under the authorization or in the absence of a state statute.

MUST   MAY   MUST NOT   DON'T KNOW

16. A school district . . . conduct a search of a student, without the assistance of police, if it has reasonable suspicion (but not necessarily probable) cause to believe that the student has violated or is violating the law or school rules.

MUST   MAY   MUST NOT   DON'T KNOW

17. A school district . . . refuse to provide clean-intermittent-catheterization for handicapped students who need this service to attend school.

MUST   MAY   MUST NOT   DON'T KNOW

18. A school district . . . deny enrollment in their public schools to children who are "illegal aliens" in the United States.

MUST   MAY   MUST NOT   DON'T KNOW

19. A school district . . . allow the union that is the exclusive bargaining agent sole access to its interschool mail system and teacher mailboxes, severely limiting access by unrecognized unions and any other groups.

MUST   MAY   MUST NOT   DON'T KNOW

20. A school district . . . pay attorney's fees to the prevailing plaintiff in suits arising under the Education of the Handicapped Act.

MUST   MAY   MUST NOT   DON'T KNOW

The answers to the quiz items are as follows: 1.—MAY, 2.—MUST NOT, 3.—MUST NOT, 4.—MUST NOT, 5.—MAY, 6.—MUST NOT, 7.—MUST, 8.—MUST NOT, 9.—MAY, 10.—MAY, 11.—MUST, 12.—MAY, 13.—MUST, 14.—MUST, 15.—MUST, 16.—MAY, 17.—MAY, 18.—MUST NOT, 19.—MUST NOT, 20.—MAY. In assessing your results, you may want to consider that the items are grouped as follows with regard to their primary focus: items 1 through 5—funding or religion, items 6 through 11—employees, items 12 through 17—students. A brief explanation for the basis of each item is given below along with the citations for the relevant Supreme Court decisions.

1. In *San Antonio v. Rodriguez,* 411 U.S. 1 (1973), a class representing minority or poor students residing in school districts with a low tax base challenged the constitutionality of the system for funding public schools in Texas. Under this system almost half the revenues were derived from a statewide minimum foundation program. A significant proportion of the remaining revenues were generated from a local property tax. As a result, large discrepancies existed in per pupil expenditures between rich and poor districts. Using equal protection analysis under the Fourteenth Amendment, the Court did not require a strict, compelling justification from the govern-

ment because: (1) there was no suspect class since students of all races suffer alike depending on the tax base of the district in which they attend school; and (2) there was no fundamental right since education in itself is not constitutionally protected. Thus, the Court required only that the financing system be rationally related to a legitimate state purpose which it found in the tradition of local control of education. The Court noted that some state constitutions may have stricter standards, presaging a subsequent body of varying case law at the state level.

2. In *Illinois ex rel. McCollum v. Board of Education,* 333 U.S. 203 (1948), a local taxpayer challenged the "released time" program of an Illinois school district which allowed the representative of various religions to come into the schools during school hours to offer religious instruction to interested students. These students had submitted written consent forms from their parents and were excused from their regular schedule for that part of the day. The other students remained in their regular classes. The Court ruled that the program violated the establishment clause of the First Amendment because it failed to maintain the required separation of church and state. Subsequently, in *Zorach v. Clauson,* 343 U.S. 306 (1952), the Court sustained the constitutionality of a released time program that was essentially the same except that the religious instruction was held elsewhere in the community rather than in the school district's facilities.

3. In *Stone v. Graham,* 449 U.S. 39 (1980), a local taxpayer challenged the constitutionality of a Kentucky statute that required the posting of a copy of the Ten Commandments, which had been provided by private contributions, on the wall of each public school classroom in the state. The statute also provided that each poster contain a small disclaimer stressing the secular nature of the Ten Commandments, as the basis for our legal code and common law. Using the first part of the tripartite test, which has been developed for establishment clause cases, the Court ruled that the statute did not have a secular purpose and thus was not constitutional. The Court distinguished the case from the use of the Bible for the appropriate study of history, civilization, ethics, comparative religion, or the like.

4. In *School District of Grand Rapids v. Ball,* 105 S.Ct. 3216 (1985), taxpayers filed suit claiming that the local district's "Shared Time" and "Community Education" programs were unconstitutional. Under these programs, the district provided remedial instruction for nonpublic school students in classrooms located in and leased from the nonpublic schools. Using the tripartite test, the Court found the programs to have a primary effect of advancing religion and therefore to violate the First Amendment's establishment clause. In a companion case, *Aguilar v. Felton,* 105 S.Ct. 3232 (1985), the

Court also declared unconstitutional programs similar to those in *Grand Rapids* but which outlined a system for monitoring the religious content of publicly funded classes in religious schools. The Court noted that although the supervision might assist in preventing the advancement of religion, the supervisory system would result in excessive entanglement of church and state, thus violating the third prong of the tripartite test.

5. In *Wisconsin v. Yoder,* 406 U.S. 205 (1972), members of the Old Order Amish religious community refused to send their children to any formal public or private school beyond the eighth grade, and consequently were convicted of violating Wisconsin's compulsory attendance law. They challenged the constitutionality of this law as applied to them. The Court used the balancing analysis appropriate to First Amendment free exercise cases. Although regarding an educated citizenry as a generally compelling state interest, the Court weighed the balance here in favor of the Amish parents because, among other things, (1) they comprised a long standing self-sufficient community, (2) they restricted the exemption to only the last two years of compulsory secondary education, and (3) they provided an informal educational program for their children. In subsequent years, lower courts have generally interpreted this "Amish exception" narrowly in other compulsory education cases.

6. In *Cleveland Board of Education v. LaFleur,* 414 U.S. 632 (1974), female teachers in two different school districts challenged the constitutionality of their respective maternity leave policies which both required pregnant teachers to stop working several months (four in one district, five in the other) before the expected date of birth. The policy in one of the districts also had an absolute return date several months after the date of birth. The Court found these policies to violate substantive due process under the Fourteenth Amendment because the early absolute cutoff and (late absolute) return dates constituted an "irrebuttable presumption." The Court warned that individualized early and late absolute cut off dates may not violate this presumption.

7. In the companion cases of *Board of Regents v. Roth,* 408 U.S. 564 (1972) and *Perry v. Sindermann,* 408 U.S. 593 (1972), two nontenured teachers at public institutions of higher education challenged their respective nonrenewals, arguing that they had "de facto" tenure under the Constitution. The Court ruled that under the Fourteenth Amendment they would be entitled to the procedural protections equivalent to tenure only under limited circumstances. Pointing to the due process clause of the Fourteenth Amendment, the Court identified the alternatives of loss of "property" or "liberty." For "property," the teacher would have to show a legitimate objective, not just unilateral expectation of continued

employment under state law. For "liberty," the teacher would have to show a stigmatization of reputation foreclosing educational employment elsewhere. Although lower courts have read this ruling as applicable to teachers in public institutions on the elementary and secondary as well as higher education levels, they have interpreted the liberty or property tests to relatively narrow circumstances.

8. In a series of cases beginning with *Adler v. Board of Education,* 342 U.S. 485 (1952) and ending with *Connell v. Higginbotham,* 403 U.S. 207 (1971), the Court struck down a variety of local and state loyalty oath requirements for teachers and other public employees. Although varying in their wording, these requirements were either vague, broad, or arbitrary, thus violating the void-for-vagueness, over-breadth, and substantive due process doctrines under the First and Fourteenth Amendments. For example, some of the loyalty oath statutes in this series of cases conditioned public employment on membership in a subversive organization. To be valid, the Court suggested that such statutes must be limited to knowing, active members who pursue the illegal goals of the subversive organizations. Further, in part of *Connell* and subsequently in *Cole v. Richardson,* 405 U.S. 676 (1972), the Court upheld the constitutionality of loyalty oaths that required affirmation of the state and federal constitutions.

9. In *Connick v. Myers,* 461 U.S. 138 (1983), an assistant district attorney in New Orleans challenged her dismissal, claiming that it was in retaliation for her criticism of office operations. Alluding to the first part of the First Amendment analysis under *Mt. Healthy City School District Board of Education v. Doyle,* 429 U.S. 274 (1977), by which a public employee must show that his conduct was constitutionally protected expression and that it was a substantial or motivating factor in his dismissal (if this is so, the burden shifts to the public employer to prove that it would have dismissed him anyway), the Court limited constitutionally protected expression to public issues. It is the content rather than the context that is of primary importance at this first step; for in *Givhan v. Western Line Consolidated School District,* 439 U.S. 410 (1979), the Court had held a teacher's private criticism concerning a public issue to be protected expression. This continuing line of cases, which started with the balancing test of *Pickering v. Board of Education,* 391 U.S. 563 (1968), applies to public employees generally, including teachers. However, based on the recent interpretations by lower federal courts, *Connick* serves as a significant stumbling block for these employees when they challenge dismissal or other discipline on the grounds of First Amendment freedom of expression.

10. In *Hortonville Joint School District No. 1 v. Hortonville Education Association,* 426 U.S. 482 (1976),

teachers in a Wisconsin school district went out on strike after bitter, protracted negotiations with the school board. That state's statute authorizes collective bargaining for, but prohibits strikes by, public school teachers. After holding a hearing for the striking teachers, the board terminated them. The teachers contended that their terminations violated the due process clause of the Fourteenth Amendment, claiming that the board, which had been their bitter adversary in its negotiating role, could not be an impartial decision maker in its quasi-judicial role concerning the same situation. The Court disagreed with the teacher organization's position, ruling that the board could validly serve in the latter role to terminate the teachers in this situation unless their decision was shown to be based on personal, pecuniary, or antiunion bias. This decision would not apply in a state where teacher strikes, under certain circumstances, are legal.

11. In *Madison v. Wisconsin Employment Relations Commission,* 429 U.S. 167 (1976), the board of education and the teachers' union, which was the exclusive bargaining agent, were in the process of negotiating a new contract. One of the issues on the bargaining table was an agency shop provision, by which all teachers in the unit would be required to pay a "fair share" fee even if they were not members of the union. During the open session of a school board meeting, one of the nonunion teachers voiced opposition to the fair share proposal. The union then filed an unfair labor practice charge against the board. The state's employment relations commission agreed with the union, ordering the board to cease and desist from permitting any employee other than the exclusive bargaining agent to speak at board meetings, and thereby in effect to negotiate with the board, on matters subject to collective bargaining. The Court overturned this decision, ruling that the board's action was in violation of the individual teachers' First Amendment rights to speak, as citizens, at open meetings of the board concerning education-related issues of public concern. This issue, like the one described in the preceeding item, is moot in the minority of states where collective bargaining is not permitted or required.

12. In *Grayned v. City of Rockford,* 408 U.S. 104 (1972), a student who had been arrested for demonstrating in front of an Illinois high school challenged the constitutionality of the ordinance under which he was convicted. The Court ruled that the provision of the ordinance which prohibited all non-labor picketing within 150 feet of the schools while they are in session was unconstitutionally overbroad. Harking back to its decision in the student armband case, *Tinker v. Des Moines Independent Community School District,* 393 U.S. 503 (1969), the Court pointed out that substantial disruption must be imminent, and the judgement as to the likelihood

of disorder must be made on an individualized basis rather than on the broad, undifferentiated basis encompassed by the anti-picketing ordinance in this case. At the same time, however, the Court sustained the constitutionality of that part of the ordinance that prohibited the willful making of noise incompatible with normal school activity as long as the ordinance was limited as to time (while school is in session) and place (adjacent to the school). This part of the ordinance was not overbroad because it punished only actually or imminently disturbing conduct on an individualized basis. Nor was this part of the ordinance unconstitutionally vague, concluded the Court, because it was properly limited as to time, place, and scope.

13.   In *Lau v. Nichols,* 414 U.S. 563 (1974), a group representing 1300 Chinese-speaking pupils challenged the failure of the San Francisco public schools to provide them with remedial English language instruction. The Court ruled that the school district had an affirmative obligation to provide specialized instruction to such students based on administrative regulations implementing Title VI of the Civil Rights Act of 1964. However, the Court carefully steered away from basing its decision on the Constitution (namely, the equal protection clause of the Fourteenth Amendment) and from prescribing the specific form of instruction (specifically, referring to bilingual education as a possible, not the necessary, answer). Further, in a concurring opinion, two of the justices limited their decision to situations where there are substantial numbers of limited English proficient, national origin minority children. The results of subsequent court decisions have been mixed in terms of bilingual education, with the majority finding such a requirement under Title VI or the more recent Equal Educational Opportunity Act. This requirement is much more specific and strong in states that have legislatively mandated bilingual education.

14.   In *Goss v. Lopez,* 419 U.S. 565 (1975), nine high school students who were suspended for ten days without a hearing of any kind challenged the constitutionality of their suspensions. State legislation authorized the principal to summarily suspend students for up to ten days as a disciplinary measure. The Court held that the statute violated the students' Fourteenth Amendment right to procedural due process. Finding a "property" interest based on the state's compulsory education law and a "liberty" interest based on the stigma to the students' reputation, the Court ruled that public school students who are suspended for up to ten days are entitled to oral or written notice of the charges and, if the student objects, an explanation of the charges and an opportunity to tell his side of the story. Further, the Court concluded, these procedures should take place prior to the suspension unless the student poses a threat to persons, property, or the academic program. These informal requirements are, however, not to be confused with more formal procedures, like the right to confront and cross examine witnesses and to be represented by an attorney. Lower federal courts and some state legislatures or education agencies have required the more formal procedures for exclusions from school that exceed ten days.

15.   In *Ingraham v. Wright,* 430 U.S. 651 (1977), two students had been punished by being hit with a flat wooden paddle. As a result, one student required medical attention and missed eleven days of school, while the other reported the loss of the full use of his arm for seven days. The students argued that the paddling was cruel and unusual punishment in violation of the Eighth Amendment and a deprivation of liberty under the Fourteenth Amendment. The Court disagreed with both arguments, ruling that the Eighth Amendment applies to prisons, not public schools, and that traditional common law remedies obviated the need for procedural due process (i.e., notice and a hearing). Although the Court thus rejected these constitutional bases, some subsequent federal court decisions noted that there may be a substantive due process limit on shockingly excessive corporal punishment. Further, a few states have legislatively prohibited corporal punishment, and several others have built in procedural requirements on the statewide or local level. Finally, the traditional legal remedies remain, such as civil or criminal proceedings for battery and administrative proceedings for dismissal, where such punishment is not reasonable or allowable.

16.   In *New Jersey v. T.L.O.,* 105 S.Ct. 733 (1985), a student who had been disciplined for the sale of marijuana in school sought to have the evidence and her resulting confession excluded from the record. She had been caught violating the school's no-smoking policy. When she denied the charge, the assistant principal searched her purse, finding a pack of cigarettes. Also finding some rolling paper, he then conducted a more thorough search of her purse which yielded evidence implicating her in marijuana dealing. The student argued that in the absence of a warrant or probable cause, the search violated the Fourth Amendment. The Court disagreed, ruling that the strict requirement of probable cause does not apply to school searches conducted by school officials without police assistance. Rather, the standard in such circumstances, the Court concluded, is reasonable suspicion that the student violated or is violating the law or school rules. The search, however, must be limited in two ways: (a) the measures which are adopted must be reasonably related to the objectives of the search, and (b) the search must not be excessively intrusive. Three factors are used to determine excessive intrusiveness: the student's age, sex, and the nature of the infraction. Lower courts have generally read *T.L.O.* as

providing school officials with some latitude in conducting student searches. Nevertheless, strip searches are not looked upon favorably by the courts, and police-assisted searches have been viewed by some courts as requiring probable cause.

17. In *Irving Independent School District v. Tatro,* 104 S.Ct. 3371 (1984), the parents of a child with spina bifida who needed to be catheterized every 3–4 hours, argued that the school district was responsible for providing that service. The school district maintained that this service was medical rather than educational and thus not within its responsibilities. Based on the requirement for "related services" in the Education for All Handicapped Children Act and its implementing regulations, the Court held that the school district must provide clean intermittent catheterization to those who need this service to attend school. It is not a medical service, the Court concluded, because it does not need to be performed by a physician. Lower courts have interpreted *Tatro* to require other seemingly noneducational services, like psychotherapy provided by mental health professionals other than psychiatrists, for handicapped students who need them for educational benefit.

18. In *Plyler v. Doe,* 457, U.S. 202 (1982), a class representing school age children of Mexican origin who could not establish that they had been legally admitted into the United States challenged a state statute which permitted the exclusion of these children from public school. The statute also withheld from local school districts state funds for the education of children who were considered "illegal aliens." The Court ruled that the statute violated the equal protection clause of the Fourteenth Amendment because the state's interest in preserving its limited resources for the education of its lawful residents was not a sufficient rational basis for discriminating against illegal aliens. The Court did not apply the more stringent compelling interest test because: (1) resident aliens are not considered a suspect class, and (2) education is not considered a fundamental right requiring constitutional protection.

19. In *Perry Education Assn. v. Perry Local Educator's Assn.,* 460 U.S. 37 (1984), a union which was not the exclusive bargaining agent for the teachers in a school district challenged the constitutionality of a collective bargaining agreement which allowed the representative union exclusive access to the interschool mail system and teachers' public mailboxes. The Court ruled that preferential access to a school mail system does not violate the First Amendment because an interschool mail system is not a traditional public forum. Therefore, the school district has no constitutional obligation to let any organization use the system. The Court also ruled that the equal protection clause of the Fourteenth Amendment was not violated because the school district policy of differential access was rationally related to a legitimate state purpose: enabling the representative union to perform its obligations as exclusive representative of all teachers.

20. In *Smith v. Robinson,* 104 S.Ct. 3457 (1984), parents of a handicapped child requested attorney's fees after successfully bringing suit against a school district for their decision to no longer fund the child's placement in a special education program. By agreement between the parties, attorney's fees were awarded against the school district. The parents then sought fees and costs from the state for the hours spent in the state's administrative process. Based on statutory interpretation of the Education for the Handicapped Act, the Court ruled that parents were not entitled to attorney's fees under the provisions of that act. Currently, an amendment is pending in Congress (in special committee) that would largely reverse this decision.

REFERENCES

Abegglen, William P. (1985). Knowledge of United States Supreme Court decisions affecting education held by selected Tennessee public school personnel. Doctoral dissertation, East Tennessee State University.

LaMorte, Michael W., and McCollum, Patricia M. (1986, April). A re-examination of the liberal/conservative attitude of the Burger Court toward educational issues. Paper presented at the annual meeting of the American Educational Research Association in San Francisco.

Reutter, E. Edmund, Jr. (1982). *The Supreme Court's Impact on Public Education.* Bloomington, Ind.: Phi Delta Kappa and NOLPE.

Zirkel, Perry A. (1978a). *A Digest of Supreme Court Decisions Affecting Education.* Bloomington, Ind.: Phi Delta Kappa.

Zirkel, Perry A. (1985, July). Educators' knowledge of school law. *NOLPE Notes, 20* (7), 3–5.

Zirkel, Perry A. (1982). *Supplement to a Digest of Supreme Court Decisions Affecting Education.* Bloomington, Ind.: Phi Delta Kappa.

Zirkel, Perry A. (1978b). Test on Supreme Court decisions affecting education. *Phi Delta Kappan, 59,* 521–22, 555.

Chapter 4
Urban Education for the 1980s: Trends and Issues
A. Harry Passow*

Crystal-ball gazing regarding the future of education is always perilous, but it is especially chancy in the area of urban education. Among the many factors complicating predictions concerning urban education are Reaganomics and the Reagan Administration's policies regarding human services and education. Will they cripple our urban school systems, erasing whatever gains have been made over the past decade and more? To what extent will recession, budget cuts, the reduction or elimination of categorical grants, and the conversion to block grants affect the precarious funding of urban schools? How will the Administration's stance on desegregation, human services, civil rights, and the appropriate role for the federal government affect the functioning of urban schools?

In 1963, in *Education in Depressed Areas,* I observed that about two-thirds of the U.S. population lived in the 189 areas designated, by virtue of population size and density, as metropolitan, and that, in the decade from 1950 to 1960, 80% of the total population growth took place in those areas. At that time, almost one out of every six elementary and secondary school children attended public school in one of the 16 largest U.S. cities. However, as I pointed out:

Statistics do not depict the physical and economic deterioration of the central-city gray areas, the movement of the middle class to the suburbs, the transiency and instability of the in-migrant families, the concentration and intensification of social problems in depressed areas. City slums have existed for generations, even though their tenants have changed with each migration. Ethnic, racial, and socioeconomic groups have coalesced in areas of the city, creating de facto segregation in schools even where laws imply nonsegregation. School buildings in the depressed urban areas seem to house the greatest array of educational problems.[1]

At the time, I felt that the outlook was both discouraging and hopeful—"discouraging in terms of its size, com-plexity, bitterness, and the human cost involved . . . hopeful in the forces which are being mobilized to dissect and resolve this wasteful, destructive problem of displaced citizens in a rejecting or ignoring homeland."[2]

Several years later, writing in *Urban Education in the 1970s,* it seemed to me that the crisis in urban education had grown even more intense in all of its dimensions:

Since then (1962), having spent billions of dollars on compensatory education, initiated thousands of projects (each with its own clever acronym title), completed hundreds of studies of uneven significance and even more disparate quality, entered numerous judicial decisions and rulings, experienced dozens of riots and disorders, and generated whole new agencies and educational institutions, the nation's urban schools continue to operate in a vortex of declining achievement.[3]

The 1970 national census confirmed that the largest population growth had been in suburbia, with the segregation and isolation for the poor and minority groups becoming even more intense in central cities. Middle-class blacks and other minority groups had joined the march to the suburbs—leaving the poor behind.

Looking Back at the Seventies

The decade of the 1970s saw a number of positive and negative developments affecting urban school systems in the U.S. On the negative side, a number of large-city school systems (e.g., Cleveland, Detroit, and New York), along with their municipal governments, teetered on the brink of bankruptcy and had to slash their budgets, reduce staff, and cut services in order to remain solvent. In addition, several urban school systems (e.g., Boston, Los Angeles, and Columbus) were under court order to desegregate their schools. The disruption and violence in

*Dr. A. Harry Passow is a Jacob H. Schiff Professor of Education at Teachers College, Columbia University, New York, NY. Reprinted with permission of the author and *Phi Delta Kappan*, April, 1982.

Boston was front-page news for months. In 1978 Los Angeles began a mandatory busing program amid considerable controversy; the busing ended in the spring of 1981 by order of the California State Supreme Court. The impact on white flight, with fewer than 20% of Los Angeles pupils affected, was difficult to assess. In fact, both the white and the black populations continued to decline, but the number of Hispanic and Asian pupils increased rapidly in the same period. School desegregation continued to disrupt urban schools more than a quarter century after the *Brown* decision.

School violence and vandalism were a bitter part of urban schooling throughout the Seventies. Although reliable data on violence and vandalism are elusive, a study of school crime and violence in 15 major cities revealed that, from 1970 to 1975, weapon and drug violations increased in every one of the cities except Oakland.[4] (Differences in classification and methods of reporting criminal incidents make it difficult, however, to trace trends from city to city or over a long period of time.) A study of school principals in 1975-76 showed crime and vandalism to be "serious" in 15% of the large-city schools and 11% of those in small cities. Only 8% of the suburban schools and 6% of school in rural areas had similarly severe problems.[5] Among the findings of this study by the National Institute of Education (NIE): "Risks of assault and robbery to urban youngsters aged 12-19 are greater in school than out. Most of this disparity is accounted for by 12- to 15-year-olds, whose risks at school are much higher than elsewhere."[6] Urban schools are perceived as unsafe schools by public, staff, and students alike.

With respect to the real business of the schools—academic achievement—urban schools have not been at the top of the scale for some time. Because urban school districts are now serving sharply increased proportions of children from low-income families, from racial and ethnic minorities, and from non-English-speaking backgrounds, there is greater need for compensatory education programs. Compensatory education has been delivered primarily through Title 1 of the Elementary and Secondary Education Act ($2.735 billion in fiscal year 1978) and through state funds (approximately $490 million in some 17 states during fiscal year 1978).

How effective has compensatory education been? Have various compensatory education programs and provisions reversed the trend of academic failure found among children from disadvantaged backgrounds? In his message to Congress in 1970 on educational reform, President Richard Nixon commented on the "series of ambitious, idealistic, and costly programs for the disadvantaged, based on the assumption that extra resources would equalize learning opportunity and eventually help eliminate poverty"; he observed that a few such programs had dramatically improved educational achievement, many had provided important auxiliary services such as better nutrition and medical care, and some programs may have helped prevent some children from falling even further behind. He concluded, "However, the best available evidence indicates that most of the compensatory education programs have not measurably helped poor children catch up."[7]

In 1978 the NIE published the results of a study of the purposes and effectiveness of compensatory education programs, which consisted of a nationwide survey of compensatory programs, special demonstration projects in 13 school systems, and case studies of particular aspects of the Title I program.[8] The study sought to determine if Title I funds were being distributed as Congress had intended, that is, to help school districts provide services to areas with high concentrations of low-income families.

The NIE analysis revealed that Title I was superior to other federal and state programs "in terms of its capacity to increase educational spending at the local level rather than being used to replace local expenditures," but it went on to say that, at the local level, Title I funds were not concentrated solely on the lowest-income schools. The study concluded:

> In general, NIE's findings do not show that Title I is effective everywhere or that past problems with the quality and stability of instructional services have been solved. But the results do indicate that school districts can create conditions necessary to make compensatory instructional services effective.[9]

The study suggests, though, that "Title I has succeeded in providing additional educational services to those students whom the schools usually serve least well."[10] The portion of the NIE study that examined the instructional effects of Title I revealed that, in three out of four cases, achievement test scores of students in regular classrooms were higher than those of students in so-called "pull-out" classrooms. There is some disagreement on the effectiveness of compensatory education programs, however.[11]

Some Recent Positive Signs

Since the mid-1960s early childhood education (including preschool) has been viewed as a significant component of compensatory education. Thousands of disadvantaged; young children have participated in the Head Start and Follow Through programs as well as in hundreds of other preschool programs. The Westinghouse Learning Corporation study on the impact of Head Start set the tone for many subsequent reports; it concluded that preschool education may help disadvantaged children in some ways but has no real impact on academic achievement.

Consequently, the report of the Consortium for Longitudinal Studies title *Lasting Effects After Preschool* provided a fresh perspective. The consortium comprises 12 groups involved in longitudinal studies on the outcomes of early childhood education programs. The report details the findings from analyses of longitudinal studies of low-income children who had participated in experimental infant and preschool programs begun in the Sixties. Some 3,000 low-income children who had participated in various intervention programs or who had served as controls for such programs were reexamined in 1976-77. The implications drawn from the findings were as follows:

> High-quality early education programs are likely to benefit both low-income children and the larger society by: reducing the number of children in later cost special education programs in schools, helping children avoid grade failure, increasing children's math achievement scores at fourth grade and I.Q. scores at least up to age 13, and influencing aspects of children's and mothers' achievement orientation.[12]

In fiscal year 1979 federal spending for early intervention programs totaled $1.58 billion and served approximately 1.9 million preschool children.[13] Although not all of those low-income students are located in urban centers, they do constitute a sizable population for whom, as one project report put it, "preschool education can be part of the solution, but it is only a part."[14]

In July of 1981 Atlanta, Boston, New York City, Philadelphia, and Washington, D.C., all reported "sharply higher scores" on standardized tests of reading and mathematics. New York City reported that for the first time since 1970 more than half of the elementary school students scored above the national average. Atlanta reported that 43% of students in grades 1 to 8 were above the national average—up from 31% in the previous year. Forty-seven percent of Atlanta's elementary pupils topped the national average, up from 33% a year earlier.[15]

Roy Forbes, the director of the National Assessment of Educational Progress (NAEP), observed that students in cities larger than 200,000 seem to be gaining slightly more than students in smaller cities in reading and mathematics achievement. Thirteen-year-olds in cities dropped 4% in reading between 1971 and 1975 but gained 2.6% in the four years following 1975. The NAEP reported that the largest gains during the 1970s had been among students where federal money, particularly Title I money, had been concentrated. The large-city gains seem not to have been sustained beyond the ninth grade. Forbes said, "Students are getting a better foundation in the basics

but have declined in the more complex skills. We need to focus our attention on the high schools now."[16]

In the 1960s researchers began to examine the factors that governed educational effectiveness and that may contribute to schools' attaining unexpectedly high scores. Ronald Edmonds has identified what seem to him to be seven of "the most tangible and indispensable characteristics of effective schools" for the urban poor.[17] This line of research is not without its skeptics and critics, of course, primarily because of its school-centered view of the determinants of achievement.[18] But the research findings could be extremely helpful to urban educators.

Another study, the three-year Urban Education Studies project, attempted "to identify, and to impart impetus to, strategies and developments which seem likely to contribute to the revitalization of educational institutions, personnel, and practices."[19] Between 1977 and 1980 the project staff gathered information on promising programs and developments in 16 large cities, looking particularly at those factors and conditions that promised systemwide improvement. The study "revealed that in all of these systems there are many excellent schools, many dedicated, highly competent teachers and other staff members, and serious efforts to improve educational performance at every level."[20] Francis Chase, the project director, found 10 factors that appeared in one form or another in all 16 urban school systems. These included:

- the formation of partnerships of other collaborative relationships between schools and other community agencies and organizations;
- active involvement of parents and other citizens in educational planning, curriculum development, and instruction;
- the establishment of new types of schools that offer alternatives to neighborhood elementary schools, middle schools, and comprehensive high schools;
- extended provisions for early childhood education;
- new emphasis on the teaching of basic skills;
- the introduction of bilingual and multicultural programs;
- the initiation of new programs for the handicapped;
- broadened roles for the creative and performing areas;
- the installation of instructional management systems; and
- the initiation of approaches to systemwide planning, management, and evaluation.

Three trends were found in all 16 cities: (1) participation in educational decision making by significantly larger numbers of minority groups and the poor, (2) increased attention by school boards and administrators to advice from individuals and groups outside the profession, and (3) unprecedented collaboration between schools and nonschool agencies.

Urban Education in the 1980s

Recently Egon Guba listed 13 difficulties facing urban educators in the 1980s, a listing that was by no means exhaustive, "any one of which is sufficient to undermine the commitment of all but the most determined individuals": money, pressure for desegregation, demands for efficiency, negative public perceptions, the cross-fire generated by differing values, inadequate plant, political pressures, union demands, dissatisfied teachers, struggle for federal/state dollars, revolving-door programs, unresponsive students, and declining enrollments.[21] Although these problems are not limited to urban school systems, they take on a particular intensity and/or complexity in urban centers. But Guba concluded with a note of hope:

> Despite the fact that many of the reasons for today's state of affairs are beyond the school's control, they have not avoided making every effort to respond. Good use is being made of adversity that now confronts them, and a variety of interventions have been constructed—process interventions such as R&E planning, management, and special projects, and substantive interventions such as program innovations, new materials, organization strategies, community involvement, financing strategies, cooperative efforts among districts, teacher/administrator retraining, and marketing of the schools—that give reasonable promise of success.[22]

The range and diversity of programs and strategies employed by urban schools to tackle their multitude of problems are impressive. They focus on different target populations, on different kinds of treatments and services, on various components of the educational system, and even on diverse goals and objectives. The "success" of urban school programs varies, depending on the goals that are sought. The concept of "equality of educational opportunity," for example, has many different meanings and could be attained in one sense and not in others.

What should urban schools be doing to be considered successful? If the urban poor were at or above grade level in the basic skills of reading and arithmetic—the goal of many Title I programs—would that be sufficient? If we provided high school youths with marketable skills or increased the college-going rate, would that remove some of the pressure from our urban schools? If we closed the gap between the children of the poor and of minorities and children of the middle class majority—assuming there was agreement on the nature of the gap—would urban programs be considered successful?

Urban education continues to be a euphemism for education of the disadvantaged, the poor, and the racial and ethnic minorities. To ignore the diversity of population, of course, can only result in an intensification of the problems urban schools face, and educators must keep in mind that middle-class, majority students present their own challenges—related and yet distinct.

Cities constitute rich environments for educating individuals of all ages. The urban environment contains cultural, educational, social, economic, physical, and natural resources that influence the development of its inhabitants. Urban education, when it consists only of that which takes place at that site called "school," is clearly too limited and limiting.

More than a decade ago the Urban Education Task Force of the Department of Health, Education, and Welfare, in examining problems and solutions related to urban schooling, urged the development of master plans, arguing that such plans

> . . . must concomitantly deal with causes and symptoms, must be *conceived within a framework of overall urban problem solving rather than education per se,* and must encompass all educational levels....Moreover, this plan must reflect a considerable expansion and enrichment of what constitutes "education." Within the educational plan, there must be stress on developing and implementing appropriate curricular designs, consumer participation, staff development programs for *all* concerned, supportive services, and evaluation. *Finally, it must be interrelated with other facets of the larger urban problems, such as housing, employment, recreation, and health.*[23] (Emphasis added)

The various programs, projects, and activities that have occupied our urban schools during the past two decades may have taken us as far as we can go. It was not all that long ago that our urban school systems were, in fact, the elite of U.S. education. The large-city schools excelled on all criteria used to judge the quality of education and schooling. It is only as the so-called "urban crisis" evolved in the 1930s that urban education began to decline, for education was an integral part of the overall urban crisis.

The shape of urban education in the 1980s will be determined by the extent to which education planners and decision makers relate their activities to other facets of "the larger urban problems" and conceive their plans "within a framework of overall urban problem solving." To do otherwise will be to restrict development to goals that are achievable but fall short of what we are capable of becoming.

FOOTNOTES

1. A. Harry Passow, *Education in Depressed Areas* (New York: Teachers College Press, 1963), p. 1.

2. Ibid., p. 351.

3. A. Harry Passow, *Urban Education in the 1970s* (New York: Teachers College Press, 1971), p. 1.

4. Martha R. Asner and James Broschart, eds., *Violent Schools—Safe Schools: The Safe School Study Report to the Congress* (Washington, D.C.: U.S. Government Printing Office, 1978), p. 34.

5. Ibid., p. 38.

6. Ibid., p. 74.

7. Constantine Menges, *The Effectiveness of Compensatory Education: Summary and Review of the Evidence* (Washington, D.C.: U.S. Government Printing Office, n.), p. 14.

8. National Institute of Education, *The Compensatory Education Study: Executive Summary* (Washington, D.C.: U.S. Government Printing Office, 1978), p. 2.

9. Ibid., p. 12.

10. Ibid., p. 13.

11. See, for example, David R. Caruso and Douglas K. Detterman, "Intelligence Research and Social Policy," *Phi Delta Kappan,* November 1981, pp. 183-86; and Lawrence J. Schweinhart, "Comment on 'Intelligence Research and Social Policy,' " *Phi Delta Kappan*, November 1981, p. 187.

12. Irving Lazar and Richard B. Darlington, eds., *Lasting Effects After Preschool* (Washington, D.C.: U.S. Government Printing Office, 1979).

13. Lawrence J. Schweinhart and David P. Weikart, *Young Children Grow Up: The Effects of the Perry Preschool Program on Youths Through Age 15* (Ypsilanti, Mich.: High/Scope Press, 1980), p. 84.

14. Ibid., p. 86.

15. "Scores Up Because of Hard Work, Big City School Administrators Say," *Education USA,* 6 July 1981, p. 345.

16. Ibid., p. 350.

17. Ronald Edmonds, "Effective Schools for the Urban Poor," *Educational Leadership, October 1979,* pp. 15-24. Some of these characteristics of effective schools may be found in Daniel U. Levine, "Successful Approaches for Improving Academic Achievement in Inner-City Elementary Schools," *Phi Delta Kappan,* April 1982, p. 523.

18. Ralph Scott and Hebert J. Walberg, "Schools Alone Are Insufficient: A Response to Edmonds," *Educational Leadership,* October 1979, pp. 24-27.

19. Francis S. Chase and William E. Bell, "Introduction: The Urban Education Studies, 1977-1980," in Francis S. Chase, ed., *Educational Quandaries and Opportunities* (Dallas: Urban Education Studies, 1980), p. 1.

20. Francis S. Chase, "Educational Revitalization: A Search for Promising Developments," in *Educational Quandaries and Opportunities,* p. 33.

21. Egon Guba, "Challenges to Public Education," in *Educational Quandaries and Opportunities,* pp. 10–17.

22. Ibid., p. 32.

23. HEW Urban Education Task Force, *Urban School Crisis: The Problem and Solutions* (Washington, D.C.: National School Public Relations Association, 1970), p. 45.

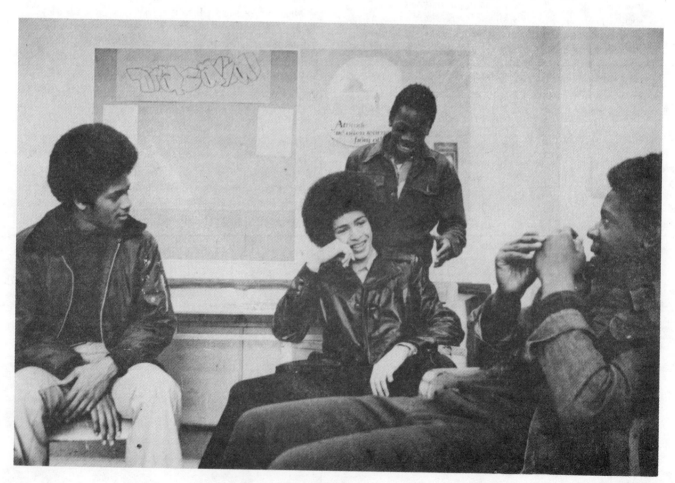

Ellen Meltzer

Chapter 5
The Great American Schooling Experiment
John I. Goodlad*

In the summer of 1983 a group of educators from western European ministries visited President Reagan and discussed comparative issues and problems of schooling. They were deeply interested in the recommendations of *A Nation at Risk,* released a few months earlier, and in what this report boded for schooling in the U.S.

In particular, they wondered about the practical implications of a fresh emphasis on excellence. Was this to be excellence for a few, or the academic elite? Might they anticipate some shift away from America's primary concern with universal education? Such a shift would not go unnoticed in their countries, which are now experiencing rapid enrollment increases in secondary education, comparable to those that took place in the U.S. between the two world wars.

The substance of this White House discussion illustrates one of the most striking features of schooling in America and of the continuing debate, here and abroad, that has marked the "Great American Schooling Experiment" since it first began. Martin Trow put the matter well:

> The role of public education in American thought and popular sentiment, and its perceived connection with the national welfare and individual achievement, have, at least until recently, been greater in America than in any other country. . . . The commitment of America to equality of opportunity, the immense importance attached to education throughout American history, the very role of education as an avenue of mobility in a society where status ascribed at birth is felt to be an illegitimate barrier to advancement—all of these historical and social psychological forces are involved in the extraordinary American commitment to mass secondary and high education.[1]

The effort to match a system of comprehensive schooling to these beliefs and expectations has brought with it the inevitable charge that excellence has been overwhelmed by mediocrity—in recent years a "rising tide of mediocrity," according to the National Commission on Excellence in Education. And so the debate always comes down to whether we can have mass secondary education and excellence, too.

In recent years, the *Kappan* has provided a useful forum for the scholarly, data-based portion of this debate. In his cross-national analysis, Burton Clark argued that "the dream of universal education, in the form of the comprehensive school . . . is a huge burden on the school system." While he acknowledges that the "democratic idealism" implicit in this concept has helped to integrate our society, he nevertheless contends that "the perceived failure of the U.S. secondary schools is, to a considerable degree, the result of a short-fall in outcomes when they are measured against the expectation that the comprehensive school . . . can be helpful to all students from all types of backgrounds."[2] Others have argued that the top students in U.S. schools are still a match for those of any other nation, despite our national goal of universal education.[3]

The question that rises out of this debate is this: What, specifically, is wrong with the American system of education? If something is wrong, let's fix it.

There is no doubt that much in the system needs fixing, and I agree with Clark that many of the needed changes are organizational, a fact that most of the commission and task force reports of the past few years have evaded.[4] Many of the problems in American education have become features of educational systems throughout the world, most of which try to be comprehensive at some level.[5]

Clark pinpointed the cause of "the distinctively American problem posed by universal education" as "an

---

*Dr. John I. Goodlad, former dean of the Graduate School of Education at the University of California, Los Angeles, is a professor of policy, governance, and administration in the College of Education at the University of Washington, Seattle. Reprinted with permission of the author and Phi Delta Kappan, December, 1985.

excess of hope."[6] This hope is the expectation that all members of an age group will remain in school for 12 years and graduate with some kind of diploma.

There it is. The essence of our problem is "an excess of hope"—a condition that defies quantitative analysis. Hope eludes stratification by economic or social class, by race, or by creed. It is appropriately democratized; it is everybody's problem.

How, then, do we deal with this problem? Two alternatives suggest themselves. We could work to reduce our hope, though doing so may inadvertently cultivate despair and cynicism. Still, the payoff could be a reduction in disappointment. Or we could devote more attention to clarifying those aspects of our diverse array of hopes that have some prospect of being achieved through education. Then we could set our expectations accordingly. This approach would deal practically with the problems of schooling. It then becomes possible to estimate what the cost of addressing these problems will be and to determine whether we are willing to pay the price. Diane Ravitch looks unblinkingly at just where we stand with regard to this second approach:

> Every nation gets the schools that it deserves, and we have today a system that reflects our own conflicts about the relative importance of different social and educational values . . . and it is obvious that we do not yet have a philosophical commitment to education that is strong enough to withstand the erratic dictates of fashion.[7]

To what degree are our expectations for schools inflated? What are the prospects of and strategies for achieving a balance between expectations and what is reasonable to anticipate?

Hope cannot be measured. It cannot be counted or weighed, and, therefore, it is difficult to judge what is too much or too little. What we can do by way of analysis is to describe what we hope for and see how widely our hopes are shared. If we find our hopes are widely shared, it would be irresponsible to judge them idiosyncratic. If they are persistently shared, it would be unwise to judge them ephemeral. Are there any hopes for education and schooling that are widely and persistently shared?

Nothing that has transpired in the last four decades suggests that Americans are abandoning their broad and comprehensive expectations for schooling. In today's enormously complex society, however, the difficulty comes in translating expectations into actual programs. The idea of going "back to basics," for example, seems to be relatively straightforward. In practice, it is anything but straightforward. In the mid-1970s, some legislators, school board members, and educators took the media-driven message that the schools should "get back to the

basics" as a directive to expunge from the curriculum virtually everything except the three R's. Some school boards seriously considered reintroducing the McGuffey Readers into their school systems. It was difficult for me to believe that this activity could be anything other than short-lived or that parents had jettisoned a large portion of the hopes they held for the education of their children.

My graduate students and I devoted part of a yearlong seminar to describing the hopes of parents and defining any consensus that ran through them. We found that academic expectations expanded steadily from a few simple learnings in the 17th century to include virtually all the domains of knowledge by the end of the 19th century. Meanwhile, vocational and citizenship goals were added, and, in the 20th century, schooling was to be not only for the development of responsible parents, citizens, and workers, but also for the cultivation of the self.[8]

Were these ever-broadening expectations for schooling to be cast aside? We studied the goal statements of all 50 states. There they were again: academic/intellectual, social/citizenship, vocational, and personal goals, with subgoals defining them further and with admonitions regarding the importance of *every* student. We used the language of these documents in seeking to define each goal area for a questionnaire we administered to nearly 18,000 students, 8,600 parents, and 1,350 teachers. All four goal areas were judged to be "very important" or "essential."

When forced to choose only one area to be given top priority, our respondents were not in agreement. Each goal area received a substantial portion of the votes. The most surprising finding was that only 50% of the parents chose the academic/intellectual area as their top priority—approximately 57% of the parents of elementary school students and 46% of the parents of high school students. Other data gathered revealed an expectation for safety in the school environment, for one's child to be known and supported in school, and for individual attention. Drawing primarily on documentary evidence, Ernest Boyer reached the same conclusion, and he and I titled chapters that dealt with Americans' expectations for schooling in our respective books, "We Want It All."[9]

These expectations tend not to be lowered for long. Each apparent retreat from them has been followed rather quickly by a resurgence of interest (usually for too short a time and with too small an allocation of resources) and a fresh resolve to make the reality of schooling live up to our goals. A consensus on hopes and aspirations is quite a different matter from a consensus on the kind and amount of formal education our children should have and on the organization and conduct of schooling. Is there a *working* consensus at this practical level? I believe there is, as long as we bear in mind that a working consensus is always ragged around the edges.

What schools require to function is that the sum of fragmentation be somewhat less than the central core of agreement.

In the early years of this century, the working consensus was the translation of hopes and aspirations into a common school: an elementary school of seven or eight grades; free education until graduation from this school; common attendance; and a common curriculum. The common school was a terminal institution, and only one in 10 students went on to secondary education.[10] The pressure on elementary schools to pay more attention to their preparatory function would not come until more students continued on to secondary school.

That change was not long in coming. Whereas the high school population rose from 6.7% of the age group in 1889 to 15.4% in 1909, the growth in the next three decades was phenomenal, reaching 73.3% by the end of the 1930s. The elementary school was no longer viewed as terminal. With this transformation came complaints, particularly from high school personnel, that students were being passed along to the high schools ill-prepared; complaints also came from educators, employers, and citizens generally that completion of grade school no longer meant anything. The obvious answer was a matriculation examination, from which the ablest students were often excluded, and repetition of the final year of elementary school became more common.

The secondary school enjoyed the advantage of being considered a terminal school for several decades. The Great Depression effectively closed entry into the labor force to graduates of elementary schools and contributed to the raising of the school-leaving age to 16. Because there were no jobs to be had, there was little motivation to leave school. The high school, therefore, modified and expanded its curriculum to accommodate large numbers of students who had little motivation for study but even less reason to leave. Many of the problems of secondary education that Clark labeled an "embarrassment" today were in the making in the postwar years. With nearly 90% of the age group attending secondary school in 1958, it was often said that nobody knew anymore what a high school education meant.

In our society, the more commonly things are possessed, the less they are valued. This is particularly true when the thing possessed is seen as instrumental to other things perceived to be even more valuable.

The rapid growth of higher education following World War II approximated the rapid growth of secondary schooling during the decades between the two world wars. The force behind this growth was the same that produced near-universal elementary schooling by the turn of the century and near-universal secondary schooling a half-century later: namely, the interaction of

changes in the hopes and aspirations of the people and changes in the society at large. The secondary school was transformed once again from a terminal institution to a preparatory one. Completing high school became the passport for entry into the labor force or into higher education. Both by definition and in fact, the high school became the upper portion of the common school.

The problems of secondary schooling emerge less from an excess of hope than from impatience and frustration over our inability to properly cultivate the fruits of our hopes. The words on one of Corita's serigraphs come to mind: "We harvest the fruit of hope in order to begin again to hope." Near-universal secondary education is merely a prelude to near-universal higher education, both the fruits of our hopes.

"There is no reason to believe," Martin Trow wrote, "that the United States will stop short of providing opportunities and facilities for nearly universal experience of some kind in higher education."[11] Trow wrote these words nearly a quarter of a century ago, noting as he did so the intense criticism of secondary education stemming from the juxtaposition of preparatory and terminal functions within the same institution. Critics, especially university professors, stressed the need for a different guiding philosophy for secondary schools; the defenders of secondary education pointed to the needs of the many students who did not go on to college. And this issue remains at the center of the current debate over secondary schools.

This debate, however, obscures the way in which changing circumstances and changing hopes have combined to produce a core of consensus that is larger than the sum of the ragged edges. The essence of this consensus is that all students, whether or not they intend to go to college, *require education that is at least equivalent in function to what the common elementary school provided at the turn of the century.* In short, this means a secondary education, for the lack of a high school diploma is generally recognized as a serious, lifelong handicap.

A somewhat smaller part of this consensus is currently growing: the idea that a substantial segment of the curriculum should be common to all students. On this, virtually all the recent commission and task force reports agree. This interest in a common curriculum has been strengthened by reports of the growing gap between high school vocational training and the job market. Although we are not at all clear on how technology will affect our lives or our vocations in the years to come, the fact that only 10% to 12% of the workforce will soon be producing *all* the food we eat and *all* the goods we use cannot be ignored. More and more people are concluding that there are no significant differences between the kind of formal schooling required to prepare for entry into higher education and the kind required to prepare for entry into the workforce.[12]

If we are indeed at a point at which we want to make the level and kind of schooling essentially the same for the college-bound and the non-college-bound, then the distinctions between the terminal and preparatory functions of secondary education become meaningless. The possible differences would have to be in the areas of social/citizenship goals and of personal goals. But to deliberately set out to differentiate in the schooling of the college-bound and the non-college-bound in these areas surely would embarrass us more than the fact that many students graduating from our high schools read and write poorly.

If the success of the "Great American Schooling Experiment" is judged on the criterion of universal secondary education, then we are well on our way. The U.S. high school is where the elementary school was several decades ago. The first set of problems that stems from this advance has to do with our ambiguous attitudes. We are not at all sure about whether what we have wrought is good or bad. We become particularly nervous during times of declining confidence in ourselves, in our economy, or in our place in world affairs, because we have connected these matters intimately to schooling. Moreover, we accept uncritically whatever negative comparisons are made between our schools and those in Japan, Germany, or Switzerland.

Despite this nervousness, we are not about to abandon our drive toward universal secondary schooling. Minnesota is proud of its front-rank status with respect to the retention of young people in high school (86%), while Mississippi (61.8%) is envious.[13] Yet, when we compare the quality of schools, we look almost exclusiveily at the achievement test scores of the students still in them. Were we not so ambivalent in our attitudes toward schools, we would compile data both on dropouts and on those pushed out of school, and we would make use of these data in judging a school's quality.[14] Instead, we seem to look the other way. As of 1984, "virtually no state passed 'reform' legislation that contained specific plans to provide remediation to those who did not meet the higher standards on the first try," and, in 1985, several reform-minded states "moved up the high jump bar from four to six feet without giving any additional coaching to the youth who were not clearing the bar when it was set at four feet."[15]

The second set of problems growing out of our goal of nearly universal secondary education stems from not clearly articulating the means to achieve it. Our commitment to this ideal was implied in many of the state documents on expectations that my students and I examined. But the prose in these documents was cautious and tentative. There was little in them to inspire state, district, or

school responsibility for advancing all students through those common learnings thought necessary for responsible citizenship, for entry into the workforce or higher education, and for personal growth and satisfaction. Furthermore, there is little or nothing in our present demands for accountability that is likely to call attention to our neglect of this commitment.

And so we sidestep the questions that must be answered if our hopes are to be truly realized. We brush aside such questions as, What are the learnings—both knowledge and ways of knowing—that should constitute the common core? Merely specifying four years of English, three of mathematics, two of history and government, and so on is clearly a cop-out. If our goal is universal secondary education, then the high school is a terminal institution and should be regarded as the final chance to give everyone the general education that our goals imply we want them to have. Defining what constitutes this education becomes imperative. Similarly, defining the structural arrangements, the pedagogy, and the substance of teacher education become imperatives.

If there is a consensus on our hopes—including universal secondary education, a core of common learnings, and equal access to knowledge (the most ragged part of the fabric)—then certain practices become suspect. High on a list of suspect practices comes the sorting of students into high, middle, and low tracks, in which, with disturbing frequency, course content, teacher enthusiasm, and other opportunities are clearly differentiated in favor of the upper tracks.[16] The evidence suggests that tracking is a convenient, if sometimes discomforting, way to get around a troublesome problem. Why tackle something more difficult if the articulation of educational policy fails to make clear that the provision of two different kinds of learning opportunities—one for the future banker and one for the future street cleaner—is simply unacceptable?"[17]

This brings me to the third and most troublesome set of problems growing out of progress toward universal secondary education. We simply do not have generation after generation of grauduates from all segments, and socioeconomic levels of society. Consequently, we have large numbers of parents who are more uneasy than their children about desegregated schools. And some of them, as well as many other parents, cannot give their sons and daughters the kind of support that yesterday's principals and teachers could take for granted. Only recently has a body of literature emerged on how schools might work effectively to support rather than discriminate against minority students.

With regard to much of secondary education, we are, in effect, still in the experimental stage; we are going around for the first time. However, there is nothing experimental about the concept of universal secondary education. It is here to stay, warts and all. Controversy will continue over how to remove the warts—and especially over which warts mask malignancies.

I have no misgivings about our ability to deal with both the warts and the malignancies. I do worry about the price of simultaneously cultivating an educated elite and a comprehensive system of education—both goals that we are extremely unlikely to abandon. Torsten Husén has drawn the following conclusion:

> An elite *can* be cultivated within a comprehensive educational system. Whether or not the elite produced in such a system is worth its price is another question. One should, however, recognize that, in selective systems, the high standard of the elite is bought at the price of more limited opportunities for the majority of students.[18]

Individualism runs deep in American culture. Political leaders at times speak eloquently about "community," but in recent years the spoils have gone more to those who have touched our sense of individuality. The system of comprehensive schooling we have today has fewer common elements than did its predecessor, the common elementary school, largely because of the way individuality of interest has intruded on it. As community has withered to become "people of my race, my neighborhood, my economic class,"[19] support for a common school, commonly attended, has declined.

We have been highly successful in broadening our sense of community in times of national emergency. The National Commission on Excellence in Education may have done us a favor with its liberal use of war-time figures of speech. Concern over our schools grew to crisis proportions soon after the release of *A Nation at Risk*.

However, we have been unable to come up with an agenda for reform that is even close to matching this sense of crisis. I think this may be because we view change primarily in terms of how it will affect "me and mine." Thus we suffer not so much from an *excess* as from an *imbalance* of hope. We seem to view hope as finite. That is, the more widely we spread it around, the less there will be for each of us. John Dewey's ideal for the schools, though widely cited, remains as elusive today as ever: "What the best and wisest parent wants for his own child, that must the community want for all of its children."

The astonishing growth of both secondary and higher education in this country may have blinded us to the fact that our experiment in schooling is unfinished. As long as our poor and minorities are distinctly in the minority, we seem unlikely to work ourselves up into a crisis mentality over the fact that 40% of Hispanic students do not complete high school or that enrollments of black and His-

panic students in higher education are falling. Even what Husén sees as the worldwide possibility of "a new educational underclass"[20] arouses us only a little.

What may stir us to transcend self-interest could be the sudden awareness that the problem worrying Husén is our problem, too. The aging of the adult population has helped to obscure the rapidly changing demographic picture of the school-age and early childhood population. In 1984, 36% of the babies in the United States were born to members of minority groups. Large numbers of these children are the offspring of teenage mothers who have no guaranteed source of income. Many of these mothers did not enjoy the good nutrition and prenatal care thought necessary for a healthy baby. The children of these mothers are likely to be more difficult to educate than the average child. Combine these facts with other data on births out of wedlock, divorce, and the like, and we have a picture of a future in which the nuclear family, working together with the school to educate a child, will be the exception.

I find it difficult to believe that these data imply either business as usual or a lessening of our commitment to schooling. Instead, they seem to point to an even greater need to find creative alternative ways to organize and teach so that schools will be attractive and so that the common learnings that bind us together as a society will be learned. I reject the idea that one of these ways is the early sorting of children into categories that harden into self-fulfilling prophecies.

We will be in much need of hope, especially the kind of hope that embraces an ever-expanding concept of community. Along with hope, however, we must also have commitment not to lower our standards but to increase our effort to realize our hope. We can learn a few things, of course, from our history and from the experience of other countries, especially from the way other countries see us. The educators from foreign ministries expressed concern for the future of the Great American Schooling Experiment. But, no doubt, they were even more concerned for the future of the Great American Experiment in Democracy. So must we be.

FOOTNOTES

1. Martin Trow, "The Second Transformation of American Secondary Education," *International Journal of Comparative Sociology,* September 1961, p. 147.

2. Burton R. Clark, "The High School and the University: What Went Wrong in America, Part I," *Phi Delta Kappan,* February 1985, pp. 395-96.

3. See Torsten Husén, "Are Standards in U.S. Schools Really Lagging Behind Those in Other Countries?," *Phi Delta Kappan,* March 1983, pp. 455-61; and Harold L. Hodgkinson, "What's STILL Right with Education," *Phi Delta Kappan,* December 1982, pp. 231-35.

4. Burton R. Clark, "The Hgh School and the University: What Went Wrong in America, Part 2," *Phi Delta Kappan,* March 1985, p. 472.

5. See Thomas F. Green, *Predicting the Behavior of the Educational System* (Syracuse, N.Y.: Syracuse University Press, 1980).

6. Clark, Part I, p. 392.

7. Diane Ravitch, *The Schools We Deserve* (New York: Basic Books, 1985), pp. 46, 74.

8. This research is reported in John I. Goodlad, *What Schools Are For* (Bloomington, Ind.: Phi Delta Kappa Educational Foundation, 1979).

9. Ernest Boyer, *High School* (New York: Harper & Row, 1983); and John I. Goodlad, *A Place Called School* (New York: McGraw-Hill, 1983).

10. Lawrence A. Cremin, *The Transformation of the School* (New York: Alfred A. Knopf, 1961), p. 291.

11. Trow, p. 152.

12. See National Academy of Sciences, National Academy of Engineering, and Institute of Medicine, *High Schools and the Changing Workplace* (Washington, D.C.: Report of the Panel on Secondary Education and the Changing Workplace, National Academy Press, 1984).

13. Statistics reported in Harold L. Hodgkinson, *All One System: Demographics of Education, Kindergarten Through Graduate School* (Washington, D.C.: Institute for Educational Leadership, 1985), p. 11.

14. For further discussion of the usefulness of this kind of contextual appraisal in improving schools, see Kenneth A. Sirotnik and John I. Goodlad, "The Quest for Reason Amidst the Rhetoric of Reform: Improving Instead of Testing Our Schools," in William J. Johnston, ed., *Education on Trial* (San Francisco: Institute for Contemporary Studies, 1985), pp. 277–98.

15. Hodgkinson, pp. 11–12.

16. Jeannie Oakes, *Keeping Track: How Schools Structure Inequaltiy* (New Haven, Conn.: Yale University Press, 1985).

17. Over 60 years ago, after conducting a detailed study of selectivity in American education, George Counts raised the same question and gave the same answer. See George S. Counts, *The Selective Character of American Secondary Education* (Chicago: University of Chicago Press, 1922).

18. Husén, p. 473.

19. Robert M. Hutchins, "The Great Anti-School Campaign," *The Great Ideas Today* (Chicago: Encyclopedia Britannica, 1972).

20. Husén, p. 461.

Chapter 6
Vouchers: The Hoax Is Transparent
Mary Hatwood Futrell*

The Reagan Administration recently unveiled a plan to radically revise the federal program that targets the special educational needs of disadvantaged youngsters. This program—Chapter 1—currently delivers nearly $3.2 billion to local school districts for services to improve the basic academic skills of millions of poor children.

The Administration's new plan would halt this process. Chapter 1—arguably this nation's most successful federal aid-to-education effort—would be converted into a voucher system and administered like Green Stamps. Parents of disadvantaged children would receive government coupons, then redeem them at a school of their choice, public or private.

This Reagan Administration plan to "voucherize" education aid for the disadvantaged is the latest attempt to introduce vouchers into education. But vouchers, in whatever form, are no answer to the problems of education in the United States today. Vouchers are a hoax, and that hoax can be illustrated quite clearly by closely examining the Reagan Administration's voucher plan for Chapter 1.

The Reagan Administration's Chapter 1 voucher plan is based on the assumption that a voucher worth $600 will provide parents greater freedom in choosing a school for their children. The evidence indicates, however, that for many parents there would be little "choice" if the Administration's voucher plan were enacted. The obstacles would be many.

Financial Obstacles

Some public school districts now allow students to transfer in from other districts without paying tuition. Other school districts have made arrangements for tax fund transfers between districts. But most public school systems charge high tuition for out-of-district transfer students—tuitions that would dwarf any $600 voucher. Some examples:

- Parents wishing to transfer a child to suburban White Plains, New York, would face a bill of $7,000 for the tuition the school system charges nonresidents to attend its public elementary schools.
- Parents of children in kindergarten through 8th grade in Bieber, Oklahoma can expect to pay $2,000 to transfer to nearby Forgan.
- According to local school officials in Long Beach, California, transfer students are either required to pay $3,000 tuition or—as is much more likely the case—to persuade their home district to agree to pay Long Beach the $3,000. Unless the individual can pay $3,000, therefore, the choice of transferring districts most often belongs to the *district* rather than the individual.
- The Reagan Administration's voucher proposal would allow students to transfer to non-public schools. Tuition at most independent private schools hardly makes them a viable option for low-income families.
- Tuition in Washington, D.C. independent schools, for example, ranges from $800 per year to $8,700 per year, with a median of $2,300.
- The nationwide median tuition for independent schools ranges from $3,310 for pre-school to $5,338 for grade 12 students.

Financially, the most likely option for parents of Chapter 1 students appears to be the Catholic school system, which accounts for 56 percent of all non-public enrollment. Tuition at 54 percent of Catholic grade schools is below $500 per year. But the median tuition at Catholic high schools is $1,230 per year.

Parochial schools would be the only remotely affordable alternative for Chapter 1 students under the Administration's voucher plan. But the use of public funds to subsidize religious institutions raises serious constitu-

*Mary Hatwood Futrell is President of the National Education Association.

tional questions. The First Amendment guarantees the separation of church and state, a principle that has been repeatedly upheld by the United States Supreme Court. The high court's 1973 decision in *Committee for Public Education and Religious Liberty v. Nyquist* specifically found that a New York statute providing income tax benefits to parents of children attending nonpublic schools violated the First Amendment because it had the "impermissable effect of advancing the sectarian activities of religious schools."

Transportation Obstacles

Transportation would also present a major problem for parents of Chapter 1 students if the Reagan Administration's voucher plan were enacted into law. If students did decide to transfer under the Administration's plan, how would they get to and from a school in another district, or even to a different school in the same district?

Some school systems have agreements where neighboring schools arrange for bus transportation for transfer students. But many others either have no arrangements or, even worse, do not *allow* buses from one district to pick up students in another district.

Classroom Space Obstacles

The Reagan Administration's voucher plan also assumes that students would be allowed to transfer into programs of their choice in neighboring schools. But many of the specialized programs that are most likely to serve Chapter 1 students are already overcrowded. In many urban areas, schools are also bound by formulas for racial balance and not allowed to accept transfer students. In either case, the "choice" opened up by the enactment of the Administration's voucher plan would, in reality, be very limited.

Some specific examples:

- Cleveland schools have several special programs, magnet schools, and honors programs. Many of these programs consider achievement tests, grades, and performance evaluations in selecting their students. All transfer students are considered on a first-come, first-served basis. Although transferring from one school to another is accepted in theory, the practice is uncommon. The special programs are already overbooked, and there are not enough funds available to expand those programs. To compound this problem, Cleveland is under court order to maintain racial balance in the schools, which severely inhibits movement from one school to another.
- In Long Beach, California, the magnet school specializing in international commerce is an attractive

choice for many local students—and potentially for transfer students. It is currently overcrowded, however, and can accommodate only a fraction of those students that apply.

The obstacles to the successful implementation of the Reagan Administration's voucher plan raise deep questions about the proposal, questions of equity.

Not everyone would share equally in the new "freedom of choice" that the Reagan Administration claims its voucher plan would bring. The "choice" of families in urban areas would be restricted severely by tuition costs, overcrowding, and desegregation plans.

Those who appear to be most likely to benefit from the Reagan Administration's voucher proposal are families who would send their children to religious schools anyway and those families who live in areas where the public school tuition is lower than $600, such as the rural and deep South. The Reagan Administration's plan would not provide greater opportunity for lower-income Americans. Instead, there exists the very real possibility that this voucher plan would serve to reinforce economic, religious, and racial segregation.

The Reagan Administration has ignored these questions of equity. It has made no convincing case that vouchers would cure any of the ills that currently ail America's public schools. The administration's failure to detail the ailments that its voucher medicine is designed to cure stems from one simple fact: the voucher scheme wouldn't cure *anything*. It's a medication in search of a disease.

Let us test this hypothesis. In the most recent Gallup Poll of attitudes toward the public schools, the American people identified discipline and student drug use as problems of crisis proportions. Would vouchers have even a negligible impact on these problems? Surely not. Troubled students—rich *and* poor—seldom find a welcome mat awaiting them at the doors of private schools. Poor families with troubled students will confront that tough reality the moment they try to cash in their vouchers. Private schools choose their clientele. Public schools have been—and remain—the only schools that accept the challenge to educate *all* youngsters.

Where are the problems to which the voucher "solution" corresponds? Will a voucher plan help any of the 80 percent of Hispanic students, the 72 percent of Black students, and the 50 percent of white students currently dropping out of New York City's schools? Will it halt this tragic waste of human potential that is a fact of life in virtually every major American city? The *New York Times* commentary on the Administration's proposal is right on the mark: To give children of poverty a voucher is not to help them—it is to taunt them. It is also to taunt millions of caring and devoted parents.

An Administration committed to these parents and their children would cherish Chapter 1 and strive to expand its scope. Sadly, the current Administration has chosen the opposite course: It has abandoned needy children, systematically slashing Chapter 1 funds. As a result, the program now serves 900,000 fewer students than it did in 1980.

Substituting vouchers for what remains of Chapter 1 signals further retreat. The intent of the Adminstration's proposal is not to improve but to impoverish public schools, to weaken the very institutions that have most helped the most needy. Vouchers, in short, are a cover for funneling public monies to private schools. When this strategy is defended on the grounds that it will unleash the potential of 11 million disadvantaged children, the hoax is more than hypocritical. It is cruel.

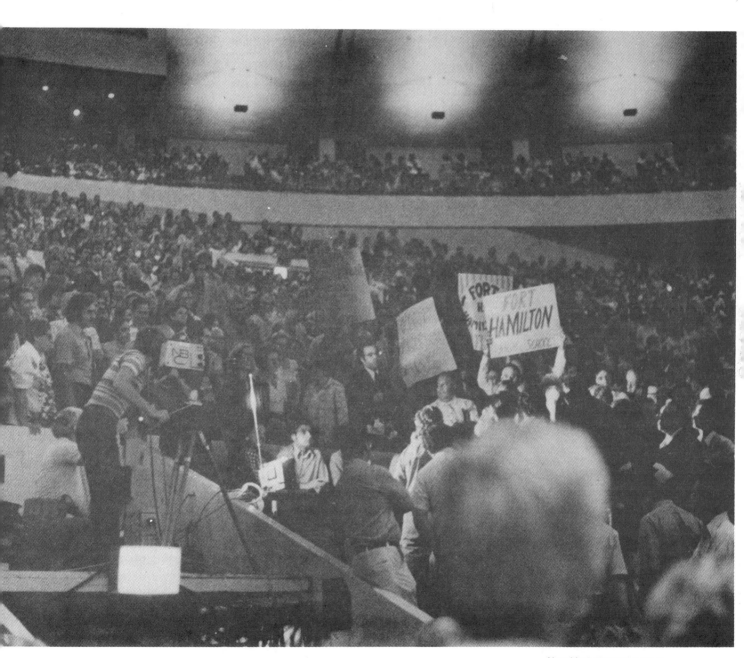

New York Teachers' Staff

Section II
School Climate and Behavior
Introduction by Brian M. Austin*

The articles in Section II focus on the societal conditions that have given rise to the challenges confronting adolescents as they strive toward adulthood and on the strategies educators can use to facilitate this developmental process. Grant and Briggs, in their paper "Today's Children are Different," chronicle the social conditions that gave rise to the social status of "adolescence" over the past four decades. Increased legal rights without corresponding responsibilities contribute to the confusion many adolescents experience.

Bronfenbrenner's "Alienation and the Four Worlds of Childhood" addresses fundamental shifts in societal institutions; he discusses the potential effects of single-parent and dual-career families. Both of these social changes, in certain circumstances, can create a family environment that encourages a sense of alienation in students. Bronfenbrenner believes schools must create a curriculum that intentionally teaches citizenship. Students must learn to care for others. Adult mentoring appears to hold promise as a means to teaching the art of caring.

In their paper, "The Name of the Game is Discipline," Alschuler, Dacus, and Atkins appear to agree with Bronfenbrenner about the importance of trust and rapport in creating a learning climate in the classroom. Their work on teaching "social literacy" to inner city students and teachers suggests that a cooperative classroom atmosphere depends on all participants understanding the rules of negotiation, contracting, and conflict resolution. The authors offer an interesting approach to helping students learn self-discipline.

Glasser, in his article "A New Look at Discipline," also has as a theme the fostering of self-discipline by teaching "social literacy." He focuses on the unmotivated and disruptive student and offers specific steps that can be taken to help students learn how to control their own behavior. In contrast to the contingency management system suggested by Glasser, McDaniel offers a set of eclectic guidelines for motivating undisciplined students. His emphasis is on building motivation that will capture the interest of student and teacher.

The final article in this section cautions educators to remain sensitive to the distinctions between criminal violence and school discipline. The current political climate has blurred these differences, according to the author. In "The Politics of Violence In School," Wayson argues that violence is not a frequent school occurrence and discipline policies should not be unduly influenced. He identifies factors that produce good school discipline and offers guidelines to create a school climate conducive to the purposes of educating today's youth.

*Dr. Brian M. Austin is Assistant Vice President of Student Affairs, Wake Forest University, North Carolina.

Chapter 7
A New Look at Discipline
William Glasser*

Tommy is your discipline problem. It's now December, and despite frequent conferences with the principal, the school psychologist and Tommy's parents, nothing seems to work.

Perhaps Tommy comes from a broken home or has a physical handicap; perhaps he is an only child or the last of a large family. Likely he has barely learned to read. He may never have had a consistently good school experience. But whatever his problems, you have him in your class for a school year, and if you can't get him to cooperate, he will suffer and your life will be miserable.

Here are ten steps to follow in dealing with your behind-in-his-work, disruptive, doesn't-listen, never-on-time, always-picking-fights Tommy (or Susan). I believe if you doggedly follow them, you may help him change into someone who, though far from perfect, is enough improved to reward your efforts. No miracles will occur; this is hard, slow work. A month is probably your minimum time commitment; certainly you're not likely to see progress before that. But if the slow progress tempts you to give up, consider this question: What do you have that is better?

1. List Your No-No's

What you are doing with him now isn't working. This isn't criticism; your techniques may have worked with others. But if they haven't worked with Tommy by now, they probably aren't going to, so it seems only logical to change your approach. To start, sit down tonight in a quiet place and jot down the essence of what you do when Tommy upsets you. Forget the things you might have done or wanted to do. Do you talk to him? Yell at him? Threaten him? Ignore him? Have you asked him what's bothering him or how he feels? Be honest and list the pattern of the efforts you are making to help him right now.

For the next four weeks, try to refrain from doing anything you have put on tonight's list—unless it coin-cides with one or more of these ten steps. When you are tempted (and you will be) to return to old patterns, pull out the no-no list and ask yourself: "If they didn't work in the past, what chance do they have now?"

2. Start Fresh

Now promise yourself that tomorrow, no matter how disruptive Tommy is, you will try to act as if this is the first time he has behaved badly. Don't say, "O.K., you're doing it again" or "I have had enough of that." Don't do anything that reminds him that this is repetitive behavior. On the other hand, if he does do something good, whether he's done it before or not, reinforce him: "Tommy, it's great when you sit still" or "I appreciate that." Tell him he was good, pat him on the head, give him some verbal and even physical recognition for good behavior. If you'll start fresh with him tomorrow and each day for the next month, you may be pleasantly surprised.

3. A Better Day Tomorrow

This gets harder. I want you to figure out at least one thing you can do for Tommy, to Tommy, about Tommy that can help him have a better day tomorrow. It doesn't have to be much; a little goes a long way. One thing I have seen and done that fills the prescription is to pat him on the back as soon as he comes in and say, "Good to see you, Tommy." This brief greeting can be amazingly effective. Twenty seconds of unexpected recognition can mean a lot to him. Yes, he may wonder if you've suddenly gone crazy, but he'll still appreciate the simple, warm gesture. (And it will probably make you feel better, too.)

Or maybe a note has to be run to the office. Though you never in a million years would have asked Tommy, how about trying it tomorrow? "Hey, Tommy, would

*Dr. William Glasser is President of the Institute for Reality Therapy in Canoga Park, CA. Reprinted with permission of the author and *Learning Magazine*, December, 1974.

you do me a favor and take this down to the office and then come right back?'' Say it calmly and matter-of-factly as if he has done it many times before. He may astonish you.

Commit yourself to do this or something like it each day for the next four weeks. You are trying to give Tommy a new idea: that he has some value in your class. His only recourse for recognition for far too long has been to disrupt. You are trying to break that cycle, and these first three steps are the way to start. Continue to implement them as often as possible in the next month; they are prerequisites for the steps that follow.

The first three steps suggested changing your attitude and resolving to start fresh. The next set of steps suggests nonpunitive responses to Tommy when he breaks the rules—at least nonpunitive in the sense that they eliminate emotion-laden blaming and threatening. Keep the tone cool and crisp until Tommy gives some recognition of the rules and makes some effort to comply; at the same time, continue the effort of the earlier steps to inject some warmth and recognition into his day.

4. Quiet Correction

All too soon, you are almost certain to have a disruption. Despite some success with the first three steps, at some point, Tommy's going to mess up. I am sure that just mentioning this has you apprehensively nodding your head. Perhaps when you ask the class to line up he continues sitting at his desk, or for the hundredth time he messes with the paints and spills some on the floor. Let's say this time he busts the line to find the place he wants and starts a fight in the process. Try to act as if it is the first time he has ever done this (step two) and ask him to stop fighting and go to his place in line. If this doesn't work, then try the scenario that follows, no matter what he replies or doesn't reply.

You: What did you do, Tom?
Tom: What?
You: What did you do, Tom?
Tom: Nothing.
You: Please Tom, I just asked you what you did. Tell me.
Tom: Well, this is my place in line and they won't let me in.
You: What did *you* do, Tom?
Tom: It's my place so I pushed my way in.

Then, with no further discussion, you take him by the hand and walk him to his correct place, and stay with him, maybe still holding his hand.

You: Can you walk quietly now?
Tom: What are you going to do?
You: I just asked if you can walk quietly now; we'd all like lunch.

Tom: O.K., I'll try.

If he doesn't agree to try, don't give up; you still have six more steps.

You are trying to establish that, while he must take responsibility for doing something wrong, you are willing to correct him and that, if he accepts the correction, that ends it. Also, your calm demeanor suggests confidence in him. You are not blaming, not threatening or yelling, not doing any of the things you used to do. If step four works and he goes quietly, say nothing more about the incident except to give him a little reinforcement like a pat or ''I was sure you could do it.''

5. Make a Plan

Unfortunately, we must anticipate that before long there may be a situation for which step four won't work. Try it first, but if it doesn't here is the scenario for step five. Let's continue with the scuffle in line, but as you walk toward him, Tommy dashes to the playground. He was supposed to go with the class to the cafeteria and he knows he's breaking the rules. But his need for attention is so great that he cares nothing about the rules. Your job is to get him to care, so get someone to take your class—perhaps appoint a monitor—and follow him, saying quietly, ''Come here, Tommy, I want to talk with you.'' Don't chase, just walk quietly after him. When eventually you get to him:

You: Tom, what did you do?
Tom: I'm just swinging: I'm not hurting anybody.
You: Tom, where are you supposed to be?
Tom: Here; I'm not hungry anyway.
You: What's the rule?
Tom: I don't like that rule. Why should you have to eat if you're not hungry? Why can't I swing? There's no one here. Who'm I hurting?
You: Tom, was it against the rules? (Keep plugging away.)

You have to be very insistent. You are telling Tommy he broke the rules, and he is evading this issue in every possible way. Through all his evasions, you have to stick to a focus on rules. Ultimately, he will say, ''Well, so what?'' or he'll say nothing, which is a tacit admission that he is beginning to face the issue. Continue then:

You: Well, Tom, can you make a plan to follow the rules?
Tom: What do you mean? You mean go to lunch? Jeez, look how long the line is.
You: Are you willing to go to lunch (Doggedly.)
Tom: What happens if I won't?
You: You'll have to leave the swings and take a rest. (To be explained.)
Tom: Do I have to go to the end of the whole line?

You: Not the whole line, just at the end of our class. After lunch, you can swing all you want.

I'm afraid I'll lose some of you here, because this takes time and, of course, it may not work. Or you'll worry that Tommy may think it's weak and silly. This early in the game, you may be right. But remember, you've admitted that what you usually do doesn't work. Besides, you're only at step five. It *may* work, and anytime something works, Tommy has experienced a success—and so have you. This is how he, how everyone, learns discipline.

6. Conference Time

In steps four and five you were warm and supportive but did not talk much. Here, you bring Tommy to the point of a conference. Suppose you have trouble on the swings again: he won't take turns and kicks others away.

You: You want to use the swings, but we have rules. Can you make a plan with me so that you can get a fair turn on the swings and still give others their chance? You can't kick the others away.

Tom: Well, none of them like me; they never give me a turn. If I don't push, I never get a chance. You going to send me to the office?

You: No, Tom, I just want to make a plan with you. Let's try to work it out.

Tom: Heck, I don't like the swings much anyway. I like kickball but those rats never let me play.

You: That's funny; you used to play.

Tom: Yeah, but now they won't let me. They don't like me.

You: When you used to play. I heard them yell at you to follow the rules.

Tom: Big deal. I got mad once, and now they won't let my play.

You: I tell you what, Tom; why don't we take some time and maybe talk this over. You're not having too much fun and I think I can help.

Tommy may be leery at first, believing that a conference just delays his ultimate punishment. All you can do is tell him he won't be punished and that you'd like to help him work it out. You listen to his complaints, talk, joke a little, get to know him better and then try to work out a plan for him to follow the rules. Don't rehash old faults but stress that rules are important and that you have faith he can follow them. Finally you'll work out a plan either for the swings or to get him back at kickball. You may want to put it in writing; sometimes a contract helps the commitment. You are saying to Tom that *he has the power to make a good plan.* It takes time, sure, but it takes a lot out of you to yell and get excited, too.

The last four steps are a graduated series of "benching" techniques. In effect Tommy is interfering so seri-

ously that he has to be taken out of the game to cool off. Once again, these steps come into play only if the earlier ones have failed; rather than acting out of instinct, the teacher by now should have a rather clear idea that it's time to move to the next level of response.

7. Off to the Castle

Now you need to create a place in your room where you can separate Tommy from the class. Not a dunce's seat or a punishment corner, this is an enrichment spot whose occupants can sit comfortably but separately from the class. Get together some books, coloring materials, puzzles and quiet games, so that normally a child wouldn't mind being here for a while. Maybe you could discuss the idea in a class meeting and make a project out of it. This retreat is not only for disruptive children but is a place for others who on occasion want a quiet, separate place. However, the disrupters have priority in the "Castle" or whatever you decide to call it.

If Tommy disrupts, and you are by now sure none of the earlier steps are going to work, then say, "Look, Tom, go sit in the Castle." Don't do or say anything else. Take only a moment and send him firmly there, with no discussion. In the castle, he can see and hear what's going on, but he is separated. Casually observe him, but pay no obvious attention to him. Don't worry if he spends several hours or most of the day there. The isolation has a way of making the normal class routines look more attractive. More important, *he has to learn that he can be nondisruptive,* and the way to learn is through experience.

Eventually, as nice as the Castle is, he'll want to rejoin the class. He may indicate his readiness by being a little restless. Don't take this necessarily as more disruption. Be ready to work out a plan.

When you believe he has settled down, ask him if he is ready to return to his regular seat and take part. If he answers yes, then in your next break go over the class rules briefly and ask him to make a plan to follow them. The plan may be as simple as "O.K., I'll try" or "If you seat me over there away from Johnny, we won't hassle so much." But he has to have some sort of plan.

Try to keep these mini-confrontations as light as possible. Laughter is a magic aid to this whole procedure. If you can keep your sense of humor, he'll have much less tendency to resist. When trouble arises, try to start with a step that will work at that time, but don't be too concerned at this stage if you think it right to start with the Castle. Don't be anxious to get him back to class. Count on the fact that he probably knows best what he can and can't handle. Again, be patient. You're trying to teach him something in a month that he hasn't yet learned in five years.

8. Off to the Office

If Tommy still disrupts, despite steps one through seven, then he must be removed from class. You've put up with a lot, you've bent over backwards, but now you have had it. You can't continue to teach with a constantly disruptive child; it's not fair to you or to the other children. When that point is reached, say, "Tom, go down to the office and take a rest." You take a rest, too. You've earned it.

Your principal must help you now in setting up the office rest place. Here again, it's a comfortable spot: perhaps an old donated couch the kids can scrunch down into. Have some books around, comic magazines, perhaps some peanuts or raisins for Tom and his conferees to munch on. In short, make him comfortable in an atmosphere that shows you care and that you don't want to hurt him.

This nonpunitive atmosphere may be hard for you and your principal to accept, but look again at that list from step one; you can see he's been in the "old" office plenty, with no results. Our task is to get him to change, and new surroundings as well as new methods are necessary. So get together with your principal and perhaps the rest of the faculty to establish this new office rest place. As with the Castle, it should be open to nondisruptive children as well, though Tommy has priority.

Here is sample dialogue from the office (almost repeating step seven):

Principal: What did you do, Tom?

Tom: Well, old Miss Green, she kicked me out of the room. She's mean! I wasn't doin' nothing.

Principal: Well, this is what she said you did, here on this note.

Tom: Then what did you ask me for?

Principal: Because what you say is important. Look, let's work out a plan.

Tom: Oh, God, a plan. Is that all you do around here?

Principal: We always do it when you're here in the office.

You shouldn't be punitive in act or demeanor. You, as principal, let him sit there comfortably while you get the facts. When he sees you're not about to paddle him or call his mother, he'll settle down. Once you have his story, move into the make-a-plan phase to get him back to class. If he complains about Miss Green and won't make a plan, tell him that it's his class and that, while you'll help him get along there, thats where he has to go. Let him sit there comfortably until he's ready to make a plan. Don't be concerned if he sits there a while. This whole scheme is aimed at reducing the alternatives, at getting him to realize that he really only has two choices: to be in class and behave, or to be outside and sit. Pretty soon, class will begin to look better, but he'll need some help with the plan. Help him. You're trying to convey to him that he has to follow reasonable rules, or he's out. But while he's out, you're not going to hurt him or reject him, which would let him rationalize his misconduct on the basis of his dislike for you.

9. A Tolerance Day

If he is totally out of control and can't be contained in the office rest-spot, then a parent will have to be called in to take him home. This is the first time in this trial month you've contacted his parents (and if you follow steps one through eight, it shouldn't happen too often). Now is the time to put him on a "tolerance day," if possible. This means that he comes to school in the morning and stays until you've reached step nine. You don't have to start at one, but start as far back as you can. If he's quiet in the office, hold at step eight. Perhaps you or the principal could make a graph to show him his daily progress in tolerating more of school. But if he can't be helped in school at all, then he'll have to stay home, which means either a home tutor or, if no parents are at home, going on to step ten.

10. Where There's Life There's Hope

If school can't contain him, either he stays home or some other agency in the community will have to take him. Even juvenile hall is a possibility as a last resort. Though it sounds harsh, you must remember that sometimes this will finally jolt him awake, and he'll then be ready to plan. If he is in the hall, perhaps the judge can be persuaded to try letting him come back to school on a tolerance day from there. He can return from home, hall or from any other agency if he seems ready, reentering at the lowest step possible depending on his behavior. Remember that step ten is for a very rare child, but when a child can no longer make it in school, this step must be used.

We all agree that discipline must be learned. I believe these steps outline an effective way to teach it early. The child who learns it very likely learns it for the rest of his life. As far as I'm concerned, there is no learning more valuable; steps like these should be built into the curriculum.

While this program is in use now, and works well, more feedback is needed to work out various contingencies. I would like very much to hear from an elementary school teacher who puts this plan into effect for at least four weeks. Write me in care of *Learning,* 530 University Avenue, Palo Alto, CA 94301, and tell me what happened, good or bad. Ask me questions—I'm sure there'll be plenty. I'll try to read every word, and after a number of queries have come in, I'll work up a cassette and send it back. [*Editor's note:* Dr. Glasser will charge only cassette and mailing costs for this service.]

Chapter 8
The Name of The Game Is Discipline

Alfred Alschuler, James Dacus, and Solomon Atkins*

The Name of the Game Is "Discipline"

To learn anything, students must be in physical and psychological attendance. Even Pavlov remarked in his scientific diary that his dogs wouldn't condition when they weren't paying attention, i.e., when they had bored, flopped-down ears. In junior high school, most activities, materials, and personnel are directed toward capturing students' attention and focusing it on the subject matter: truant officers, bells, hall passes, tardy notes, role-taking, P.A. announcements ("May I have your attention?"—a superfluous question, considering the inescapable electronic volume), hall monitoring, assignments; coaxing, cajoling, enticing, and threatening.

In competition with this impressive array of external forces there are a number of forces within each student, an array of inner concerns: clothes, "face" (pride, self-respect, sense of control), friends, "playing the dozens" (the ancient game of mutual insult), active student resistance (the parade to the pencil sharpener all during class), and passive resistance (daydreaming and unashamed dozing, e.g., one boy we observed frequently tires in the middle of class, pulls his coat around him like a tent and speeds to dreamland). Attempts to eliminate these distractions and instead focus students' attention on the mandated curriculum are only partially successful.

The ubiquitous battle is a standoff. By a systematic observation method,[1] we discovered that on the average, students are paying attention to learning about one-half of a normal class period. The best name for this continuing battle for students' attention is "the discipline problem," because (1) when students refuse to let their attention be controlled, teachers and administrators are forced to engage in *disciplinary* actions; (2) the subject-matter *discipline* is failing to sustain students' attention (3) the external attempt to control stu-

dents' attention is not an effective way to teach students *discipline* (internal self-regulation); (4) the battle between teachers and students is antagonistic to developing and maintaining the respect and affection characteristic of *disciplined* relationships (the original, root meaning of being "disciplined").

In a series of continuing observation and reflection sessions, we have finally been able to more fully name the obvious. The discipline problem is a game, a contest between teachers and students in which each side develops tactics and strategies and tries to win. Although each side has a basic repertoire of moves that becomes familiar to the opponents through exposure and experience, the game plans are never publicly shared.

In order to understand the discipline problem, we have had to discover the rules of the game. Our first step in attempting to discover these rules has been to make a list of the basic moves of teachers and students. For example, teachers' moves include taking attendance, bantering, body language directions, tunnel vision, waiting and staring, making rules, sarcasm, threatening, mini lectures on goodness and evil; students' moves include talking, put-downs, complaining, getting up, conspiracies, making noise, forgetting materials, solitary escapes, refusals, rebellions, fighting. Teachers and students combine these moves with nearly

*Dr. Alfred Alschuler, Professor of Education, University of Mass.; James Dacus, Doctoral Student, University of Mass.; Solomon Atkins, Doctoral Candidate, University of Mass. A very similar version of this article appeared in *Learning Magazine*, August-September 1974.

Editor's note: Fifteen years ago Dr. John Deady and Dr. John Shea of the Springfield School System invited Professor Alschuler to establish a collaborative working relationship in order to help solve some of the pressing educational problems in this urban school system. This article by the principal members of the University team reports their progress.

blinding speed in chain reactions to each other. We are calling these cycles "discipline games." We found that there are a finite, actually rather limited set of discipline games with a seemingly endless number of variations on the basic games depending on the moment and the styles of the teacher and student involved, much like the variations on basic plays in football. A brief analysis of one discipline game will clarify this approach.

— The bell rings.
— *Students* group around the teacher with questions and comments: "I forgot my homework." "Can I get a drink of water?" A few students talk in the corner of the room.
— The *teacher* asks each student individually to sit down.
— Other *students* come up who didn't hear, or pretend not to have heard, the teacher's request.
— The *teacher's* voice rises so that the whole class can hear the command, "All right! Everybody sit down. C'mon."
— *Students* move ever-so-slowly to their seats, as if only an intermission warning bell had sounded. They chat leisurely as they move.
— The *teacher* becomes impatient since it's difficult to take attendance. Often a threat occurs here.
— Still some *students* get up, this time to sharpen pencils or deliver a note.
— The *teacher* stops, stares, warns, or gives a detention notice.

This "milling game" happens so regularly we would think something was wrong if one day everyone were in his or her seat quietly eager to begin the lesson when the bell rang. The purpose of the milling game is to delay the opening of class (i.e., decrease attention to learning). If we were to create a rulebook for new teachers and new students on "How to Win the Milling Game" it would be short and simple.

To new teachers
— Answer as many requests as possible within reason.
— It's not fair to get mad at one person.
— Be sure to distinguish between the players and the real learners.
— Don't get hooked into turning your back on the class.
— Beware of questions about your favorite topic that have nothing to do with the course.
— Anger is O.K. to a degree, but you lose points if the students get to you.

To new students
— Never, ever mill alone!
— Never move farther or faster than you absolutely have to.
— Always ask questions as if you really wanted to know the answers.
— Provoke the teacher, but not enough to get punished. You get points for how close you come to the cliff without getting shoved of.

What's the payoff? Why do teachers and students play the milling game every day in almost every class? There must be some extremely meaningful "points." As best we can determine, students get to be part of a team, enjoy beating the system, and get attention from both their peers and the teacher, though for different reasons. Teachers want to be responsive, to feel competent, to have students' respect and, most of all, they want to help students get what students want. Notice, almost *all* of these needs are virtuous, innately human and usually inoffensive. But, when the milling game is the context, these needs are placed in opposition, become mutually antagonistic and often destructive, most of all for the students who get kicked out of class.

Junior-High-School Justice

It should be obvious by now that it takes at least two people to play discipline games. This fact, when traced to its conclusion, has revolutionary implications. Our habitual patterns of thinking place the discipline problem in students, *not* in the rules of the game. If it is true that the discipline problem is *in the game,* not in the students or teachers, then the games must be changed if the discpline problem is to be solved. Futhermore, (and this realization still send chills down our spines) if the problem is not in the students, then it is patently unjust that only the students are punished and countless times students are unfairly punished by being sent to the front office.

Hundreds of studies have been conducted that ask questions like, "What are the characteristics of problem students?" We asked that question last year[2] and found out that such students are more often boys than girls; proportionately more in the ninth than the eighth than the seventh grades; disproportionately black, with lower I.Q. scores, lower reading scores, and from the lower social classes. What do such "results" mean? You could decrease the number of referrals to the front office by expelling all lower-class black males in the ninth grade with low I.Q.'s, right? Yes, but in doing so we would punish the victim. This solution is absurd because the question is misleading. We can find only *individual* characteristics when that's all we look for.

As social scientists we must begin to look at characteristics for *relationships that break down* and look at how the system sets up those dysfunctional relationships. Then the obvious leaps out. For instance, a friend of ours, Peter Kuriloff, a professor at the University of Pennsylvania, has also been studying junior-high-school discipline. He told us that he identified the ten worst "teacher-killers" in the seventh grade, the students no one could handle. He interviewed them to see whether the popular assumption of "underlying psychological pathology" was justified. Only two of the students seemed to warrant such a diagnosis. The other eight so-called "teacher-killers" had *relationship problems,* not the least of which was a reputation that preceded them, scared teachers, and led to super-fast crackdowns.

Peter then studied the school's "killer-teachers." He discovered that six of thirty-five teachers in the seventh grade accounted for over sixty percent of the discipline referrals to the front office. Then something bizarre happened. The referral rate of the worst "killer-teacher" in the school dropped almost to zero overnight. Amazed, Peter decided to find out what happened. Actually it was quite simple. The principal asked the teacher to join three other teachers in a team approach to individualize instruction. No longer forced to control an entire class by lecturing (in retrospect, obviously not her strongest asset), she was spared the student irritations caused by her lecturing. She worked with individual students, which both she and the students enjoyed much more. There simply was no cause any longer to throw kids out of class. Now, where was the discipline problem? Not in the kids, and we must grieve for the hundreds of previous victims of that situation. Nor was the problem in the teacher, though God knows she also suffered from the daily battle. The problem was in the relationship—in the systems of informal rules defining the teachers' relationships to students. Changing the relationship rules eliminated the cause of the problem and stopped the daily injustices to students.

Actually, the discipline problem victimizes everyone, especially those students who suffer unconscionable injustices. But teachers are also victimized by unpleasant relationships. Assistant principals, chosen for their outstanding records as teachers, are victimized in one school we studied by having to spend an average of twenty-two minutes per referral for nearly one thousand referrals per semester. The assistant principals would have to be mentally ill to enjoy spending twenty-two thousand minutes punishing kids each semester. And the principal is victimized by such preoccupation with discipline that he can't devote the time he would like to get curriculum reform off the ground. Even the

taxpayers are victimized by what seems to be fifty-percent wasted class time and a cost of over thirty-thousand dollars a year in the school we studied to administer corrective actions for problems *created* by the system.

Social Literacy[3]

Literacy is the power to name, analyze, and transform reality. For instance, quantity is a fundamental aspect of the world. In math classes in primary grades children learn to *name* different quantities (numbers) and to *analyze* basic relationships between those quantities (more than, less than, included in). They also learn *transformation* rules (multiplication, division, subtraction, addition, raising to a power, etc.). Not only can children play with numbers abstractly, they can apply these names, relationships, and transformation rules to reality. They are literate with numbers every time they name the reality of their bank account balance, analyze the upcoming additions and subtractions, and manipulate reality by either saving or spending. Without this basic numeracy (being literate with numbers), we would be less powerful in solving all kinds of problems from carpentry to the use of census data in planning more adequate transportation facilities.

There is massive illiteracy in our junior high schools—social illiteracy. We teach students to be literate with words, with numbers, with chemicals, and even with their bodies—but not with their social relations. Teachers and administrators are social illiterates too. There are no established methods of analyzing relationships, no shared formal vocabulary and no public transformation rules. Unable to name, analyze, or transform our social relationships, they are powerless and remain victimized. It is the proper role of public schools to raise the social literacy level along with other types of literacy.

It is a tremendous job first to become literate ourselves by creating an alphabet, syntax, and grammar, and then to develop a social literacy curriculum to teach others. However, because our goals are clear, it is possible to define our curriculum objectives.

Objective I: Teach everyone in our school that the system of social relations can be seen as a game.

We engage in social relationships without seeing the patterns, naming them, etc., just as we speak long before we read and write the symbols for spoken words. The transition from mere spoken language to literacy is as great as the transition from being in social relationships to being socially literate. The first step in that transition is becoming aware that there are regularities, moves, games, and rules in social relations—analogous to learning that spoken language has a system of letters, words, grammar, and syntax.

Objective II: Name the basic moves and social games in the classroom.

This is equivalent to learning the alphabet and recognizing words. However, it's not clear yet that we have adequately named the moves or the games. A good deal of our work at the present time is devoted to developing an excellent, basic vocabulary.

Objective III: Analyze classroom discipline cycles.

Essentially this means figuring out with our students the answers to a number of questions about each discipline cycle: How does the cycle start? What are the rules of this cycle? When are moves offensive? Defensive? How do you get points? From whom? What are you trying to protect? How do you feel? What position do you play? How do you go from "I win—you lose" cycles to "we both win" cycles? How can we change the game so that everyone gets more points?

Objective IV: Transform discipline games through negotiated changes in the rules into the Discipline of learning.

The object is to decrease the amount of mutual victimization and disciplinary activity by collaboratively making new social relationship rules, rules that adapt the subject-matter discipline to mutual interest, that increase teachers' and students' internal self-regulation (discipline), and that increase discipleship.

Objective V: Generalize from this experience in social literacy to the study of national and international liberation movements.

One way to view world and national history is as shifting patterns for domination and liberation. The process of coming to believe in the possibility of change, of naming reality, analyzing it, and collaboratively transforming it is, in miniature, the basic process of cultural and national liberation movements. Obviously there are important differences between libera-

tion in junior high schools and national liberation. However, the direction of new social studies curricula would start with experience in the classroom and generalize these insights to international history.

The work we have reported in this article is in progress. At present we are entering the fourth year of a collaborative relationship with the Springfield School System, in particular with Van Sickle Junior High School. With the support of a small grant from the Dexter Foundation, this year is devoted to the creation of dialogical methods and social literacy lessons. A few of the units we developed last year include MALT, a systematic observation method for determining the amount of Mutual Agreed Learning Time in a class period; the "Name It Game," a format for teaching the basic vocabulary; The Disclipline Game, a board game that simulates the discipline problem in school, helps identify game rules that can be changed, and provides students and teachers practice in negotiating mutually acceptable changes; IBM's, a method in which students and teachers make contracts for Interdependent Behavior Modification.

Before we train vast numbers of social-literacy teachers we want to be reasonably certain that our analysis is accurate, and that our methods work. Based on normative data collected and available over the last three years, we hope to verify decreases in the number of victims sent to the front office, increases in the average amount of mutually agreed upon learning time, improvements in the attentional quality of the subject matter, increases in achievement test scores, and improvement in student-teacher relationships. We are interested in promoting all these aspects of positive discipline.

FOOTNOTES

1. The observation method is systematic, but we have not conducted an extensive, systematic study of all classes.
2. The findings emerged from Mr. Bruce Irons' doctoral dissertation. "A System-Blame Explanation for Discipline Problems."
3. Our definition of literacy as well as our whole approach is modeled on Paulo Freire's work.

Chapter 9
Motivating the Unmotivated: Principles and Practices
Thomas R. McDaniel*

In contemporary classrooms—especially in urban schools—there is a crisis in student motivation. How can teachers turn reluctant learners on to learning? Fifty years ago the question was virtually ignored in teacher education programs. Teachers then were advised to "have a good lesson plan," "be enthusiastic," and "use grades and prizes" to stimulate interest. It was assumed that students wanted to learn what schools wanted to teach. Then the behaviorists developed and promoted some techniques of "extrinsic motivation" that were derived from reinforcement theory. Many of these techniques found their way into schools in the form of behavior modification programs, most notably in special education classrooms. Some urban schools adopted behavior mod strategies for regular classrooms. Following the behaviorists, humanistic educators and psychologists told teachers to focus more on "intrinsic motivation," self-concept development, and individual needs. Now we are asked to improve classroom climate, mediate transactions, and invite school success. As Hawley (1982) theorizes, "Persuasion, force, and incentives are outside forces, but motivation comes from within (p. 2)."

While we have more theories now, there are also more concerns about motivation. The new-found interest in teacher and school effectiveness, the public concern for higher achievements in the light of declining test scores, and the social problems—discipline, drugs, drop-outs—of the community and the school raise new demands that teachers and their classrooms be more motivating. How can schools expect higher productivity and achievement unless students *somehow* become more interested in and committed to their own educational improvement? This is the essential challenge of instructional motivation, and the challenge is one which confronts the classroom teacher daily.

Why a student will "move" (the etymological meaning of "motivation") toward instructional goals and how to maximize the inclinations of individuals so to move are questions that must be answered in the context of partic-

ular lessons by particular teachers in particular classrooms in particular schools. As Drew and associates (1974) suggest, "To create good learning environments, it is essential that the teacher get to know the child and the environmental circumstances that inspire his activity (p. 8)." There does appear to be an emerging set of principles to guide teacher behaviors related to effective instructional motivation, however. Principles are no better than the teachers who make them work, but the following ten principles are offered as an eclectic combination of traditional and modern, practical and theoretical, pedagogical and psychological techniques that teachers *can* make work for better motivation. Although in reality these principles are closely connected, each focuses on a given aspect of what the effective teacher-as-motivator believes, says, or does.

Principle 1:   Build an Interesting Curriculum.

The key term here, of course, is *interesting*. Students are always more motivated to school studies when those studies relate to topics, ideas, experiences, and materials that children find fascinating. When you plan your curriculum for the year, month, week, or day, start with the guiding question, "What would my students enjoy doing that will also correlate to my learning objectives?" Remember: No one hired you because you were dull. Boredom is the arch enemy of motivation; a high-interest curriculum is your greatest ally. Of course, much of any teacher's curriculum is prescribed, but every teacher has a measure of freedom in what he or she will teach and how it may be taught. Use that freedom to maximize *interest*.

*Dr. Thomas R. McDaniel is Charles A. Dana Professor and Chair of the Department of Education at Converse College. This article combines ideas developed in two earlier works by the author: "A Primer on Motivation: Principles Old and New," *Phi Delta Kappan*, September, 1984, and "The Ten Commandments of Motivation," *The Clearing House*, September, 1985.

Practices

1. Use written questionnaires to identify particular interests and areas of interest.
2. Use values strategies (e.g., "Twenty Things I Love to Do," "Values Auction") to identify and evaluate interests; watch what children do in their free time as a guide to what their true interests are; plan surprise activities and instructional games.
3. Consider how student interests can be integrated into the curriculum: starting points of lessons, examples of lesson concepts, applications of learned skills. For example, when beginning a study of mythic heroes, ask students to list their own heroes from sports, television, and contemporary affairs—or to bring to class comic books they have that revolve around "super heroes."
4. Individualize by providing choices so students have more opportunity to select assignments, activities, or projects that are, for *them,* interesting. Contracts, learning activities packages (LAPS), and centers can help provide choices.

Principle 2:   Set Clear Goals.

Educational research supports the reasonable idea that students will "move" toward goals when they know what the goals are. The goals need to be fairly specific (behavioral objectives are effective in this respect), should be challenging without being too difficult, and should be communicated as expectations for the results of learning. When you plan your curriculum, units, and daily lessons, do so not in terms of what *you* are going to "cover" but of what the *students* should be able to do when the instruction is finished.

Practices

1. Involve students in some of the goal setting for the class and for themselves individually; be sure *you* are clear about your objectives for students.
2. State goals in behavioral terms ("the student will be able to identify the three symbols used in the poem" rather than "the student will understand symbolism").
3. Communicate goals and objectives to students before *every* lesson, orally or in writing: "Listen, kids, by the end of class today, you will be able to use the color wheel to find complementary colors. You also ought to be able to select the best color combination for your painting. Now, let's get started."
4. Evaluate student progress or mastery in terms of the specified objectives.

Principle 3:   Communicate High Expectations.

While goals can be one way to help students move in purposeful directions, high expectations require teachers to communicate positive attitudes that convey confidence that students *can* learn, *can* achieve, *can* succeed. Too many students have quit trying because of a fear of failure, low self-concept, and negative expectations. As Purkey (1972) argues, teachers can motivate students by exhibiting genuine belief that every child has positive self-worth and untapped potential for high performance. Crucial here is the attitude a teacher can develop that turns high expectations from teachers into desirable self-fulfilling prophecies for students.

Practices

1. Set objectives that challenge, but do not intimidate, students.
2. Speak encouraging words like, "I know this is difficult, but you can do it."
3. Show respect for student effort; comment on progress, be a "booster": "Keep trying . . . you are almost there . . . thanks for your hard work."
4. *Assume* students want to learn and focus them on future success, not past failures ("Next time will you indent your paragraphs?" instead of "Why didn't you remember to indent your paragraphs?").

Principle 4:   Employ Positive Reinforcement.

Most teachers know that the behavioral principles of positive reinforcement can be used as a powerful extrinsic motivator. But few teachers actually *use* this principle as effectively as they might. It is so easy to get caught in the "criticism trap": a student misbehaves to get attention, the teacher reprimands the student, the student (having got his attention need met) quiets down, the teacher (having got his or her need for order met) feels satisfied with the effectiveness of the negative command. But since both student and teacher have been *positively* reinforced by a negative interaction, both are likely to *increase* their respective negative behaviors. Effective employment of positive reinforcement requires understanding, skill, and practice of the principle.

Practices

1. List all of the specific things kids do that you *want* to reinforce so that you can work consistently and systematically toward rewarding students. This will help you "look for the positive."
2. Use verbal and non-verbal reinforcers—praise, smiles, touch, attention, proximity, nods, winks,

etc.—immediately after any movement toward one of your "target behaviors." This can encourage kids to keep moving in the right direction and help you avoid the "criticism trap."

3. Remind students of specific academic objectives or social behaviors that you will be looking for and then acknowledge and show appreciation for examples you see: "I am watching to see who will be able to put the dinosaur bones in the right place. . . . Good job, Freddy! You have the leg bones joined correctly at the knees and hip joints."

4. Give *specific* praise for what you can find right and successful in students' work: Not "Clarence, you missed four out of ten spelling words—and your penmanship is awful" but, "Clarence, you got six out of ten spelling words right this time, which is an improvement—and the penmanship on the last two words is exactly what I want to see you do with all your words." Low ability youngsters with weak self-concepts are especially responsive to this motivational technique.

Principle 5:   Invite Success.

Students (as are we all) are motivated by success—and success breeds success (Purkey, 1972). Our job as teachers is to maximize each student's chances for succeeding in his or her academic work, social growth, and personal achievements. At issue in this principle is a teacher's attitude, an attitude that invites success because it says in word and deed, "I am going to teach you in ways that will encourage you to do well." Unfortunately, research shows that teachers tend to seat lower ability students further away from the teacher, give them less time and fewer opportunities to respond to questions, and interrupt their performances more often. The invitation to succeed motivates when it reaches all students, and is effective when a teacher genuinely believes that all students are capable.

Practices

1. State rules positively: "Walk in the hall" rather than "No running in the halls." Compliment students' success in complying with rules.

2. Maximize "right answers" by asking open-ended and multiple-right answer questions: "What would the United Sates be like today if Columbus had landed on the *West* Coast of America?"

3. Maximize "right answers" by changing your questions to fit the answer: "Well, 'veins' would have been a good answer if I had asked what carries blood *to* the heart; can you now tell us what takes blood *from* the heart?"

4. Challenge students with direct invitations: "This is a tough problem; who wants to give it a try?"

Principle 6:   Teach Cooperation.

Teachers know how to use competition—games, contests, rewards—to promote motivation but, as Johnson and his colleagues (1984) suggest, can also enhance motivation by actively teaching students how to cooperate in reaching academic goals. Collaborative skills do not come naturally to students, especially when many of our instructional and evaluation approaches are based on competitive assumptions and processes. For example, when students cooperate on tests they are usually reprimanded for cheating. The emphasis in schools on competition, sorting and grading students, and picking "winners" creates many "losers" as well, and losing, or even the threat of losing, is hardly motivating. Cooperation, however, can build supportive relationships and group morale, handmaidens of motivation.

Practices

1. Assign learning tasks to students in heterogeneous pairs, triads, and small groups. (You may want to give individual *and* group grades.)

2. Develop a "skill bank" of student experts (with every student an expert in *something*) who help other students in given areas of expertise.

3. Teach small group skills (differentiated tasks and roles, leader behavior, defining group goals, etc.) directly; let effective groups be models for other groups.

4. Have students evaluate their own group processes and effectiveness; discuss these findings in class: "How many groups got every member to participate? Did leaders listen to everyone's ideas?"

Principle 7:   Demonstrate Enthusiasm.

Enthusiasm is a quality that springs from the personality of the teacher but which can be developed by any instructor. We know that demonstrating a particular behavior is often the most effective way to teach it to the young; we also know that enthusiasm is both a producer and a by-product of motivation. Motivated students are enthusiastic and enthusiastic students are motivated. So much of school life is routine and mundane that teachers and students can slip into a business-as-usual rut. But enthusiasm in the classroom is the spice that brings new zest to learning for teachers as well as students.

Practices

1. Plan special events that break the routine: change the furniture, reassign seating, redecorate the room,

change the procedure for collecting homework, invent an unusual field trip, try a new teaching technique, etc.

2. Employ motivational statements that *sell* the value of your subject matter on activity: "I've got a great poem for you today, class; I want you to listen to the music in the rhyme and visualize the pictures it creates in your mind."

3. Speed up your physical movement in the classroom: be in a hurry to get on-task (the loss of "engaged time" at the beginning of most classes is a motivation damper); be "on your feet, not on your seat."

4. Enjoy your work—and let your students know you enjoy it—not only by being enthusiastic yourself but by direct statement: "I like math because. . . ." "Social studies is exciting when. . . ."

Principle 8: Personalize Instruction.

Motivation is increased when students see a connection between a subject under study and real people. Indeed, the teacher who is generally able to show students that a classroom is about *life,* not "subject matter," is a teacher who experiences few motivation problems. Teachers can ask about any lesson, "What should this mean to my students? How does this material relate to their personal lives?" One of the strongest intrinsic motivators for all of us is *ourselves.* When a teacher talks about his or her students to them instead of talking at them about the information "to be covered," watch the interest and attention snap into place.

Practices

1. Greet students at the door when they enter class: shake hands, use a "special greeting" (and expect a personal response), ask a personal question. Such personal contacts recognize the individuality of students and welcome them to the class.

2. Use touch (one of the few behaviors that consistently correlates with high ratings of effective teachers in the perceptions of students): a pat on the back, a kindly touch on the shoulder, etc. This comes more naturally to some teachers than others, of course, but to some extent is a skill that can be developed by practice.

3. Employ personal examples and illustrations in the lesson: "Now, Robby, you and Katy walked to school today; how many steps per minute do you think you took? How many steps per minute do you predict *I* would take?" Students usually like being personally involved as part of the subject matter of a lesson.

4. Acknowledge personal ownership of learning: "O.K., the first group—Eric, Lori, Sally, and

Blake—concluded that Poe's 'The Raven' is about an *imaginary* bird. Does anyone want them to defend their idea?"

Principle 9: Induce Readiness to Learn.

Often, we try to teach before the students are ready to learn. "Get out your spelling books and turn to page six" is hardly a request that motivates students to want to study spelling. Effective motivators plan specific instructional activities that create interest in a topic about to be taught. Variously termed as "set induction," "focusing events," "advance organizers," or "grabbers," such activities arrest attention and pique the curiosity of students so that they will want to pursue the subsequent learning activity, but the technique can be an important motivator because of the power of anticipation.

Practices

1. Ask thought-provoking questions that can only be answered in the activity that follows: "Who can guess how many lightbulbs Edison invented before he got one to work? Let's have some estimates. Now, let's read the story about an inventor who wouldn't give up, no matter how many times he failed. Ask yourself how long *you* would have stayed with this experiment."

2. Start with an event in the school and work backward to the lesson: "Did you hear the announcements on the speaker? What descriptive adjectives did your principal use to help you visualize the new report cards? . . . O.K., today we are going to write a paragraph of description."

3. Use cartoons, pictures, newspaper headlines, taped excerpts of television programs, records, etc., to capture attention: Show and discuss a headline about the President's China trip before a lesson on the Great Wall of China; ask students to speculate on the meaning of an editorial cartoon before you begin a lesson on tariffs; play the record of a Bob Newhart parody before reading a Twain parody.

4. Construct set induction experiences: have volunteers try to communicate an idea without talking and while blindfolded as a prelude to studying the life of Helen Keller; let all the tall people go to lunch early as a prelude to a discussion of discrimination.

Principle 10: Encourage Student Responses.

While inducing readiness is an instructional technique for initiating movement into the lesson, keeping students involved and participating requires special skill—especially in terms of questioning strategies. Students need to be encouraged to respond to questions and to interact with one another during most lessons. If you are practicing the first nine principles of motivation, you are likely to have an attitude and an orientation to the students and to instruction that will make you an effective questioner too. But there are some specialized skills that can help you be even more motivating in your interaction with students.

Practices

1. Ask questions to find out what students know, not what they do *not* know: avoid questions designed to trap, trick, punish, or accuse; ask questions that allow students to demonstrate what they know, believe, or value: "Mary Lou, you had some fascinating ideas in your essay on pollution. Can you share some of those with us?"
2. Give more "wait time" after a question is asked (the average "wait time" is only one second!); you will get longer and more thoughtful responses. If you want to motivate longer responses, probe by asking, "Can you tell me more about that?" instead of the intimidating "why?"
3. Ask questions you do not know the answer to—confess your ignorance and see how well the students can teach *you.* "Gosh, I don't know what causes 'continental drift.' Who has some information or ideas about that?"
4. Suspend judgment when students respond to questions; instead of saying "right" or "not quite so," simply move to other students and get a handful of responses before commenting (your "comment" could be a synthesis of the responses); after a response, poll the class instead of judging: "How many of you agree with Clarence?" Polling encourages students to *listen* to one another.

These ten principles of motivation, in the hands of a competent and conscientious teacher, can turn a routine classroom into an exciting one, a mundane lesson into a challenging one, and apathetic students into interested ones. Most important of all, these motivational principles can help teachers themselves become more positive and more motivated to be the best teachers they can be. Increasing student motivation is an imperative for all educators and may well be the secret to more "engaged time" and higher achievement in contemporary classrooms. To motivate youngsters a teacher has to develop those attitudes, instructional skills, and motivational

techniques that both research and experience identify as useful. And these develop only with a teacher's conscientious *practice.*

The rewards of such practice justify the effort. Wlodkowski (1984) said it well:

> Those smiling, enthusiastic faces, those moments of insight and wonder, those student expressions of completion and accomplishment, and those heads held upright and eyes wide that say "I did it. I learned something," are the force that give life to our work (p. 191).

The teacher who motivates well teaches well. The rewards of effective teaching are the intrinsic ones that motivate good teachers to stay in the classroom.

SELECTED BIBLIOGRAPHY

Ball, Samuel (ed.). *Motivation in Education.* New York: Academic Press, 1977.

Canfield, Jack; and Wells, Harold C. *100 Ways to Enhance Self-Concept in the Classroom.* Englewood Cliffs, New Jersey: Prentice-Hall, Inc., 1976.

Drew, Walter F.; Olds, Anita R.; and Olds, Henry F., Jr. *Motivating Today's Students.* Palo Alto, California: Education Today Company, 1974.

Hawley, Robert C. *The Steps for Motivating Reluctant Learners.* Amherst, Massachusetts: Education Research Associates Press, 1982.

Hawley, Robert C. and Hawley, Isabel L. *Building Motivation in the Classroom.* Amherst, Massachusetts: Education Research Associates Press, 1979.

Hyman, Ronald T. *Improving Discussion Leadership.* New York: Teachers College, Columbia University, 1980.

Johnson, David W.; Johnson, Roger T.; Holubec, Edith J.; and Roy, Patricia. *Circles of Learning: Cooperation in the Classroom.* Alexandria, Virginia: Association for Supervision and Curriculum Development, 1984.

Kolesnik, Walter B. *Motivation: Understanding and Influencing Human Behavior.* Boston: Allyn and Bacon, Inc., 1978.

Purkey, William W. *Inviting School Success: A Self-Concept Approach to Teaching and Learning.* Belmont, California: Wadsworth Press, 1978.

Wlodkowski, Raymond J. *Motivation.* Washington, D.C.: National Education Association, 1982.

———. *Motivation and Teaching: A Practical Guide.* Washington, D.C.: National Education Association, 1984.

Chapter 10
Alienation and the Four Worlds of Childhood
Urie Bronfenbrenner*

To be alienated is to lack a sense of belonging, to feel cut off from family, friends, school, or work—the four worlds of childhood.

At some point in the process of growing up, many of us have probably felt cut off from one or another of these worlds, but usually not for long and not from more than one world at a time. If things weren't going well in school, we usually still had family, friends, or some activity to turn to. But if, over an extended period, a young person feels unwanted or insecure in several of these worlds simultaneously or if the worlds are at war with one another, trouble may lie ahead.

What makes a young person feel that he or she doesn't belong? Individual differences in personality can certainly be one cause, but, especially in recent years, scientists who study human behavior and development have identified an equal (if not even more powerful) factor: the circumstances in which a young person lives.

Many readers may feel that they recognize the families depicted in the vignettes that are to follow. This is so because they reflect the way we tend to look at families today: namely, that we see parents as being good or not-so-good without fully taking into account the circumstances in their lives.

Take Charles and Philip, for example. Both are seventh-graders who live in a middle-class suburb of a large U.S. city. In many ways their surroundings seem similar; yet, in terms of the risk of alienation, they live in rather different worlds. See if you can spot the important differences.

Charles

The oldest of three children, Charles is amiable, outgoing, and responsible. Both of his parents have full-time jobs outside the home. They've been able to arrange their working hours, however, so that at least one of them is at home when the children return from school.

If for some reason they can't be home, they have an arrangement with a neighbor, an elderly woman who lives alone. They can phone her and ask her to look after the children until they arrive. The children have grown so fond of this woman that she is like another grandparent—a nice situation for them, since their real grandparents live far away.

Homework time is one of the most important parts of the day for Charles and his younger brother and sister. Charles's parents help the children with their homework if they need it, but most of the time they just make sure that the children have a period of peace and quiet—without TV—in which to do their work. The children are allowed to watch television one hour each night—but only after they have completed their homework. Since Charles is doing well in school, homework isn't much of an issue, however.

Sometimes Charles helps his mother or father prepare dinner, a job that everyone in the family shares and enjoys. Those family members who don't cook on a given evening are responsible for cleaning up.

Charles also shares his butterfly collection with his family. He started the collection when he first began learning about butterflies during a fourth-grade science project. The whole family enjoys picnicking and hunting butterflies together, and Charles occasionally asks his father to help him mount and catalogue his trophies.

Charles is a bit of a loner. He's not a very good athlete, and this makes him somewhat self-conscious. But he does have one very close friend, a boy in his class who lives just down the block. The two boys have been good friends for years.

Charles is a good-looking, warm, happy young

*Dr. Urie Bronfenbrenner is a Jacob Gould Shurman Professor of Human Development and Family Studies and of Psychology at Cornell University, Ithaca, NY. Reprinted with permission of *Phi Delta Kappan*, February, 1986.

man. Now that he's beginning to be interested in girls, he's gratified to find that the interest is returned.

Philip

Philip is 12 and lives with his mother, father, and 6-year-old brother. Both of his parents work in the city, commuting more than an hour each way. Pandemonium strikes every weekday morning as the entire family prepares to leave for school and work.

Philip is on his own from the time school is dismissed until just before dinner, when his parents return after stopping to pick up his little brother at a nearby day-care home. At one time, Philip took care of his little brother after school, but he resented having to do so. That arrangement ended one day when Philip took his brother out to play and the little boy wandered off and got lost. Philip didn't even notice for several hours that his brother was missing. He felt guilty at first about not having done a better job. But not having to mind his brother freed him to hang out with his friends or to watch television, his two major after-school activities.

The pace of their life is so demanding that Philip's parents spend their weekends just trying to relax. Their favorite weekend schedule calls for watching a ball game on television and then having a cookout in the back yard. Philip's mother resigned herself long ago to a messy house; pizza, TV dinners, or fast foods are all she can manage in the way of meals on most nights. Philip's father has made it clear that she can do whatever she wants in managing the house, as long as she doesn't try to involve him in the effort. After a hard day's work, he's too tired to be interested in housekeeping.

Philip knows that getting a good education is important; his parents have stressed that. But he just can't seem to concentrate in school. He'd much rather fool around with his friends. The thing that he and his friends like to do best is to ride the bus downtown and go to a movie, where they can show off, make noise, and make one another laugh.

Sometimes they smoke a little marijuana during the movie. One young man in Philip's social group was arrested once for having marijuana in his jacket pocket. He was trying to sell it on the street so that he could buy food. Philip thinks his friend was stupid to get caught. If you're smart, he believes, you don't let that happen. He's glad that his parents never found out about the incident.

Once, he brought two of his friends home during the weekend. His parents told him later that they didn't like the kind of people he was hanging around with. Now Philip goes out of his way to keep his friends and his parents apart.

The Family Under Pressure

In many ways the worlds of both teenagers are similar, even typical. Both live in families that have been significantly affected by one of the most important developments in American family life in the postwar years: the employment of both parents outside the home. Their mothers share this status with 64% of all married women in the U.S. who have school-age children. Fifty percent of mothers of preschool children and 46% of mothers with infants under the age of 3 work outside the home. For single-parent families, the rates are even higher: 53% of all mothers in single-parent households who have infants under age 3 work outside the home, as do 69% of all single mothers who have school-age children.[1]

These statistics have profound implications for families—sometimes for better, sometimes for worse. The determining factor is how well a given family can cope with the "havoc in the home" that two jobs can create. For, unlike most other industrialized nations, the U.S. has yet to introduce the kinds of policies and practices that make work life and family life compatible.

It is all to easy for family life in the U.S. to become hectic and stressful, as both parents try to coordinate the disparate demands of family and jobs in a world in which everyone has to be transported at least twice a day in a variety of directions. Under these circumstances, meal preparation, child care, shopping, and cleaning—the most basic tasks in a family—become major challenges. Dealing with these challenges may sometimes take precedence over the familiy's equally important child-rearing, educational, and nurturing roles.

But that is not the main danger. What threatens the well-being of children and young people the most is that the external havoc can become internal, first for parents and then for their children. And that is exactly the sequence in which the psychological havoc of families under stress usually moves.

Recent studies indicate that conditions at work constitute one of the major sources of stress for American families.[2] Stress at work carries over to the home, where it affects first the relationship of parents to each other. Marital conflict then disturbs the parent/child relationship. Indeed, as long as tension at work do not impair the relationship between the parents, the children are not likely to be affected. In other words, the influence of parental employment on children is indirect, operating through its effect on the parents.

That this influence is indirect does not make it any less potent, however. Once the parent/child relationship is seriously disturbed, children begin to feel insecure—and a door to the world of alienation has been opened. That door can open to children at any age, from preschool to high school and beyond.

My reference to the world of school is not accidental, for it is in that world that the next step toward alienation is likely to be taken. Children who feel rootless or caught in conflict at home find it difficult to pay attention in school. Once they begin to miss out on learning, they feel lost in the classroom, and they begin to seek acceptance elsewhere. Like Philip, they often find acceptance in a group of peers with similar histories who, having no welcoming place to go and nothing challenging to do, look for excitement on the streets.

Other Influences

In contemporary American society the growth of two-wage-earner families is not the only—or even the most serious—social change requiring accommodation through public policy and practice in order to avoid the risks of alienation. Other social changes include lengthy trips to and from work; the loss of the extended family, the close neighborhood, and other support systems previously available to families; and the omnipresent threat of television and other media to the family's traditional role as the primary transmitter of culture and values. Along with most families today, the families of Charles and Philip are experiencing the unraveling and disintegration of social institutions that in the past were central to the health and well-being of children and their parents.

Notice that both Charles and Philip come from two-parent, middle-class families. This is still the norm in the U.S. Thus neither family has to contend with two changes now taking place in U.S. society that have profound implications for the future of American families and the well-being of the next generation. The first of these changes is the increasing number of single-parent families. Although the divorce rate in the U.S. has been leveling off of late, this decrease has been more than compensated for by a rise in the number of unwed mothers, especially teenagers. Studies of the children brought up in single-parent families indicate that they are at greater risk of alienation than their counterparts from two-parent families. However, their vulnerability appears to have its roots not in the single-parent family structure as such, but in the treatment of single parents by U.S. society.[3]

In this nation, single parenthood is almost synonymous with poverty. And the growing gap between poor families and the rest of us is today the most powerful and destructive force producing alienation in the lives of millions of young people in America. In recent years, we have witnessed what the U.S. Census Bureau calls "the largest decline in family income in the post-World War II period." According to the latest Census, 25% of all children under age 6 now live in families whose incomes place them below the poverty line.

Countering the Risks

Despite the similar stresses on their families, the risks of alienation for Charles and Philip are not the same. Clearly, Charles's parents have made a deliberate effort to create a variety of arrangements and practices that work against alienation. They have probably not done so as part of a deliberate program of "alienation prevention"—parents don't usually think in those terms. They're just being good parents. They spend time with their children and take an active interest in what their children are thinking, doing, and learning. They control their television set instead of letting it control them. They've found support systems to back them up when they're not available.

Without being aware of it, Charles's parents are employing a principle that the great Russian educator Makarenko employed in his extraordinarily successful programs for the reform of wayward adolescents in the 1920s: "The maximum of support with the maximum of challenge."[4] Families that produce effective, competent children often follow this principle, whether they're aware of it or not. They neither maintain strict control nor allow their children total freedom. They're always opening doors—and then giving their children a gentle but firm shove to encourage them to move on and grow. This combination of support and challenge is essential, if children are to avoid alienation and develop into capable young adults.

From a longitudinal study of youthful alienation and delinquency that is now considered a classic, Finnish psychologist Lea Pulkkinen arrived at a conclusion strikingly similar to Makarenko's. She found "guidance"—a combination of love and direction—to be a critical predictor of healthy development in youngsters.[5]

No such pattern is apparent in Philip's family. Unlike Charles's parents, Philip's parents neither recognize nor respond to the challenges they face. The have dispensed with the simple amenities of family self-discipline in favor of whatever is easiest. They may not be indifferent to their children, but the demands of their jobs leave them with little energy to be actively involved in their children's lives. (Note that Charles's parents have work schedules that are flexible enough to allow one of them to be at home most afternoons. In this regard, Philip's family is much more the norm, however. One of the most constructive steps that employers could take to strengthen families would be to enact clear policies making such flexibility possible.)

But perhaps the clearest danger signal in Philip's life is his dependence on his peer group. Pulkkinen found heavy reliance on peers to be one of the strongest predictors of problem behavior in adolescence and young adulthood. From a developmental viewpoint, adolescence is a time of challenge—a period in which young people seek activities that will serve as outlets for their energy, imagination, and longings. If healthy and constructive challenges are not available to them, they will find their challenges in such peer-group-related behaviors as poor school performance, aggressiveness or social withdrawal (sometimes both), school absenteeism or dropping out, smoking, drinking, early and promiscuous sexual activity, teenage parenthood, drugs, and juvenile delinquency.

This pattern has now been identified in a number of modern industrial societies, including the U.S., England, West Germany, Finland, and Australia. The pattern is both predictable from the circumstances of a child's early family life and predictive of life experiences still to come, e.g., difficulties in establishing relationships with the opposite sex, marital discord, divorce, economic failure, criminality.

If the roots of alienation are to be found in disorganized families living in disorganized environments, its bitter fruits are to be seen in these patterns of disrupted development. This is not a harvest that our nation can easily afford. Is it a price that other modern societies are paying, as well?

A Cross-National Perspective

The available answers to that question will not make Americans feel better about what is occurring in the U.S. In our society, the forces that produce youthful alienation are growing in strength and scope. Families, schools, and other institutions that play important roles in human development are rapidly being eroded, *mainly through benign neglect.* Unlike the citizens of other modern nations, we Americans have simply not been willing to make the necessary effort to forestall the alienation of our young people.

As part of a new experiment in higher education at Cornell University, I have been teaching a multidisciplinary course for the past few years titled "Human Development in Post-Industrial Societies." One of the things we have done in that course is to gather comparative data from several nations, including France, Canada, Japan, Australia, Germany, England, and the U.S. One student summarized our findings succinctly:

"With respect to families, schools, children, and youth, such countries as France, Japan, Canada, and Australia have more in common with each other than the United States has with any of them." For example:

- The U.S. has by far the highest rate of teenage pregnancy of any industrialized nation—twice the rate of its nearest competitor, England.
- The U.S. divorce rate is the highest in the world—nearly double that of its nearest competitor, Sweden.
- The U.S. is the only industrialized society in which nearly one-fourth of all infants and preschool children live in families whose incomes fall below the poverty line. These children lack such basics as adequate health care.
- The U.S. has fewer support systems for individuals in all age groups, including adolescence. The U.S. also has the highest incidence of alcohol and drug abuse among adolescents of any country in the world.[6]

All these problems are part of the unraveling of the social fabric that has been going on since World War II. These problems are not unique to the U.S., but in many cases they are more pronounced here than elsewhere.

What Communities Can Do

The more we learn about alienation and its effects in contemporary post-industrial societies, the stronger are the imperatives to counteract it. If the essence of alienation is disconnectedness, then the best way to counteract alienation is through the creation of connections or links.

For the well-being of children and adolescents, the most important links must be those between the home, the peer group, and the school. A recent study in West Germany effectively demonstrated how important this basic triangle can be. The study examined student achievement and social behavior in 20 schools. For all the schools, the researchers developed measures of the links between the home, the peer group, and the school. Controlling for social class and other variables, the researchers found that they were able to predict children's behavior from the number of such links they found. Students who had no links were alienated. They were not doing well in school, and they exhibited a variety of behavioral problems. By contrast, students who had such links were doing well and were growing up to be responsible citizens.[7]

In addition to creating links within the basic triangle of home, peer group, and school, we need to consider two other structures in today's society that affect the lives of young people: the world of work (for both parents and children) and the community, which provides an overarching context for all the other worlds of childhood.

Philip's family is one example of how the world of work can contribute to alienation. The U.S. lags far behind other industrialized nations in providing child-care services and other benefits designed to promote the well-being of children and their families. Among the most needed benefits are maternity and paternity leaves, flex-time, job-sharing arrangements, and personal leaves for parents when their children are ill. These benefits are a matter of course in many of the nations with which the U.S. is generally compared.

In contemporary American society, however, the parents' world of work is not the only world that both policy and practice ought to be accommodating. There is also the children's world of work. According to the most recent figures available, 50% of all high school students now work part-time—sometimes as much as 40 to 50 hours per week. This fact poses a major problem for the schools. Under such circumstances, how can teachers assign homework with any expectation that it will be completed?

The problem is further complicated by the kind of work that most young people are doing. For many years, a number of social scientists—myself included—advocated more work opportunities for adolescents. We argued that such experiences would provide valuable contact with adult models and thereby further the development of responsibility and general maturity. However, from their studies of U.S. high school students who are employed, Ellen Greenberger and Lawrence Steinberg conclude that most of the jobs held by these youngsters are highly routinized and afford little opportunity for contact with adults. The largest employers of teenagers in the U.S. are fast-food restaurants. Greenberger and Steinberg argue that, instead of providing maturing experiences, such settings give adolescents even greater exposure to the values and life-styles of their peer group. And the adolescent peer group tends to emphasize immediate gratification and consumerism.[8]

Finally, in order to counteract the mounting forces of alienation in U.S. society, we must establish a working alliance between the private sector and the public one (at both the local level and the national level) to forge links between the major institutions in U.S. society and to re-create a sense of community. Examples from other countries abound:

- Switzerland has a law that no institution for the care of the elderly can be established unless it is adjacent to and shares facilities with a day-care center, a school, or some other kind of institution serving children.
- In many public places throughout Australia, the Department of Social Security has displayed a poster that states, in 16 languages: "If you need an interpreter, call this number." The department maintains a network of interpreters who are available 16 hours a day, seven days a week. They can help callers get in touch with a doctor, an ambulance, a fire brigade, or the police; they can also help callers with practical or personal problems.
- In the USSR, factories, offices, and places of business customarily "adopt" groups of children, e.g., a day-care center, a class of school children, or a children's ward in a hospital. The employees visit the children, take them on outings, and invite them to visit their place of work.

We Americans can offer a few good examples of alliances between the public and private sectors, as well. For example, in Flint, Michigan, some years ago, Mildred Smith developed a community program to improve school performance among low-income minority pupils. About a thousand children were involved. The program required no change in the regular school curriculum; its principal focus was on building links between home and school. This was accomplished in a variety of ways.

- A core group of low-income parents went from door to door, telling their neighbors that the school needed their help.
- Parents were asked to keep younger children out of the way so that the older children could complete their homework.
- School children were given tags to wear at home that said, "May I read to you?"
- Students in the high school business program typed and duplicated teaching materials, thus freeing teachers to work directly with the children.
- Working parents visited school classrooms to talk about their jobs and about how their own schooling now helped them in their work.

What Schools Can Do

As the program in Flint demonstrates, the school is in the best position of all U.S. institutions to initiate and strengthen links that support children and adolescents. This is so for several reasons. First, one of the major—but often unrecognized—responsibilities of the school is to enable young people to move from the secluded and supportive environment of the home into responsible and productive citizenship. Yet, as the studies we conducted at Cornell revealed, most other modern nations are ahead of the U.S. in this area.

In these other nations, schools are not merely—or even primarily—places where the basics are taught. Both in purpose and in practice, they function instead as settings in which young people learn "citizenship": what it means to be a member of the society, how to behave toward others, what one's responsibilities are to the community and to the nation.

I do not mean to imply that such learnings do not occur in American schools. But when they occur, it is mostly by accident and not because of thoughtful planning and careful effort. What form might such an effort take? I will present here some ideas that are too new to have stood the test of time but that may be worth trying.

Creating an American classroom. This is a simple idea. Teachers could encourage their students to learn about schools (and, especially, about individual classrooms) in such modern industrialized societies as France, Japan, Canada, West Germany, the Soviet Union, and Australia. The children could acquire such information in a variety of ways: from reading, from films, from the firsthand reports of children and adults who have attended school abroad, from exchanging letters and materials with students and their teachers in other countries. Through such exposure, American students would become aware of how attending school in other countries is both similar to and different from attending school in the U.S.

But the main learning experience would come from asking students to consider what kinds of things *should* be happening—or not happening—in American classrooms, given our nation's values and ideals. For example, how should children relate to one another and to their teachers, if they are doing things in an *American* way? If a student's idea seems to make sense, the American tradition of pragmatism makes the next step obvious: try the idea to see if it works.

The curriculum for caring. This effort also has roots in our values as a nation. Its goal is to make caring an essential part of the school curriculum. However, students would not simply learn about caring; they would actually engage in it. Children would be asked to spend time with and to care for younger children, the elderly, the sick, and the lonely. Caring institutions, such as day-care centers, could be located adjacent to or even within the schools. But it would be important for young caregivers to learn about the environment in which their charges live and the other people with whom their charges interact each day. For example, older children who took responsibility for younger ones would become acquainted with the younger children's parents and living arrangements by escorting them home from school.

Just as many schools now train superb drum corps, they could also train "caring corps"—groups of young men and women who would be on call to handle a variety of emergencies. If a parent fell suddenly ill, these students could come into the home to care for the children, prepare meals, run errands, and serve as an effective source of support for their fellow human beings. Caring is surely an essential aspect of education in a free society; yet we have almost completely neglected it.

Mentors for the young. A mentor is someone with a skill that he or she wishes to teach to a younger person. To be a true mentor, the older person must be willing to take the time and to make the commitment that such teaching requires.

We don't make much use of mentors in U.S. society, and we don't give much recognition or encouragement to individuals who play this important role. As a result, many U.S. children have few significant and committed adults in their lives. Most often, their mentors are their own parents, perhaps a teacher or two, a coach, or—more rarely—a relative, a neighbor, or an older classmate. However, in a diverse society such as ours, with its strong tradition of volunteerism, potential mentors abound. The schools need to seek them out and match them with young people who will respond positively to their particular knowledge and skills.

The school is the institution best suited to take the initiative in this task, because the school is the only place in which all children gather every day. It is also the only institution that has the right (and the responsibility) to turn to the community for help in an activity that represents the noblest kind of educating: the building of character in the young.

There is yet another reason why schools should take a leading role in rebuilding links among the four worlds of childhood: schools have the most to gain. In the recent reports bemoaning the state of American education, a recurring theme has been the anomie and chaos that pervade many U.S. schools, to the detriment of effective teaching and learning. Clearly, we are in danger of allowing our schools to become academies of alienation.

In taking the initiative to rebuild links among the four worlds of childhood, U.S. schools will be taking necessary action to combat the destructive forces of alienation—first, within their own walls, and thereafter, in the life experience and future development of new generations of Americans.

FOOTNOTES

1. Urie Bronfenbrenner, "New Worlds for Families," paper presented at the Boston Children's Museum, 4 May 1984.

2. Urie Bronfenbrenner, "The Ecology of the Family as a Context for Human Development," *Developmental Psychology,* in press.

3. Mavis Heatherington, "Children of Divorce," in R. Henderson, ed., *Parent-Child Interaction* (New York: Academic Press, 1981).

4. A.S. Makarenko. *The Collective Family: A Handbook for Russian Parents* (New York: Doubleday, 1967).

5. Lea Pulkkinen. "Self-Control and Continuity from Childhood to Adolescence," in Paul Baltes and Orville G. Brim, eds., *Life-Span Development and Behavior,* Vol. 4 (New York: Academic Press, 1982), p. 64–102.

6. S.B. Kamerman, *Parenting in an Unresponsive Society* (New York: Free Press, 1980); S.B. Kamerman and A.J. Kahn, *Social Services in International Perspective* (Washington, D.C.: U.S. Department of Health, Education, and Welfare, nd.); and Lloyd Johnston, Jerald Bachman, and Patrick O'Malley. *Use of Licit and Illicit Drugs by America's High School Students—1975–84* (Washington, D.C.: U.S. Government Printing Office, 1985).

7. Kurt Aurin, personal communication, 1985.

8. Ellen Greenberger and Lawrence Steinberg, *The Work of Growing Up* (New York: Basic Books, forthcoming).

Chapter 11
Today's Children Are Different
Gerald Grant and John Briggs*

In contrasting ourselves with our children or our grandparents, we tend to exaggerate change. For instance, maturation now occurs earlier—perhaps a year or so—but nothing on the order of magnitude previously assumed.[1] Yet the relationships between young and old have changed, as well as the way we socialize the young. It is these changes, rather than the shift in maturation rates, that are most important.

Socialization strongly influences the kinds of persons we become and the attitudes we have, including our attitude toward biological change. I would like to reflect on those changes by comparing what adolescent life was like for my father and myself and is now for my son, a 16-year-old high school sophomore.

My son lives only a mile from the house where my father was born in 1899 and two miles from the neighborhood in which I grew up. He attends the public schools of Syracuse, as we did. Of course the Syracuse that my father knew was a small but bustling city less than a fifth its current size. Barges came through town on a canal that has been filled in, paved over, and renamed Erie Boulevard. The center of the city is relatively dead today—the action, especially for adolescents, is in the suburban malls, where they shop for electronic gear, sports equipment, and designer jeans, and then return home to talk about their forays, possibly on their own telephone.[2]

My grandfather, James Grant, a Scot who was part owner of Master's and Grant Livery, fell on hard times and into hard drinking and died when my father was 13. Mary Duffy Grant moved her five children to a flat over Madigan's butcher shop, where my father went to work after he completed grammar school in 1912. An older brother was "placed out" with relatives in Cleveland, a common practice in the 19th century. He was the only one of the five to complete high school, not far from the average in 1900 when the nation was still three-fifths rural and 10 percent completed high school. My father's work experience typified the shift that was occurring in an urbanizing nation. He had some apprentice-like jobs in the stable and butcher shop, where adult supervision was close but informal. At 18 he went to work in a new steel factory, where relationships were more hierarchical and the work took on the specialized character of the industrial era.

Most males went to work at 14 and learned what they needed to know in face-to-face relationships on the job. One learned by watching and imitating, picking up skills according to one's interest, effort, and opportunities. From the age of 13, my father turned over his earnings to his mother. He took us on tours of his old neighborhood, pointing out the flats in which he had lived and at what rent—he remembered because he had paid it. This, too, was typical throughout the 19th century, when children aged 12–18 supplied a third of the family income. It was a time when the young were expected to do the work of adults but were treated in most respects as children until 18, when those in rural areas might leave home for a boarding house in the city. Although one was not legally an adult until 21, most were emancipated informally by 18.

"Adolescence" Is Born

By the mid-20th century adolescent culture had been born and given a name by G. Stanley Hall. The adolescent was neither expected to do the work of an adult nor treated as an adult. Adolescence was a moratorium from adult responsibilities and privileges with the exception of those "dropouts" (and the term was just then coming into use) who went to work, bought a car, and weren't kids any longer. Sociologists wrote about

*Dr. Gerald Grant is a sociologist and Dr. John Briggs is an historian in the Department of Cultural Foundations of Education and Curriculum, Syracuse University, Syracuse, NY. Reprinted with permission of the Association for Supervision and Curriculum Development and the authors. Copyright © 1983 by the Association for Supervision and Curriculum Development. All rights reserved.

the overwhelming power of the per group as the high school became the major socializing institution for most youth.

In *Adolescent Society,* James Coleman described Syracuse Central, the kind of high school from which I graduated in 1955. It was a place in which rating and dating games rivaled the formal academic curriculum. The curriculum was "tracked" and the path to maturity was partly affected by whether one was preparing for real work on graduation or continuation of the dating game in college, which then had such old-fashioned requirements as curfews and separate dormitories for boys and girls.

The adults in the school had more real power: we students could parody the uptight principal but we were careful when we did so because we knew he could throw us out. We generally observed the rules and believed that completing school was important to our occupational futures, but our strongest emotional commitments were to the values of the peer group. We did not feel the need to challenge adult culture as youth were to do in the 60s; we tended to give it superficial compliance while attending to our own pursuits—within bounds allowed by adults. Those bounds included the acceptance of chaperones at school events, and in the lower middle class neighborhood where I grew up, adults on the block felt free to correct a misbehaving child on the street.

Within my peer group culture, coke was something that went with french fries. Marijuana or any hallucinogenic drugs were unknown. Beer was regularly smuggled to parties after junior year but hard liquor was rarely seen. The fine gradations of petting dominated sexual discussion and "going all the way" was generally forbidden. Pregnancy meant disgrace and automatic marriage; abortion was rare except among the wealthy. The technology of birth control was limited to the male condom and it was more for show than use.

The school was still perceived as a powerful social escalator. For families like ours, it worked. Whereas my father had gone only as far as eighth grade, three of his sons finished college; two of them are professors. But it was a world much less fair to women and blacks. My sister went to business school, not to college (later she because a nurse). Although Syracuse Central abutted what was then a black ghetto, it enrolled few blacks, and most of them left or were pushed out by the end of compulsory schooling at age 16. Those who could not afford to go to college usually didn't. There was no community college and virtually no free public higher education with the exception of state teachers colleges.

High School Evolves

By the 1980s school had become a more open institution. On the way into my son's high school you will pass students in wheelchairs taking a last drag on a cigarette before classes begin. The enrollment is about 55 percent black and includes a variety of new immigrants, including some Cambodian refugees. More than 90 percent graduate. Paradoxically, while graduation no longer gives one an advantage in the competition for jobs, those labeled dropouts pay a penalty. Youth are increasingly granted adult rights but few expect them to bear adult responsibilities. Many work part-time but it is a rare parent who expects any contribution to the family purse. Teen income goes for teen consumer items—one's own stereo has become a birthright.

The adult keepers often feel stripped of most of their former powers. The courts have held that teenage girls can obtain birth control services over their parents' objection, and the children's rights movement has won new due process rights for young teenagers. In Washington, D.C., regulations forbid a teacher from barring a door to a pupil no matter how late he or she arrives, since pupils have a right to an education (presumably on their terms).

Some schools, particularly larger urban high schools, have taken an adversarial turn. In the face of elaborate due process procedures, adults shrink from instituting charges because of the demands it would make on their own time or because they fear they lack evidence that would "stand up in court." Instead, they look the other way.

The reasons for these shifts are complex and it is impossible to assign precise weights to them. To a considerable degree, our problems have been a function of our successes. We have laid a great burden on American public schools: namely, to be the principal avenue of creating a more equal and just society. We have attempted to right some great wrongs and have carried out a social revolution in the schools. Schools have become larger and more diverse. Perhaps there never has been a true consensus on the socializing and moral functions of the schools, but simply an agreement among the elite whom the schools predominantly served in an earlier era.

Now nearly everyone is in the school tent and feels he or she has an equal voice in deciding what kind of show should go on. Specific court decisions, especially on the Supreme Court decision re Gault, were interpreted as placing strong limits on the discretionary power of principals and teachers, and subject any disciplinary decision to quasi-appellate review. The children's rights movement has exploited these decisions, and concern about genuine child abuse has created the machinery for children to challenge parents in the much more doubtful area of "emotional abuse." There has been a significant shift from the traditional American attitude of independence, absorbed from the cradle, of "ain't nobody the boss of me" to adolescents who have gone a step further. "Don't touch me or I'll have you arrested."[3]

The radical wing of the movement has stressed the oppression of youth, as in this excerpt from the Youth Liberation of Ann Arbor:

Our lives are considered the property of various adults. We do not recognize their right to control us. We call this control adult chauvinism, and we will fight it. We quickly begin to learn that these schools and families are part of a whole system that is sick.[4]

In addition to the pull of children's rights from below, so to speak, some parents appear to be giving push from above by relieving themselves of the burdens of parenthood. In recent decades there have been increases in divorce rates, in children living with one parent, in two-career families as well as shifts in attitudes about the responsibilities of parents. Survey data indicate parents are now less altruistic, for example, with 66 percent feeling they "should be free to live their own lives even if it means spending less time with their children." And 63 percent say they have a right to live well now "even if it means leaving less to the children."[5]

There is also evidence that parents have withdrawn from efforts to supervise children, taking a more passive role in relation to their children's curriculum choices (math, science, and foreign language enrollment have fallen markedly), and a 1978 poll showed that nearly three-fourths of all parents had no regular rules limiting television watching.[6] When the students themselves were asked whether teachers demanded enough of them, 57 percent said they were not asked to work hard enough.[7]

Increased Affluence

In part, the shifts I am describing reflect the increased affluence of the nation as a whole. My father spent his youth in the working class, whereas my son enjoys upper middle class status. Similarly, some of the privileges that were once extended to a few youth in the 19th century now are enjoyed by a broad middle and upper class. But there has been a shift in the nature of those privileges and in the kinds of relationships that

exist between adolescents and adults. At least five significant trends differentiate my father's world from my son's:[8]

1. *From being known to being on one's own:* In the world my father knew, children came into fairly intimate contact with a variety of adults in work and apprenticeship relations. Today, the separate culture of the adolescent has been accentuated by the extension of many formal rights to adolescents. The young act on their own with respect to many fundamental decisions, which they make in isolation from adults and adult responsibilities.

2. *From obvious necessity to seemingly arbitrary authority:* The necessity for doing the task was self-evident in an apprentice-like world. Now reasons are more obscure—learn calculus this term so that you'll be able to do advanced economics later and thus get a good job someday. Adult roles cannot be readily discerned, and the connections between what you are required to do now and might do ten years from now are often difficult to understand.

3. *From a world of likely success to one of possible failure:* In a society in which schooling played a less dominant role, you were seldom asked to do much beyond your evident abilities. If you could not repair the roof, you could clean the barn. This matching of person to task was less harsh than the sorting and grading that occurs in school where one is tested frequently and faced with the possibility of being stamped a failure. Compulsory schooling requires some to continue at frustrating tasks. Grade inflation and a general reduction in academic standards have been unsatisfactory solutions to this problem.

4. *From shared parenting to teenagers in opposition to parents:* In large families with children aged five to nineteen, older siblings shared parenting tasks and responsibility for discipline was more diffuse. With the advent of modern family planning techniques and the tendency to have fewer and more closely spaced children, the modern teenager is more likely to feel a member of a cadre in opposition to adults.

5. *From early contributors to long-term borrowers:* Until the end of the 19th century and part way into the 20th, the period of dependency was short and children became significant contributors to the family purse by age 14. Financial dependency now is longer (even to the late 20s for many graduate students) and increases during the late teenage years when many parents must take out a second mortgage to cover college costs.

From the adolescent side of the relation, then, adults seem more distant and less intimately knowledgeable about the talents and capabilities of the young. Adults appear more arbitrary about what they expect the young to do, and they are more inclined to administer tests and to exercise social control through bureaucratic arrangements. In the family, us-them feelings are stronger and adolescents may resent rather than feel grateful for the long-term dependency that the costs of extended formal education usually require.

From the adult side, there are fewer opportunities for the rewards of nurturance that occur in mentoring relationships. Like the young, adults struggle with the lengthened drain on the family purse and the tension that this often produces.

Adults in Transition

Contemporary adults are confused and less certain of their own authority.[9] Many who lived through the cultural revolutions of the 1960s took drugs themselves, participated in the sexual revolution, and experimented with the new "lifestyles." Guilt and pain over increased divorce rates and family breakup is widespread. Those who are internally divided sometimes mask their tension by adopting an authoritarian posture (and both authoritarian sects and schools are on the increase). But the more likely response is to withdraw from the responsibility of enforcing a standard or to let someone else do it. In many cases, that someone else is the adolescent, operating under a new system of rules and rights. The adolescent experiences this not as true freedom—for they yearn for the presence of strong adults who care enough to hold them to worthwhile standards—but as the withdrawal of adults from responsibilities that are properly theirs. I agree with B.C. Hafen that the indiscriminate growth of the children's rights movement could have disastrous consequences: "It would be an irony of tragic proportion if, in our egalitarian zeal, we abandoned our children to their 'rights' in a way that seriously undermined their claim to protection and developmental opportunity."[10]

Daniel Offer and his colleagues have argued persuasively in a recent study[11] that psychologists have overemphasized the supposed turmoil that characterizes relationships between healthy adolescents and adults. Yet his data also show that teenagers have grown much less trusting in the last two decades. Comparing responses by teenagers in the early 1960s with those in the late 1970s, he concluded that "with respect to almost every self-image dimension teenagers in the 1970s felt worse about themselves than did teenagers in the 1960s." Teenagers describe themself as less able to take criticism without resentment (dropping from 70 to 57 percent), and more likely to "get violent if I don't get my way" (5 percent then, 17 percent now). Increases in

teenage worries about their health and feeling "empty emotionally most of the time" corroborate other data showing increased drug use and suicide rates among adolescents.

The loss of trust is quite marked. Nearly twice as many (13 vs. 25 percent) say, "If you confide in others, you ask for trouble." The share of those who believe, "An eye for an eye and a tooth for a tooth does not apply to our society" has fallen from 67 to 40 percent. More now "Blame others even when I know I was at fault." Sidetaking and an adversarial posture are more evident in their views of their own families as well, with a doubling of those who believe, "My parents are almost always on the side of someone else" (14 to 32 percent).

No Ideal Past

That loss of trust is related more to withdrawal on the part of adult socializers than to changes in children or in their basic needs. The proper response to our contemporary dilemma is neither to seek the restoration of some supposedly ideal past nor to "liberate" children from supposedly oppressive adults. It is rather to accept our responsibilities for having brought children into the world, to counter the current trends toward withdrawal from those responsibilities, to pursue an honest dialogue about the nature of those responsibilities, and to come to some agreement about what share of the responsibility the school should bear. Adults need to summon courage, conviction, and compassion in order to connect with adolescents even at the cost of painful confrontations and temporary rejections.

We also need to share socializing tasks with young adults as they begin to exercise more responsibility. We should give serious attention to mandating a year or at least a semester of voluntary service for all high school students. They could help feed the elderly in nursing homes, improve parks and public lands, care for the young in preschool centers, tutor poor readers in elementary schools, assist disabled students and those teachers who are trying to make mainstreaming work, improve food service operations in school cafeterias, paint and repair schools (including the teachers' lounge), coach grade school soccer teams, and minister to the needs of the terminally ill, to suggest a short list.

The young would have an opportunity to learn more by giving more, to develop other sides and aspects of themselves in a noncompetitive environment, to gain dignity and a heightened sense of self-worth by being useful to others, and to build a wider network of mentoring relationships with adults. A volunteer year would help to create a world in which adolescents would have more opportunities to be contributors and not just borrowers, to be known in relationships where authority is less arbitrary, and to feel less a cadre in opposition.

FOOTNOTES

1. See V.L. Bullough, "Age at Menarche: A Misunderstanding," *Science* 213 (July 17, 1981): 365-366. It appears that the alleged steep decline in the average age of menarche from 17 to 12.5 years was based on an atypical sample of Norwegian girls. We are grateful to Christine Murray for pointing out this article to us.

2. A poll of its high school readers by *Highwire* magazine shows 37 percent own their own phones, 71 percent have a stereo system, and 84 percent a radio/cassette. "Students and Their Money," *Highwire* 2,5 (Fall 1982): 20-23.

3. For a more extensive analysis of these influences, see Gerald Grant, "Children's Rights and Adult Confusions," *The Public Interest* 69 (Fall 1982): 83-99.

4. Youth Liberation of Ann Arbor, "We Do Not Recognize Their Right to Control Us," in *The Children's Rights Movement: Overcoming the Oppression of Young People,* ed. Beatrice Gross and Ronald Gross (New York: Anchor Press/Doubleday, 1977), p. 128. In the introduction to the volume, the authors write: "A good case can be made for the fact that young people are the most oppressed of all minorities. They are discriminated against on the basis of age in everything from movie admissions to sex. They are traditionally the subjects of ridicule, humiliation, and mental torture by adults. Their civil rights are routinely violated in homes, schools, and institutions," p.1.

5. Daniel Yankelovich, "New Rules in American Life," *Psychology Today* 15, 4 (April 1981): 35-91.

6. National Center for Educational Statistics, *The Condition of Education,* Washington, D.C.: Government Printing Office, 1979, p. 18.

7. Ibid, p. 72.

8. We are indebted to Joseph Kett's *Rites of Passage: Adolescence in America 1790 to the Present* (New York: Basic Books, 1977).

9. Although contemporary parental confusion may be particularly acute, it is certainly not new, as Bernard Wishy notes in *The Child and the Republic* (Philadelphia: University of Pennsylvania Press, 1968) quoting Charlotte Perkins Gilman in 1903 on the timidity and confusion of parents: "Our own personal lives, rich as they are today . . . are not happy. We are confused, bewildered," p. 121.

10. B.C. Hafen, "Puberty, Privacy, and Protection: The Risks of Children's Rights," *American Bar Association Journal* 63 (1977): 1383-1388, quoted in Bettye M. Caldwell, "Balancing Children's Rights and Parents' Rights," in *Care and Education of Young Children in America* ed. R. Haskins and S. Gallagher (Norwood, New Jersey: Ablex, 1980) p. 35.

11. Daniel Offer, Erik Ostrow, and Kenneth I. Howard, *Adolescence: A Psychological Self-Portrait* (New York: Basic Books, 1981).

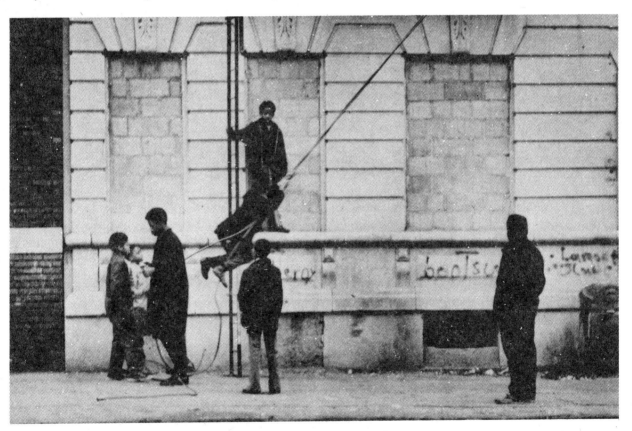

Robert Wolf

Chapter 12
The Politics of Violence in School: Doublespeak and Disruptions in Public Confidence
William W Wayson*

When people discuss school problems, someone inevitably confuses the issue of violence with the issue of school discipline.[1] In reality, violence and school discipline are separate problems, and confounding them only reduces the probability of solving either one. Violence is rare in schools. However, seemingly petty annoyances and trivial but disruptive behaviors—the kinds of activities that have characterized schoolchildren for generations—continue to pose frequent and perplexing problems for teachers.

Certain groups have a vested interest in confounding violence and school discipline. These groups include: (1) those politicians and their followers who hope to extract votes from the fearful and the ill-informed, (2) those teachers who hope that, once aroused, public indignation will bring sympathy for teachers and their plight, (3) those school boards that hope to thwart court-ordered desegregation or justify discriminatory practices by using distorted statistics to play on public prejudices against minority students or those who live on the "wrong side of town," and (4) those consultants who sell solutions designed to fix things that aren't broken. Anyone who climbs aboard the bandwagon to reduce criminal violence in the schools will show remarkable results in short order,[2] because that particular problem isn't nearly as serious as everyone seems to think.

Recently, federal agencies—including President Reagan's advisors and speechwriters—have consistently lumped together violence and ordinary discipline problems. At times the mixing seems calculated to win votes from a public already anxious about the perceived lack of discipline in the schools.[3] At other times the mixing seems designed to gain support for denying "undesirable" students their fundamental rights.[4] Sometimes the mixing seems intended to appeal to teachers who feel unappreciated. Then again, on closer inspection, the mixing appears to be a subtle attempt to undermine public confidence in the public schools in order to win support for vouchers or other measures that afford parents some choice in the schools their children attend.[5]

At the federal level, violence and ordinary discipline problems were first lumped together in a 1983 memo developed within the Education Department (ED) by a group of employees handpicked because they "supported the President's political agenda."[6] That memo, originally titled "Chaos in the Classroom: Enemy of American Education," was strongly criticized by people who were knowledgeable in the area of school discipline.[7] Since then, phrases from the report have been repeated in speeches and in articles by the primary architects of the original memo.[8]

Whatever the motive for equating school discipline problems with crime and violence, doing so does little to improve school discipline and probably leads to actions or policy stances that make the problem worse. Confounding violence and discipline problems also serves as a smoke screen, providing everyone with excuses for failing to accept personal responsibility for developing students' self-discipline. Teachers and administrators see no reason to accept responsibility when "everyone knows that the school is filled with incorrigibiles" and when no one really expects any improvement. School boards take no responsibility when they are convinced that nothing can be done with "kids like those." Students don't feel the need to take responsibility when they can tell their parents that the school is so disrupted that work is impossible.

Furthermore, the reports on school violence provide little solid data on which to base sound policy, since the reports generally rely more on opinion than on fact. It is true that Gallup Poll respondents have listed discipline as the number-one problem in the schools in

*Dr. William W. Wayson is a professor in the Department of Educational Policy and Leadership, Ohio State University, Columbus, OH. Reprinted with permission of the author and *Phi Delta Kappan*, October, 1985.

every year but one since 1969. (Interestingly, only 2% of Americans listed "crime/vandalism" as the foremost problem in 1985, while 25% put "lack of discipline" in first place.[9]) But those who use the annual Gallup Poll of the Public's Attitudes Toward the Public Schools as a basis for making policy fail to recognize that opinions and personal concerns do not prove the existence of a problem. Fifty thousand Frenchmen *can* be wrong if they agree that tomatoes are poisonous—and we should not accept their views as evidence of the toxicity of tomatoes.

When actual statistics on crime and violence in the schools are mentioned, they are often drawn from sources of questionable reliability. Figures on the incidence or frequency of occurrence of crime and violence often come from teachers' or students' responses to such questions as: Have you *or any other persons* ever been physically attacked? The responses are reported as "the number of people physically attacked" or—more accurately, but no less deceptively—as "the number of people reporting physical attacks." In such cases, one assault—even one *rumored* assault—can appear to have been 30 or more, the number increasing with each telling.

Often, little attempt is made to separate serious crime or violence from less-serious offenses.[10] Figures on "larceny" or "theft" are often derived from such questions as: Have you ever had anything taken from you in school? A stolen book or pen will count as much as a theft of $3,000.[11] By the same token, a laughable threat—"I'm going to kill you!"—from an angry third-grader will carry as much weight as the same threat from a parent or from a high school football player. Even a teacher who tells students that "sticks and stones will break your bones" is likely to respond in the affirmative to the question, "Have you ever experienced verbal abuse?," if some pugnacious primary-grader has ever cast aspersions on the teacher's ancestry. And that teacher won't even recognize that this affirmative response counts as one more case of "violence" against teachers.

A study in Boston, which confounded verbal abuse with physical assaults, is often cited as proof that assaults on teachers are common.[12] Meanwhile, in testimony before the U.S. Senate on 15 March 1984, Gary Bauer combined the number of teachers who had reported being *threatened* with the number of teachers who had reported being actually assaulted to come up with an impressive, but misleading, figure.

The fears of teachers and students are often treated as though they were grounded in reality or in direct personal experience when, in fact, they more often derive from timidity, prejudice, or displaced anxieties from other sources.[13] Even when they have absolutely no relationship to reality, such fears can be transmitted through an entire faculty or student body.[14] It is useful to know who and how many are fearful, but nothing is gained by treating all fears as though they were well-founded.

No report makes a distinction between students' fears of crime in school and students' fears that spring from the words or actions of school staff members.[15] Yet we know from Jacob Kounin's work that a "ripple effect" causes children who merely *witness* punishment to become fearful.[16] Every parent knows that a teacher who "yells" can cause high anxiety among children. Exaggerated accounts from a seemingly authoritative source can also arouse doubts or fears in those who hear or read them.

What We Know About Discipline and Violence

Though our information is flawed, we know more about school crime and school discipline than recent public pronouncements on those topics reveal. As best we know, the facts are these:

• *Any* crime or violence is too much, and no teacher or child should be subjected to crime or violence from any source. But random and unpredictable violence, though rare, is probably impossible to eradicate and should not be used to justify policies and practices that are educationally unsound.

• Most schools never experience incidents of crime or violence, and those that do seldom experience them frequently or regularly. Judging from students' and teachers' reports and from recent opinion polls, the number of incidents of violence and crime in the schools has also been decreasing of late.[17] Though relatively minor behavioral problems understandably irritate school personnel and disrupt the classrooms in which they occur, treating these problems as crimes only worsens the problems by undermining public respect for (and thus the authority of) schools and school personnel.

• Neither disruptive behavior nor crime occurs exclusively in any one kind of school or community. Similarly, safe and orderly classrooms can be found in schools and communities of every type. Disruptive behavior does not occur with equal frequency in all classrooms, either. These facts suggest that the problems do not reside within students but arise instead from factors in their surroundings.

• It is also important to note that the most serious incidents of crime and violence in the schools are committed by individuals from outside the schools.[18] School disciplinary codes and practices are unlikely to have much effect on such individuals. But several studies suggest that the students themselves will be less likely to engage in acts of violence or crime in their schools if they enjoy positive interactions with school personnel, academic success, or productive participation in school activities.[19]

• School conditions that negatively affect staff members or students are more important "causes" of disruptive behavior than any condition found within individual students.[20] Most discipline problems in schools are traceable to dysfunctions in school operations and governance, including policies and practices of teacher training institutions, state departments of education, and school boards. Those dysfunctions can be cleared up at relatively little cost, if school personnel have the insight, the will, and the incentive to do what needs to be done. Punishing students or staff members for behavior that has its roots in organizational dysfunctions is foolish and fruitless. When any organization or institution fails to win personal confidence and commitment, responsible participation also declines.[21]

• The single most important variable in determining school climate is the principal's leadership in establishing goals for the school, pursuing them aggressively, and eliciting loyal and enthusiastic commitment to those goals from staff members, students, and parents.[22] Good principals are more often hampered by the rules and practices of the local bureaucracy than by state or federal actions.[23]

• Depersonalization is most frequently suggested as a cause of disruptive behavior in schools. In buildings where disiplinary problems are rife, staff members and students do not share common understandings, a sense of belonging, or the commitment and loyalty that undergird self-disciplined adherence to mutually accepted codes of conduct.[24]

Often, schoolpeople attribute remarkable outcomes to restrictive or rigid disciplinary practices and policies,[25] when these improvements are actually attributable to other events that occurred simultaneously. In fact, any long-term improvements in a student's behavior that seem to stem from the use of restrictive, punitive disciplinary practices must derive, in reality, from other practices that improve the student's relationship with school personnel, that enhance the student's (and probably his or her parents') confidence in the school, or that reduce barriers to participation and production imposed by the school itself.[26] Unless they are accompanied by efforts to involve and serve students, restrictive policies will inevitably lead to worse disciplinary problems and, perhaps, to violence.

Too often, the students who most need and deserve an education are forced out from the schools—a practice tantamount to turning away extremely ill patients from hospitals because they need too much care. In schools with high suspension rates, most of the suspensions are for relatively trivial offenses. The most frequent offense is truancy, but some students are suspended for such "crimes" as looking sullen.[27] Expulsion—the schools' usual reaction to criminal behavior—is rare, since this response erodes public confidence in the institution.

As a justification for engaging in exclusionary or punitive practices, federal spokespersons have often misquoted and misused a study by the psychiatrist Alfred Bloch that calls teacher burnout "combat neurosis" and that likens its symptoms to those of World War I victims of shell shock.[28] The analogy has been very useful to consultants who blow into town, blow off in an entertaining way to teachers who feel oppressed, and then blow out to make another audience feel guilty if it is not suffering from burnout. But few point out that the symptoms were closely related to the teachers' socioeconomic background and lack of experience or training with minority populations. In some cases the teachers exhibited fearful, insecure personalities.[29] We will never cure teacher burnout through disciplinary programs that punish students for poor teacher training, their teachers' insecurities, or public policy that forces children to attend schools dominated by the culture of poverty.

Meanwhile, personal responsibility for teaching students self-discipline is undermined when school personnel grasp at the excuse that the courts have tied their hands and provided "too much protection" for students rights. Many faculty members who rely on this excuse don't even know what the law requires.[30] For example, one principal suspended several fourth-graders for throwing tomatoes on the school bus. Asked whether the students cleaned up the bus, he wrongly replied, "The law won't let me make them clean it up."

That principal wasn't even exercising common sense. What do children learn when someone else cleans up the messes they make? Moreover, the principal was incapacitated by his own interpretation of the law, not by any court decision. The federal government has clearly announced its resolve to protect educators who are sued or whose discretion is hampered by court decisions.[31] But it would be poor public policy indeed, if federal leadership were to placate or protect people who use the law as an excuse for incompetence, ill will, or fatigue.

In my experience, effective educators don't ask every few minutes, "What will the law let me do?" They act responsibly, relying on an abiding sense of justice. Effective educators give students more protection than the law requires. Most administrators agree with the U.S. Supreme Court that the law requires "less than a fair-minded principal would impose on himself."[32]

Factors That Produce Good School Discipline

In our study of 500 well-disciplined schools in the U.S. and Canada,[33] we identified the characteristics that seemed to make these schools orderly and safe, as well as productive. The federal government should encourage states and localities to give every child access to schools exhibiting these characteristics, for such schools develop the values, attitudes, and skills that make responsible participation in a free society possible.

In well-disciplined schools, we found that the staffs:

- did many things that good educators have done for years;
- created total environments conducive to good discipline, rather than adopting isolated practices designed to deal specifically with discipline problems;
- viewed their schools as places in which to do valuable, sucessful, and productive work;
- made most of their decisions for the benefit of the students;
- focused on causes rather than symptoms;
- emphasized positive and preventive practices, not punitive ones;
- adapted practices to meet their own needs and styles; and
- had faith in their students and themselves—and expended unusual amounts of energy to make their beliefs into realities.

In well-disciplined schools, the principals played a key role in determining how the schools operated. Each principal also suported, and was supported by, some other staff member who added to the principal's strength.

The teachers in these schools handled all or most of the routine discipline problems themselves. They had stronger-than-average ties with the parents and the communities they served. They also welcomed and used critical review from a variety of school and community sources.

Lynn Wake's master's thesis[34] shows that 11 of the 13 characteristics mentioned above clearly distinguish schools with safe, well-disciplined learning environments from schools with poor discipline. Both types of schools use practices that good educators have long used, and principals in both types of schools play a key role in determining how the schools operate. Clearly, some well-established practices are good and some are bad. Moreover, principals can make schools bad, just as they can make them good.

Approximately four of every five disruptive incidents can be traced to some dysfunction in the way we organize schools, train staff members, or run schools. Our work with 500 well-disciplined schools and our 10 years of close work with school discipline in all manner of settings have convinced us that good schools function better than bad schools with regard to eight organizational factors.[35] Good schools; (1) teach staff members to work together to solve problems; (2) spread authority for decision making and reduce status differences among both staff members and students; (3) find ways to make all students feel a sense of ownership of the school; (4) develop rules and procedures that promote self-discipline; (5) design curriculum and instruction to reach, interest, and challenge the greatest number of students; (6) deal with personal problems that affect the behavoir of both staff members and students; (7) reach out for stronger school/home cooperation; and (8) insure that physical facilities and organizational structures reinforce the practices mentioned above.

Michael Rutter and his colleagues found the same organizational features in safe British schools.[36] The Safe School Study of the National Institute of Education also confirmed these findings.[37] George Wynn found statistically significant differences between well-disciplined schools and poorly disciplined schools on all eight of these organizational factors.[38] And Thomas Peters and Robert Waterman have indicated that these organizational features also characterize effective industries and business enterprises.[39]

What Government Can Do

The U.S. must never retreat from the goal of providing a high-quality education for every child, regardless of the child's station in life or apparent willingness to be educated. Teaching every future citizen to exercise self-discipline is the most important purpose of schooling in a democracy.[40]

Intentionally or not, official doublespeak that causes unwarranted anxiety about the state of the schools or that leads to exclusionary or punitive practices is a political attack on the concept of free and universal public education. Such doublespeak undermines public confidence in the schools and simultaneously hinders true school reform.

Violence and crime should never be confused with ordinary discipline problems. Nor should violence and crime be seen as the most important deterrents to effective learning in most schools. Research—free of political purposes or distortions—must identify the real problems and assess the impact of proposed solutions. Surveys and opinion polls should be supplemented with intensive case studies that use the best interviewing techniques and anthropological approaches. These case studies should focus on identifying the causes of violence and the causes of ordinary classroom disruptions. The President should be given unbiased information and statistics, so that he can establish a national climate for policies that insure safe, just, and orderly schools.

The involvement of school staffs, students, and parents in attacking the problems unique to their own schools should be encouraged and supported by every level of government that wishes to reduce violence and disruptive behaviors in the schools. Support for better preservice preparation of teachers and administrators should yield long-term improvements in school safety and orderliness at relatively little cost. Resources should be used to help inadequately prepared school staffs to improve the learning environments in their buildings. Time or dollars spent on improving the climate for learning will yield far better results than time or money spent on establishing punitive disiplinary programs or on efforts to "cure" individual students. And efforts to improve the climate for learning are far less likely to cause more problems than they solve.

Government at all levels must protect children and adults from abuse, unwarranted accusations, and denial of their rights. School officials often make mistakes under pressure. They do not always exhibit tolerance, insight, knowledge, or good judgment. Whatever the cause, children must be protected from such events as the following, which we encountered in the course of our study:

• A principal, who regularly uses a leather strap to punish students—usually minority students—called an innocent youngster into his office and laid three hard whacks on the child's buttocks, just so that a newspaper photographer could snap a photo of "how we handle things around here."

• Three girls in one elementary school were sent home for wearing galoshes in a 1½-inch snowfall. (The school had a rule that outlawed galoshes until the snow reached a depth of two inches.)

• A seventh-grade teacher forced misbehaving students to stand in a cardboard box in the corner of the classroom.

• A high school teacher stood guard outside the boys' rest room—while inside, at the teacher's behest, a group of students punished one of their peers for an infraction of the rules.

• Suspension and corporal punishment are frequently used for trivial matters. Moreover, these disciplinary tactics are used repeatedly with the same students. Clearly, the tactics have little effect on students' behavior.

The federal government must continue to provide constitutional protection for individuals and groups that are denied equitable or just treatment in local schools. And those protections must extend to both staff members and students.

But we teach personal responsibility best by taking personal responsibility ourselves and by exposing youngsters to an institution—the school—that performs responsibly. U.S. schools today need a return to personal commitment and responsibility at all levels. Every teacher has a personal responsibility to provide each student with appropriate instruction, to communicate with parents, to protect children's rights, and to ask for help if he or she does not know how to handle these tasks. Administrators, parents, school board members, and members of the community at large all have their own parts to play. Students must be taught to assume responsibility for coming to school, for keeping the building clean, and for taking an active part in their own learning.

We educators seem to be spending most of our energy today on manufacturing reasons to shift personal responsibility away from ourselves. Yet, following the lead of Japanese managers, several U.S. corporations are finding that greater personal responsibility, and the credit and pride that accompany it, can reduce conflict and stress within an organization.[41] Our schools also need pride—the kind of pride that comes from participating and producing, not from concocting crises that promote punishment and prejudice.

FOOTNOTES

1. A good example appears in Lucia Soloranzo, "Schools Draw the Line on Troublemakers," *U.S. News & World Report,* 23 January 1984, p. 65. The caption on the story reads, "Weapons Searches, Tougher Discipline Codes Are Among Methods Used in Growing War Against Classroom Crime." Yet the story opens with this sentence: "The drive to restore discipline in the nation's classrooms is moving into high gear."

2. Note, for example, the unbelievable "turn-arounds" detailed in *The Nation Responds: Recent Efforts to Improve Education* (Washington, D.C.: U.S. Government Printing Office, 1984), a report issued by the Education Department only one year after new federal "leadership" had been infused into American schools. ED researchers termed the claims in this report "embarrassing."

3. See, for example, Alec M. Gallup, "The 17th Annual Gallup Poll of the Public's Attitudes Toward the Public Schools," *Phi Delta Kappan,* September 1985, pp. 42–43.

4. See, for example, Thomas J. Flygare, "U.S. Supreme Court Volunteers to Decide New Jersey Student Search-and-Seizure Case," *Phi Delta Kappan,* December 1984, pp. 294–95.

5. The strategy for using one's governmental office to collect "credible" data supporting vouchers and to publicize these data is outlined in *Mandate for Leadership II* (Washington, D.C.: Heritage Foundation, 1984).

6. CCHR Working Group on School Violence/Discipline, "Chaos in the Classroom: Enemy of American Education" a memorandum for the Cabinet Council on Human Resources, nd. This memorandum, released about November 1983, lists no authors but has generally been attributed to Gary Bauer, then ED deputy undersecretary for planning, budget, and evaluation.

7. The report was released by ED on 10 January 1984 under a new title, *Disorder in Our Public Schools*. For criticisms of the report, see Joseph Scherer and Jim Stimson, "Pseudo vs. Real Issues: Is School Violence a Serious Concern?," *School Administrator,* March 1984, pp. 19-20, 54. See also the testimony that led to the change of title, which can be found in *Hearings Before the Subcommittee on Elementary, Secondary, and Vocational Education of the House Committee on Education and Labor* (Washington, D.C.: U.S. Government Printing Office, 1984). The hearings on this topic took place on 23-24 January 1984.

8. Gary L. Bauer, "Restoring Order to the Public Schools," *Phi Delta Kappan,* March 1985, pp. 488-91. See articles in the same issue of the *Kappan* by Keith Baker and by George Nicholson et al.

9. Gallup, p. 42-43.

10. Scherer and Stimson, p. 19.

11. In *Violent Schools, Safe Schools: The Safe School Study Report to the Congress, Vol. 1* (Washington, D.C.: National Institute of Education, U.S. Department of Health, Education, and Welfare, 1978), the authors attempted to reduce this error by limiting stolen items to those worth $1 or more.

12. *Making Our Schools Safe for Learning* (Boston: Boston Safe Schools Commission, 29 November 1983).

13. See, for example, Ivor Wayne and Robert J. Rubel, "Student Fear in Secondary Schools," *Urban Review,* Fall 1982, pp. 197-237.

14. Study the ways in which *Disorder in Our Public Schools* makes use of findings from Gerald Grant, "Children's Rights and Adult Confusion," *Public Interest,* Fall 1982, p. 83.

15. Jackson Toby, "Violence in School," *Research in Brief,* National Institute of Justice, U.S. Department of Justice, Washington, D.C., December 1983, p. 2.

16. Jacob A. Kounin, *Discipline and Group Management in Classrooms* (New York: Holt, Rinehart & Winston, 1970).

17. Oliver Moles, "Trends in Interpersonal Crimes in Schools," paper presented at the annual meeting of the American Educational Research Association, Montreal, April 1983.

18. Toby, p. 2. See also Gary Gottfredson and Denise Daiger, *Disruption in Six Hundred Schools* (Baltimore: Center for Social Organization of Schools, Johns Hopkins University, 1979); and Douglas Wright and Oliver Moles, "Legal Issues in Educational Order: Principals' Perceptions of School Discipline Policies and Practices," paper presented at the annual meeting of the American Educational Research Association, Chicago, April 1985.

19. See, for example, David Mann and Martin Gold, "Alternative Schools for Disruptive Secondary Students: Testing a Theory of School Processes, Students' Responses, and Outcome Behaviors" (Executive Summary, National Institute of Education, Washington, D.C., June 1981); Sara Lawrence Lightfoot, *The Good High School: Portraits of Character and Culture* (New York: Basic Books, 1983); Joan

Grant and Frank J. Capell, "Reducing School Crime: A Report on the School Team Approach" (Executive Summary, Social Action Research Center, National Institute for Juvenile Justice and Delinquency Prevention, U.S. Department of Justice, August 1983); Gary D. Gottfredson et al., *Measuring Victimization and the Explanation of School Disruption* (Baltimore: Center for Social Organization of Schools, 1981); and National Diffusion Network, *Educational Programs That Work* (San Francisco: Far West Laboratory for Educational Research and Development, 1980).

20. Alfred Alschuler et al., "Social Literacy: A Discipline Game Without Losers," *Phi Delta Kappan,* April 1977, pp. 606-9; and William W. Wayson and Gay Su Pinnell, "Developing Discipline with Quality Schools," in *Citizen Guide to Quality Education* (Cleveland: Citizens' Council for Ohio Schools, 1978). See also the chapter titled "Choices" in Joan First and Hayes Mizell, *Everybody's Business: A Book About School Discipline* (Columbia, S.C.: Southeastern Public Education Program, American Friends Service Committee, 1980); Daniel Duke and Venon F. Jones, "Two Decades of Discipline: Assessing the Development of an Educational Specialization," paper presented at the annual meeting of the American Educational Research Association, Montreal, April 1983; *An Overview of the School Approach* (Washington, D.C.: National Alcohol and Drug Abuse Education Program, U.S. Department of Education, circa 1983); and James E. Cole, "What to Do About Violence," *Today's Education,* November/December 1977, pp. 58-59.

21. Wayson and Pinnell, "Developing Discipline with Quality Schools." See also Morris Janowitz, *The Reconstruction of Patriotism: Education for Civic Consciousness* (Chicago: University of Chicago Press, 1985); and James McPartland and Edward McDill, *Violence in Schools: Perspectives, Programs, and Positions* (Lexington, Mass.: D.C. Heath, 1976).

22. See, for example, Susan C. Kaeser, *Orderly Schools That Serve All Children: A Review of Successful Schools in Ohio* (Cleveland: Citizens' Council for Ohio Schools, 1979); *Why Do Some Urban Schools Succeed? The Phi Delta Kappa Study of Exceptional Urban Elementary Schools* (Bloomington, Ind.: Phi Delta Kappa, 1980); and the articles on the characteristics of effective schools that appeared in the December 1982 issue of *Educational Leadership.*

23. Ellen Jane Hollingsworth, Henry F. Lufler, Jr., and William H. Clune III, *Discipline, Order, and Autonomy* (New York: Praeger, 1984); and Wright and Moles, p. 11.

24. See citations in fn. 22 and in fns. 36-41.

25. For example, Joseph Clark, principal of Paterson (N.J.) High School, is often praised for bringing order to his school by suspending 300 students. Yet the dropout rate in the school now stands at 50%, according to Irwin Hyman and John D'Alessandro, "Good, Old-Fashioned Discipline: The Politics of Punitiveness," *Phi Delta Kappan,* September 1984, pp. 39-45.

26. See the works of Denise Gottfredson and Gary Gottfredson, staff members at the Center for Social Organization of Schools, Johns Hopkins University, Baltimore; Gay Su Pinnell et al., *An Institute to Develop Schools with Self-Discipline in Newly Desegregated Secondary Schools in Cleveland and Columbus, Ohio,* final report to the U.S. Department of Education (Columbus: Department of Educational Policy and Leadership, Ohio State University, July 1981); and idem. *An Institute to Develop Schools with Self-Discipline in Newly Desegregated Middle and High Schools*

in Columbus, Ohio, final report to the U.S. Department of Education (Columbus: Department of Educational Policy and Leadership, Ohio State University, July 1982).

27. *Children Out of School in America* (Cambridge, Mass.: Children's Defense Fund, 1974); and *School Suspensions: Are They Helping Children?* (Cambridge, Mass.: Children's Defense Fund, 1975). Though the data in these two publications are old, the general picture they present is still accurate. See also Irwin A. Hyman and James H. Wise, *Corporal Punishment in American Education* (Philadelphia: Temple University Press. 1979); and *Barriers to Excellence: Our Children at Risk* (Boston: National Coalition of Advocates for Students, 1985).

28. Alfred M. Bloch, "The Battered Teacher," *Today's Education,* March/April 1977, pp. 58-62.

29. For a discussion of personality and its relationship to stress, see Cary L. Cooper and Judi Marshall, "Occupational Sources of Stress: A Review of the Literature Relating to Coronary Heart Disease and Mental Ill Health," *Journal of Occupational Psychology,* March 1976, pp. 11-28.

30. See, for example, Lee E. Teitelbaum, "School Discipline Procedures: Some Empirical Findings and Some Theoretical Questions," *Indiana Law Journal,* vol. 58, 1983, pp. 559-62; Louis Fischer and David Schimmel, *The Rights of Students and Teachers* (New York: Harper & Row, 1982), pp. 298-327; and David G. Carter, J. John Harris, and Frank Brown, "Student and Parent Rights: What Are Their Constitutional Guarantees?," *NOLPE School Law Journal,* vol. 6, 1976, pp. 45-61.

31. See CCHR Working Group on School Violence/Discipline, *Disorder in Our Public Schools.* See also many public pronouncements on and after 10 January 1984, including

Ronald Reagan, "Excellence and Opportunity: A Program of Support for American Education," *Phi Delta Kappan,* September 1984, p. 14.

32. *Goss v. Lopez,* 419 U.S. 565 (1975). Principals' opinions are reported in Wright and Moles, "Legal Issues in Educational Order. . . ."

33. William Wayson et al., *Handbook for Developing Schools with Good Discipline* (Bloomington, Ind.: Phi Delta Kappa, 1982).

34. Lynn Wake, "A Study to Verify School Characteristics Believed to Improve School Discipline" (Master's thesis, Ohio State University, 1983). See also Wayson et al., *Handbook . . . ,* Chap. 2.

35. Wayson et al., ibid., Chap. 3.

36. See Michael Rutter et al., *Fifteen Thousand Hours* (Cambridge, Mass.: Harvard University Press, 1979); and Michael Rutter, "School Influences on Children's Behavior and Development," *Pediatrics,* February 1980, pp. 208-20, 361-62.

37. National Institute of Education, *Violent Schools, Safe Schools. . . .*

38. George Wynn, "The Development and Testing of an Instrument to Examine Organizational Design Characteristics That Impact on School Discipline" (Doctoral dissertation, Ohio State University, 1980).

39. Thomas J. Peters and Robert H. Waterman, Jr., *In Search of Excellence* (New York: Harper & Row, 1982).

40. Horace Mann advocated this goal for the schools in 1845. See Lawrence Cremin, ed., *The Republic and the School: Horace Mann on the Education of Free Man* (New York: Teachers College Press, 1957), pp. 57-59.

41. Peters and Waterman, *In Search of Excellence.*

Ken Robinson

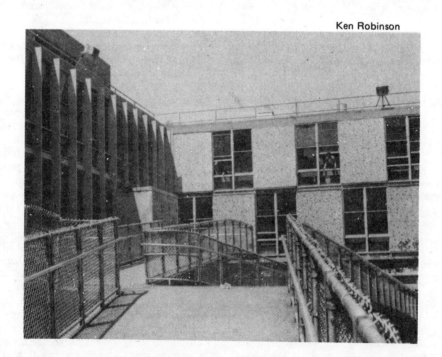

Section III
National Issues
Introduction by Gerald R. Rasmussen[*]

Since the inception of our nation, education has been a State function. Article 3 of the Ordinance of 1787 declared the importance of education and established it as a priority of that ordinance. Two years later Article X of the Bill of Rights clearly established education as a State function . . . and so it has been throughout our history. Thus, there has never been a national program of education, a national curriculum, or national certification of teachers and administrators. Each state has focused on rules, regulations, issues and programs which they feel best meet the special needs of their constituents.

At the same time, however, the Federal Government, responding to ever increasing national concerns, has had a long and significant interest in education. Legislative programs such as the Smith-Hughes Act, the G.I. Bill of Rights, the National Defense Education Act, Title IX, P.L. 94–142, and desegregation legislation have contributed to a recognition of growing national concerns which need to be addressed by public education in all states.

Other developments such as improved communication technology, population mobility, national testing, a National Teachers Examination, the changing nature of the family, and recent efforts by the University Council for Educational Administration and others to develop national criteria for credentialing school administrators through the creation of the National Commission on Excellence in Educational Administration, have led to a growing recognition of a need to focus on issues common to the nation. Section III addresses several of these issues that are currently of a national concern.

The nine articles included in Section III can be grouped under three areas: racial/ethical inequities, welfare of young people, and inadequacies of the educational program. Racial/ethnic inequities in our society and more specifically in our schools are explored in articles on desegregation (Braddock, Crain and McPartland), magnet schools (Doyle and Levine), and bilingual education (Trimarco). Concerns for the welfare of our young people are analyzed by four articles: child abuse (Elshtain), adolescent suicide (Schere), mentoring, (Silverstein, Richardson, and Lanier), and self-care issues (Holman). Two articles address inadequacies of the educational program. They focus on school finance (Godfrey), and the length of the school term (Karweit).

All of these concerns are of national interest. Educators and others interested in education of the young people of our nation must understand these issues in order to help schools meet the need of all members of our society.

*Dr. Gerald R. Rasmussen is Professor of Educational Administration, California State University, Los Angeles, CA.

Chapter 13

A Long-Term View of School Desegregation: Some Recent Studies of Graduates as Adults

Jomills Henry Braddock II, Robert L. Crain, and James M. McPartland*

The case for or against desegregation should not be argued in terms of academic achievement. If we want a segregated society, we should have segregated schools. If we want a desegregated society, we should have desegregated schools.[1]

In 1984, the 30th anniversary of *Brown v. Board of Education,* it is important to keep in mind this elegantly blunt statement by Christopher Jencks. Social scientists and educators are mistaken, if they assume that the only point—or even the main point—of the *Brown* decision was to insure that black students are given equal opportunities to learn the basic skills. Schools have a broader mission than that. Writing for the Supreme Court in *Brown,* Chief Justice Earl Warren noted:

> Today, education is perhaps the most important function of state and local governments. . . . It is the very foundation of good citizenship. . . . [I]t is a principal instrument in awakening the child to cultural values, in preparing him for later professional training, and in helping him to adjust normally to his environment. In these days it is doubtful that any child may reasonably be expected to succeed in life if he is denied the opportunity of an education.[2]

Warren's view is widely shared by both scholars and policy makers. A major goal of public education in the U.S. has always been to facilitate the assimilation of minorities; indeed, school desegregation may be the most significant example of a national policy using educational reform to achieve this end.

Yet the debate over the merits of school desegregation has virtually ignored the goal of assimilation, focusing instead on such narrow issues as whether achievement test scores rise or fall after desegregation. The evidence suggests that the test scores of minority students rise after desegregation, but this outcome is not the real test of the value of desegregating the schools. The real test is whether desegregation enables minorities to join other Americans in becoming well-educated, economically successful, and socially well-adjusted adults.

Clearly, we cannot evaluate school desegregation as if it were simply another educational innovation, akin to "new" math or to an innovative technique of individualizing reading instruction. Schools do more than teach academic skills; they also socialize the young for membership in adult society. School desegregation is not simply an educational reform; it also reforms the socialization function of the schools. For this reason, U.S. society cannot avoid the pain of decisions about school desegregation simply by improving the quality of segregated schools. Desegregation puts majorities and minorities together so that they can learn to coexist with one another, not so that they can learn to read.

Data from our work at the Center for Social Organization of Schools and from the research of a few colleagues elsewhere suggest that school desegregation is leading to desegregation in several areas of adult life. Table 1 lists the relevant studies. These studies, which have typically followed large groups of students through schools and into adulthood, are few in number because of their high cost.

Without exception, the studies listed in Table 1 show that desegregation of schools leads to desegregation in later life—in college, in social situations, and on the

*Jomills Henry Braddock II and Robert L. Crain are principal research scientists and co-directors of the Education and Work Program, Center for Social Organization of Schools, Johns Hopkins University, Baltimore, MD. James M. McPartland is co-director of the Center. Reprinted with permission from *Phi Delta Kappan*, December, 1984.

TABLE 1. Summary of

Study	Data	Independent Variable
Braddock (1980)	Survey in 1972 of black students attending four colleges in Florida (N = 253)	High school racial composition
Braddock and McPartland (1982)	Black subsample of the National Longitudinal Study (NLS) High School Class of 1972 (N = 3,119)	Elementary/secondary school racial composition
Braddock, McPartland, and Trent (1984)	Black and white subsamples of the NLS Class of 1972 merged with survey data from their 1976 and 1979 employers (blacks = 1,518; whites = 1,957)	High school and college racial composition
Crain and Weisman (1972)	Survey in 1966 of blacks living in North and West (N = 1,651)	Elementary/secondary school racial composition
Braddock and McPartland (1983)	Two-year follow-up of black subsample of NLS 1980-81 Youth Cohort (N = 1,074)	High school racial composition
Green (1981; 1982)	Ten-year follow-up of 1971 black college freshmen surveyed by American Council on Education (N = 1,400)	High school and college racial composition
Crain (1984a)	Survey in 1982 of Project Concern participants (N = 660)	Elementary/secondary school racial composition
Crain (1984b)	Survey of employers of NLS respondents (N = 4,080)	Inner-city school vs. surburban school
Pearce (1980)	14 communities	Change in school segregation indices
Pearce, Crain, and Farley (1984)	25 large cities	Change in school segregation indices

Recent Research Evidence on the Effects of Desegregation

Dependent Variable	Control Variables	Findings
Racial composition of college	Socioeconomic status, sex, high school grades, college costs and reputation, financial aid, and proximity to college	Black students from majority-white high schools are more likely to enroll at majority-white four-year colleges
Racial composition of college	Socioeconomic status, sex, high school grades and test scores, region, and proximity to college	Black students from majority-white elementary/secondary schools are more likely to enroll in and persist at majority-white two- and four- year colleges.
Racial composition of employing firm	Sex, age, public vs. private employment, educational attainment, region and community racial composition	Blacks and whites from desegregated elementary/secondary schools are more likely to work in desegregated firms; blacks from predominantly white colleges are also more likely to work in desegregated firms.
Interracial contact, neighborhood racial composition, racial composition of occupation	Socioeconomic status, age, sex, region of birth	Blacks from desegregated elementary/secondary schools are more likely to have white social contacts, live in integrated neighborhoods.
Racial composition of co-worker groups and attitudes toward white supervisors and white co-workers	Sex, age, public vs. private employment, job status, and community racial composition	Northern blacks from majority-white high schools are more likely to have white co-workers. In the South, this relationship is also positive but confounded with community racial composition. Desegregated blacks evaluate white co-workers and supervisors more positively than do segregated blacks.
Racial composition of co-worker and friendship groups	Sex, high school grades, college major, etc.	Black adults who graduated from majority-white high schools or majority-white colleges and who grew up in majority-white neighborhoods are more likely to have white work associates and friends.
Interracial contact and neighborhood racial composition	Socioeconomic status, age, and test scores	Blacks who attend desegregated schools are more likely to move into integrated neighborhoods and to have a greater number of white friends.
Employment decisions about applicants	Race, age, sex, education, and how applicant came to firm	Employers give preference to blacks from desegregated (i.e., suburban) schools.
Change in degree of desegregation in housing and in marketing policies in housing	Communities matched by size, region, racial composition	Communities with a communitywide school desegregation plan have more integration in housing and less "racial steering" by the real estate industry.
Change in housing segregation indices	City, size, racial composition, previous level of segregation	Central cities where schools are desegregated have more desegregation in housing.

job. One of the most dysfunctional aspects of racial segregation is its tendency to become self-perpetuating. Racial segregation gives birth to and nurtures a form of avoidance learning that helps to maintain the separation of blacks and whites.[3]

Prior to the *Brown* decision, blacks were educated in a dual school system that offered them putatively inferior training, especially in the South. When schools in the South began to desegregate, blacks were legally entitled to attend formerly all-white elementary and secondary schools. However, in part because of anticipated hostility from whites and in part because of the belief that prior differences in educational preparation might place them at a competitive disadvantage in desegregated schools, many blacks in the South were ambivalent about and reluctant to take full advantage of this hard-won educational opportunity.

For this reason, the Supreme Court ruled that "freedom of choice"—that is, offering blacks the opportunity to leave segregated schools for desegregated ones—is unconstitutional. The Court recognized that a century of segregation had created enormous social inertia that would, given the opportunity, maintain segregated schools far into the future.

Just as blacks who grew up in segregated schools are reluctant to send their children to desegregated schools, so they are also reluctant to place themselves in desegregated adult settings. As contact theory would predict, blacks have learned to avoid and to withdraw from interracial situations that might cause them pain or indignity. Even though the situation has changed, and the pain and indignity have lessened or disappeared altogether, many blacks remain reluctant to test the new arrangements.

Thus, as we have already pointed out, historic patterns of de jure and de facto segregation have generated a social inertia that sustains blacks' isolation from major social institutions. And this long-standing isolation of blacks has perpetuated patterns of avoidance learning and social behavior among whites that cause them to resist desegregation in the schools and in other social settings. Desegregation of elementary and secondary schools would help the U.S. to replace a self-perpetuating cycle of segregation with a self-perpetuating cycle of desegregation.

The first two research studies listed in Table 1 found that minority students who have been educated in desegregated elementary and secondary schools are more likely than their counterparts from segregated schools to attend predominantly white colleges and universities.[4] Blacks who have attended segregated schools in the South tend to perpetuate their segregation by enrolling in traditionally black four-year colleges. Blacks who have attended segregated schools in the North are more likely than their counterparts from desegregated schools to enroll in predominantly black community colleges located in urban areas.

The third study listed in Table 1 found that both blacks and whites who have attended desegregated schools are more likely than their counterparts from segregated schools to be working in desegregated settings.[5] The fourth study, by Robert Crain and Carol Weisman, used data collected in the 1960s by the U.S. Commission on Civil Rights; this study showed that blacks educated in desegregated schools are more likely than those educated in segregated ones to have white social contacts and to live in integrated neighborhoods.[6] The fifth study listed in Table 1 showed that blacks from desegregated schools are more likely than their counterparts from segregated schools to work in desegregated settings.[7]

The sixth and seventh studies listed in Table 1 found that blacks who have attended desegregated schools are more likely to work in desegregated settings, more likely to live in racially mixed neighborhoods, and more likely to have cross-racial friendships.[8] (The seventh study, conducted by Robert Crain and funded by the National Institute of Education, was a 15-year follow-up evaluation of an experimental desegregation program in Hartford, Connecticut.)

The eighth study in Table 1, also conducted by Crain, showed that a national sample of employers gives preference in hiring to black graduates of desegregated high schools.[9] And the last two studies in Table 1, which looked at entire communities, showed that those cities with desegregated schools are also more likely to have integrated neighborhoods.[10]

The studies in Table 1 show strong and consistent effects: members of minority groups who have been educated in segregated schools will generally move into segregated niches in adult society. If they have had no childhood experience with whites, members of minority groups will tend to avoid dealing with whites as adults. Sometimes they practice avoidance because they expect rejection. But this avoidance may also be explained by the fact that they have had no chance to develop effective ways of interacting and coping with whites; moreover, they have lacked opportunities in competitive situations to test their abilities against those of whites. We think it is likely, too, that the same mechanism that produces prejudice among whites from segregated backgrounds will produce prejudice among blacks who have had no contact with whites.

It seems intuitively obvious that, among blacks, the social and psychological barriers to seeking or sustaining memberships in desegregated groups should be greater for those individuals who unrealistically expect hostile reactions from whites, who have little confidence that they can function successfully in interracial situations, or who have trouble dealing with the strains that may accompany interpersonal contacts across racial lines. And indeed, Crain found, in his study of participants in the Hartford desegregation program, that minority males who had graduated from segregated schools perceived more racism, both in college and in business settings, than did males who had graduated from desegregated schools.[11] If childhood experiences in desegregated settings help blacks to break down these social and psychological barriers, the logical outcome would seem to be less avoidance or withdrawal from integrated situations in adulthood.

School desegregation also changes the attitudes and behavior of whites, by reducing racial stereotypes and removing whites' fears of hostile reactions in interracial settings. Using data on racial attitudes derived from national surveys, Richard Scott and James McPartland found that attending desegregated schools improves the attitudes of both blacks and whites toward future interracial situations.[12]

Similarly, mainstream institutions respond to school desegregation by providing more opportunities for blacks to associate with whites. Cities that have desegregated schools develop a larger quantity of desegregated housing than do cities with segregated school systems. Corporations also react more positively to black applicants who come to them from desegregated schools. Thus, even if the attitudes and behaviors of minority and majority students did not change, school desegregation would still make white-controlled institutions more open to members of minority groups, thereby creating greater opportunities for adult desegregation.

Nowhere is this result more apparent than in the two studies of the impact of schools on local housing markets.[13] We tend to think of schools simply as educational settings, but they are also major employers and respected social institutions in their communities. As such, the schools exert a powerful influence on local real estate values, and the choice of a school site is one of the most powerful city-planning tools available to local government. Cities that locate their schools and assign students to them in a manner that promotes segregation will find that they are also segregating their housing market.

An old argument, which has recently resurfaced, suggests that separate-but-equal is as good for the society as integrated-and-equal. Where the schools are concerned, at least, that argument is wrong.

Segregation in elementary and secondary schools leads to segregation in adult life—which inevitably means inequality of opportunity with regard to higher education, employment, and housing. If they wish to attend college, for example, high school graduates who are members of minority groups often have no choice but to attend a predominantly white institution. But if they have been ill-prepared by their elementary and secondary schools to cope with whites, they have been ill-prepared to cope with higher education.

Meanwhile, high school and college graduates who are members of minority groups must deal with an employment market dominated by white-owned institutions. If they lack the credentials that impress white personnel directors, these graduates are not likely to receive job offers. Moreover, researchers have found that blacks from segregated schools who have white supervisors in the workplace have more negative feelings about those supervisors than do blacks from desegregated schools.[14] Thus blacks educated in segregated schools are probably less likely to keep their jobs with white employers and to earn promotions.

Finally, in today's economy, the major portion of the average family's net worth is tied up in the family home. But those blacks who reside in the inner city have purchased homes characterized by declining property values, and they suffer serious economic losses as a consequence.

The perpetuation of segregation from childhood into adulthood might not be economically and socially harmful to minorities in a society in which minority-owned institutions provided samples opportunities for economic and social success. But U.S. society does not provide such opportunities. Therefore, segregation is harmful, because most minority-group members must find their ways into desegregated institutions if they are to achieve success as adults.

Some of the studies we have completed lend support to this statement. For example, a 1981 study by Jomills Braddock and Marvin Dawkins showed that blacks educated in desegregated high schools made better grades both in historically black colleges and in predominantly white ones.[15] Similarly, Robert Crain, Rita Mahard, and Ruth Narot found in 1983 that black males educated in segregated junior high schools in the South had much lower test scores as students in desegregated high schools than did black males educated in desegregated junior high schools in the South.[16]

By the same token, a 1978 study by Crain and Mahard showed that in the North, which has very few predominantly black four-year colleges, blacks educated in desegregated elementary and secondary schools are more likely than blacks in the South to graduate from college.[17] This seems to be the case partly because blacks in the North are more likely to chose to attend a four-year college, partly because they make higher grades there, and partly because they are less willing to drop out. Braddock and McPartland reported similar findings in 1982.[18] And Kenneth Green, in his analysis of data on black college freshmen collected by the American Council on Education, found that blacks from desegregated schools tended to make higher grades in college and to have higher college graduation rates than blacks from segregated schools.[19]

We are also beginning to accumulate some evidence that black graduates of desegregated schools have better employment opportunities than do their counterparts from segregated schools. In a study done nearly 20 years ago, Crain and Weisman found that black males from desegregated schools had better jobs and higher incomes than their peers from segregated schools.[20] Analyses by Braddock,[21] Braddock and McPartland,[22] Mickey Burnim,[23] and Harold Brown and David Ford,[24] using four different samples of data, all showed that black graduates of predominantly white colleges and universities enjoyed some degree of income advantage over their counterparts who had graduated from predominantly black institutions. If we combine these findings with those of Crain, from his study of employer stereotypes of blacks from segregated schools,[25] and with those of Diana Pearce in 1980 and of Pearce, Crain, and Reynolds Farley in 1984 on housing opportunities in cities that have desegregated schools,[26] we have considerable evidence that school desegregation is a necessary step to insure equality of economic opportunity to minorities in U.S. society.

Additional research remains to be done, however. We need more studies of how whites relate to blacks as a result of their own segregated or desegregated schooling. Nor is there yet a good study, using up-to-date data, to replicate the Crain and Weisman finding that black graduates of desegregated elementary and secondary schools enjoy higher incomes than their counterparts from segregated schools.

Nonetheless, the evidence already in hand tells us that the initial conception of the impact of school desegregation, as expressed in 1954 in the *Brown* decision, has been borne out. The schools are the place in which a society socializes its next generation of citizens. The research findings that we have presented here suggest that the U.S. cannot afford segregated schools, if this nation is genuinely committed to providing equality of opportunity to every citizen.

FOOTNOTES

1.   Christopher Jencks et al., *Inequality* (New York: Basic Books, 1972). p. 106.

2.   *Brown v. Board of Education,* 347 U.S. 483 (1954).

3.   Thomas Pettigrew, "Continuing Barriers to Desegregated Education in the South," *Sociology of Education,* Winter 1965, pp. 99–111.

4.   Jomills Henry Braddock II, "The Perpetuation of Segregation Across Levels of Education: A Behavioral Assessment of the Contact-Hypothesis," *Sociology of Education,* July 1980, pp. 178–86; and Jomills Henry Braddock II and James M. McPartland, "Assessing School Desegregation Effects: New Directions in Research," in Ronald Corwin, ed., *Research in Sociology of Education and Socialization, Vol. 3* (Greenwich, Conn.: JAI, 1982), pp. 259–82.

5.   Jomills Henry Braddock II, James M. McPartland, and William Trent, "Desegregated Schools and Desegregated Work Environments," paper presented at the annual meeting of the American Educational Research Association, New Orleans, 1984.

6.   Robert L. Crain and Carol Weisman, *Discrimination, Personality, and Achievement* (New York: Seminar Press, 1972). See also U.S. Commission on Civil Rights, *Racial Isolation in the Public Schools, Vols. I and II* (Washington, D.C.: U.S. Government Printing Office, 1967).

7.   Jomills Henry Braddock II and James M. McPartland, *More Evidence on Social-Psychological Processes That Perpetuate Minority Segregation: The Relationship of School Desegregation and Employment Segregation,* Report No. 338 (Baltimore: Center for Social Organization of Schools, Johns Hopkins University, 1983).

8.   Kenneth Green, "Integration and Attainment: Preliminary Results from a National Longitudinal Study of the Impact of School Desegregation," paper presented at the annual meeting of the American Educational Research Association, Los Angeles, 1981; idem, "The Impact of Neighborhood and Secondary School Integration of Educational Achievement and Occupational attainment of College-Bound Blacks" (Doctoral dissertation, University of California-Los Angeles, 1982); and Robert L. Crain, "Desegregated Schools and the Non-Academic Side of College Survival," paper presented at the annual meeting of the American Educational Research Association, New Orleans, 1984.

9.   Robert L. Crain, *The Quality of American High School Graduates: What Personnel Officers Say and Do About It,* Report No. 354 (Baltimore: Center for Social Organization of Schools, Johns Hopkins University, 1984).

10.   Diana Pearce, *Breaking Down the Barriers: New Evidence on the Impact of Metropolitan School Desegregation on Housing Patterns* (Washington, D.C.: National Institute of Education, 1980); and Diana Pearce, Robert L. Crain, and Reynolds Farley, "Lessons Not Lost: The Effect of School Desegregation on the Rate of Residential Desegregation in Large Central Cities," paper presented at the annual meeting of the American Educational Research Association, New Orleans, 1984.

11.   Crain, "Desegregated Schools. . . ."

12.   Richard Scott and James M. McPartland, "Desegregation as National Policy: Correlates of Racial Attitudes," *American Educational Research Journal,* vol. 19, 1982, pp. 397–414.

13.   Pearce, *Breaking Down the Barriers. . . . ,* and Pearce, Crain, and Farley, "Lessons Not Lost. . . ."

14.   Braddock and McPartland, *More Evidence on Social-Psychological Processes. . . .*

15.   Jomills Henry Braddock II and Marvin Dawkins, "Predicting Black Achievement in Higher Education," *Journal of Negro Education,* vol. 50, 1981, pp. 319–27.

16. Robert L. Crain, Rita Mahard, and Ruth Narot, *Making Desegregation Work* (Cambridge, Mass.: Ballinger, 1983).

17. Robert L. Crain and Rita Mahard, "School Racial Composition and Black College Attendance and Achievement Test Performance," *Sociology of Education,* vol. 51, 1978, pp. 81–101.

18. Braddock and McPartland, "Assessing School Desegregation Effects. . . ."

19. Green, "The Impact of Neighborhood and Secondary School Integration. . . ."

20. Crain and Weisman, *Discrimination, Personality, and Achievement.*

21. Jomills Henry Braddock II, "College Race and Black Occupational Attainment," paper presented at the annual meeting of the American Sociological Association, Detroit, 1983.

22. Jomills Henry Braddock II and James M. McPartland, "Some Costs and Benefits for Black College Students of Enrollment at Predominantly White Institutions," in Michael Nettles and Robert Thoeny, eds., *Qualitative Dimensions of Desegregation in Higher Education* (San Francisco: Josey-Bass, forthcoming).

23. Mickey Burnim, "The Earnings Effect of Black Matriculation in Predominantly White Colleges," *Industrial and Labor Relations Review,* vol. 33, 1980, pp. 518–24.

24. Harold Brown and David Ford, "An Exploratory Analysis of Discrimination in the Employment of Black MBA Graduates," *Journal of Applied Psychology,* vol. 62, 1977, pp. 50–56.

25. Crain, "The Quality of American High School Graduates. . . ."

26. Pearce, *Breaking Down the Barriers . . .* , and Pearce, Crain, and Farley, "Lessons Not Lost. . . ."

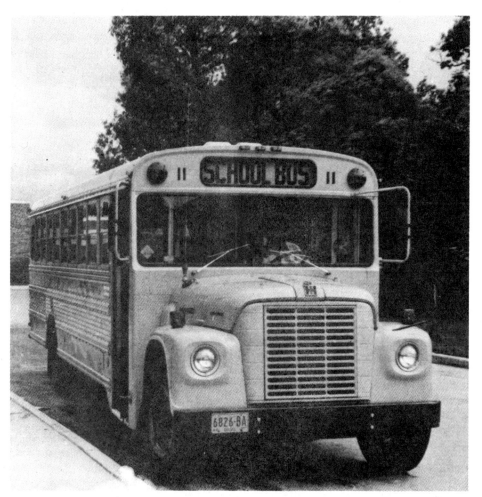

David Morenberg

Chapter 14
Magnet Schools: Choice and Quality in Public Education

Denis R. Doyle and Marsha Levine*

For generations, place of residence and a continuing search for the "one best system" have been major forces that shaped U.S. schools. In determining which school a given child would attend, "geography was destiny"; individual differences among students had no bearing. Yet assignment by neighborhood began as an administrative expedient without roots in pedagogical theory.

Although the U.S. tradition of local control has been strong, a "common school culture" has been equally strong, producing an educational system in which individual schools are surprisingly similar. The major difference between public schools is qualitative; for example, a fast-track school may set higher academic standards for its students, but its organization does not differ appreciably from that of other schools serving the same age group. Both kinds of schools: (1) divide the day into periods during which teachers lecture and students respond, (2) group children by age, (3) assign letter grades, and (4) offer courses for fixed time periods (usually semesters) instead of for the time it takes students to master the material. This common school culture reflects a strong belief in the existence of a "one best system."

The continuing quest for this "one best system" led James Bryant Conant to propose in 1959 that U.S. high schools be comprehensive.[1] American educators quickly adopted his proposal, and the pressures for uniformity in schooling increased. However, the comprehensive neighborhood high school has two important limitations: it reflects residential patterns, which isolate groups by race and socioeconomic status, and its broad curriculum lacks the depth and intensity that a more sharply focused curriculum affords.

These limitations of the comprehensive high school gave rise to today's magnet school movement. A magnet school reflects a central academic or vocational theme and stresses voluntary participation. Since students come from across the city, a magnet school promises social integration. Since students *choose* to attend a magnet school, their motivation is likely to be high. Since the curriculum of a magnet school reflects a central theme, students' studies are likely to be more focused and their performance (as measured by standardized tests) will often be higher than that of their counterparts in other kinds of schools.

Early Magnet Schools

Neighborhood schools have been the norm in the U.S. for decades. But the nation has always had a few schools that fit the description of magnet schools (though they did not originally bear that label). The best known of these schools compose an honor roll of U.S. education; the oldest is Boston Latin School, founded in 1635 (a year before Harvard University). Others include Lowell High School in San Francisco, Central High School in Philadelphia, Bronx High School of Science in the Bronx, Aviation High School in Queens, Lane Tech in Chicago, and the New York High School of the Performing Arts in Manhattan.[2]

These and similar schools represent a striking departure from the tradition of attendance by neighborhood. But selective schools that rely on voluntary enrollment have had a checkered history. Frequently accused of elitism, such schools have sometimes had to fight for their survival. For example, three selective academic high schools in New York City found that they needed special legislation to protect them from bureaucratic

*Denis P. Doyle is a Senior Research Fellow at the Hudson Institute. Marsha Levine is Associate Director, Education Issues Department, American Federation of Teachers. This article is adapted from a paper commissioned by the Pfizer Corporation; the original first appeared in *Educating Americans for the 21st Century* (Fall 1983), a publication of the National Science Board Commission on Precollege Education in Mathematics, Science, and Technology. The authors wish to thank Deborah Rogal for her assistance with the research on which this article is based. Reprinted with permission of *Phi Delta Kappan*, December, 1984.

intervention and even extinction. Nor have all selective schools been as fortunate as these three. In the mid-Fifties a bleak fate befell Dunbar High School in Washington, D.C., an institution widely perceived as the nation's premier public high school for blacks.

Despite the limitations imposed on it by a racist society, Dunbar had flourished prior to the mid-Fifties. It stood for high standards and excellence, and generations of graduates, parents, and faculty members took great pride in the school. Though it did not formally bear the label, Dunbar was a magnet school of its day, drawing able black students from across the city. Indeed, many youngsters who were not residents of Washington, D.C., moved in with friends or relatives who were, so that they could attend Dunbar. Writing in the New York Times, Fred Hechinger noted that "among Dunbar's illustrious alumni were Benjamin O. Davis, the first black general in the United States Army; Dr. Charles Drew, who devised the method of storing blood plasma and set up the first blood bank for the American Red Cross; and former Housing Secretary Robert Weaver, the first black Cabinet official."[3]

Ironically, the Washington, D.C., school board converted Dunbar into a neighborhood high school in response to the 1954 *Brown v. Board of Education* decision. This Supreme Court ruling spelled the end of fast-track public education in Washington, D.C., for both blacks and whites. Only in the past few years have magnet schools reappeared in that city—though in attenuated form.

The Issue of Elitism

From the beginning, the charge of elitism has plagued selective schools and, by extension, magnet schools. The argument is twofold: first, that separation of children by ability is undemocratic and thus intrinsically wrong; and second, that selective schools skim off the brightest children, forcing other schools to deal solely with mediocre and below-average students. Research on these issues is virtually nonexistent, but several theoreticians have made provocative statements about selective schools.

Perhaps the most powerful of these statements appeared in *Exit, Voice, and Loyalty,* by Albert Hirschman.[4] Hirschman argued that quality-conscious consumers will not tolerate the inferior products of monopolies. Although he focuses initially on the state-owned railroad in a West African nation, he later extends his discussion to include public and private schools. According to Hirschman, quality-conscious parents will not tolerate low-quality public schools—but neither can the public schools (a monopoly) tolerate the continual complaints of a small but vocal group

of discontented parents. Thus an accommodation is reached that allows quality-conscious parents to avail themselves of such high-quality alternatives as private schools. The parents are happy with the better education that these alternatives afford; meanwhile, the public schools tolerate the competition to be rid of these parents' complaints. Public magnet schools serve some of the same functions as private schools, but they do so within the public sector. More important, they contain within themselves the seeds of system wide improvement.

This analysis raises an implicit challenge to a view of education that is seriously flawed: the notion that, when the brightest children are skimmed from the population and sent to selective schools, the rest of the school system suffers. This notion is a logical (albeit wrong-headed) extension of Americans' deeply ingrained belief in the existence of a "one best system" of education—and, although it is not supported by evidence, it has strong face validity and thus requires a response.

First, the notion is based on erroneous assumptions about what makes a good school. Private schools run the gamut from Quaker institutions to military academies, from Waldorf schools to Jesuit schools, from international baccalaureate schools to institutions modeled on A.S. Neill's Summerhill. For example, New York City has three selective public high schools that focus on academics—Stuyvesant, Bronx Science, and Brooklyn Tech. These schools compete with one another, as well as with three equally selective public high schools with different focuses—Music and Art, Performing Arts, and Aviation—and with the private schools in the city. These six public schools are extraordinarily diverse. But their differences spring from differing pedagogical emphases, not from intellectual disparities among their students. Moreover, these schools clearly reveal that "good education" for one student or teacher may be quite different from "good education" for another student or teacher. Indeed, does anyone's experience suggest otherwise?

However, treating magnet schools as though they were synonymous with selective schools is both politically and pedagogically limiting—politically limiting because it raises the issue of elitism unnecessarily; pedagogically limiting because it makes too much of selectivity. In reality, rational selectivity is difficult to implement, except in extreme cases. Further, it would appear that choice is even more important than selectivity in making a difference in quality education.

Take the three academically selective high schools in New York City as examples. As many as 15,000 children take the entrance examinations each year, vying for the approximately 2,500 openings in these three schools. Only the 2,500 highest-scoring applicants are accepted. But what of the next 2,500—and the 2,500 after that? The few points on entrance examinations that separate the top 2,500 candidates from the runners-up do not represent appreciable intellectual differences. The obvious solution is to open other special schools, so that the runners-up will have choices as well. And this is precisely what is now starting to happen.

Magnet Schools Today

Magnet schools can reflect a policy of *inclusion* rather than exclusion—opening their doors to any student who cares to attend. No longer unwilling "victims" of schooling, students in open-access magnet schools become willing and eager participants in their own education.

Magnet schools also afford choices to youngsters who have differing learning styles and differing interests. Magnet schools that focus on music and art, on vocational education, on the humanities, on science and mathematics, or on any of a number of other areas make good sense, both pedagogically and socially.

Moreover, magnet schools have an ambiance that has a positive effect on personal behavior. Thus magnet schools can set standards of dress and behavior that would be impossible to enforce in comprehensive high schools. For example, a magnet school could easily require community service as a condition of graduation, whereas such a requirement would be intrusive and onerous if it were expected of all students in a given school district.

Equally important, magnet schools offer a setting in which teacher-generated reforms can take place. Think, for example, of how schools might implement the reforms suggested by Theodore Sizer.[5] Sizer has proposed, among other things, the grouping of students by ability or achievement instead of by age. How might such a change be put into effect? Should a state board of education impose it by fiat? Should the federal government support pilot projects at selected demonstration sites? Should some court order the reform—or, perhaps, forbid it? Clearly, the most intelligent and humane way to implement such an idea is for a caring and interested school community to decide to try out. Magnet schools provide just such opportunities.

We know that the reasons for establishing magnet schools vary greatly. In some communities such schools have been opened to facilitate racial integration; in others, to provide special instruction for gifted and talented students or to offer cost-effective vocational training.

All magnet schools reflect the special resources of their host communities. The New York High School for the Performing Arts, for example, is located close to the theater district. Its new $45 million campus, which opened in September 1984, is situated across from Juilliard, across from the New York Library of Music, and just behind Lincoln Center. Similarly, Houston's School of Engineering Professions reflects that city's stake in high technology.

Although we have always understood the philosophy and the purposes of magnet schools, much of what we have known about their real workings has been anecdotal and idiosyncratic, stemming as it did from personal access to information. Systematic study of magnet schools was limited, for two reasons: (1) until recently, there were not many magnet schools to study; and (2) magnet schools generated little interest because they ran against the cultural grain. However, today's policy makers are no longer reduced to anecdote and myth, common sense and prejudice—a combination certain to frustrate informed decision making. A body of data on nonselective magnet schools is emerging, and these findings are very interesting.

The Findings

What specific information do we have on magnet schools? And with what degree of confidence can we make assertions?

First, let us examine the numbers. A recent Department of Education study conducted by James Lowry & Associates indicates that there were 1,018 such schools in operation in 1981–82—601 of them elementary magnet schools; 173, middle or junior high magnets; and 244, magnet high schools. Of the total, 259 magnet schools were funded through the Emergency School Aid Act (ESAA).[6]

Classifications of magnet schools are not well developed, because magnet schools are a relatively recent phenomenon and have not been the object of sustained research. The few categories that do exist are obvious: admissions requirements (selective versus nonselective), grade levels served, source of funding, and special theme (e.g., basic skills, bilingual, Montessori, vocational, career).

Research has also revealed some outcomes that theory would predict for magnet schools: high levels of motivation among both teachers and students, high levels of student achievement, fewer behavioral problems than in other kinds of public schools, greater job satisfaction among magnet school teachers than among their counterparts in other school settings, reasonable costs, and successful racial integration. The most welcome finding is that magnet schools need be neither divisive nor elitist.

Several other findings have also come to light. For example, magnet schools change the behaviors and attitudes of both teachers and students. Greater commitment is the key; in this respect, magnet schools resemble independent private schools. Clearly, the *voluntary* association of students and teachers in magnet schools produces this powerful side effect. Even in nonselective magnet schools, students are committed to extra effort by the simple act of voluntarily enrolling. And this extra effort translates into higher achievement. In the jargon of the social scientists, a "black box" effect exists. The school makes a difference; enrolled here, the student learns more than he or she would learn in a conventional school setting.

This outcome also legitimizes the demands of the school. Moreover, since the school is able to ask more of both students and their families, teachers can forget about discipline and concentrate on teaching effectively.

Meanwhile, both anecdotal and empirical evidence suggest one curious characteristic of the magnet school movement, past and present. For reasons that remain obscure, there seems to be a naturally occurring upper limit to the number of magnet schools that any given school district will support. In most instances, the school board simply refuses to open more magnet schools, even if parental demand is high and existing magnet schools have lengthy waiting lists.

This is not a matter of clever marketing; contemporary school managers simply seem unwilling and unable to expand beyond a certain number of magnet schools. Although some school districts may be moving in this direction, no district has yet adopted a strategy that calls for every school to be a magnet school. Buffalo, New York, currently has the largest proportion of magnet schools; 37% of all schools in that city are magnets.

The Future

Are the successes of magnet schools explainable solely by the intelligence of their students, or are there also "school effects"?[7] The question is not trivial, given the problems that the rest of U.S. education faces.

The characteristics of magnet school programs are predictable: an orderly and humane learning environment, high expectations for students and teachers, required homework, a low incidence of absenteeism, and virtually no vandalism, truancy, or general incivility. In magnet schools, students enjoy the respect of teachers and vice versa. Principals of magnet schools seem to pattern their behavior after that of British headmasters; indeed, in many magnet schools the principals still teach occasionally, an activity of symbolic importance.

Perhaps the single most important dimension of magnet school programs is intangible, however: students are expected to meet their responsibilities to the school and to themselves. Learning is recognized as hard work that requires diligence and enterprise. Students in magnet schools feel real pressure to perform well. The magnet schools can apply this pressure because students are attending of their own volition.

Of course, pride and satisfaction spring from genuine accomplishment—and magnet schools maintain high standards for their students. A well-executed biology experiment cannot be faked; the same goes for a well-executed ballet solo. Advanced Placement mathematics is a no-nonsense course; so is constructing a fabric-covered airplane wing.

Are there any lessons that magnet schools can teach the U.S. that might help solve the many problems of its schools? The most important lesson is also the most obvious: motivation, like intelligence, is randomly distributed in the population. Every major city and region in the U.S. could support, staff, and operate magnet schools. Indeed, in those cities without magnet schools, the only option available to parents who desire high-quality education for their children is to buy it, either through paying tuition at private schools or through purchasing a house in the suburbs.[8]

Recent research, both in the U.S. and abroad, confirms what most parents, teachers, and students already know: the crucial ingredient in school success is the school "ethos"—an umbrella term for the sense of purpose and the reciprocal expectations that schools and their communities have for one another. When principals, teachers, students, and parents have a clear sense of purpose and know what is expected of them, they can deliver. The real power of magnet schools is their capacity to create a community of scholarship and shared interests, springing as much from the students' high level of motivation as from their high intelligence.

Our long history of compulsory attendance and school assignment by neighborhood has led us to believe that these arrangements are eternal verities that have educational or social significance and meaning. They have neither. Both compulsory attendance and assignment by neighborhood were historical accidents that bear little relationship to any legitimate pedagogical objective. Assignment by neighborhood began in the 19th century as an administrative convenience, but it has since become an American virtue. Indeed, faced with the prospect of school desegregation, many Americans have made neighborhood schools an article of faith. Yet neighborhood schools today make neither administrative nor pedagogical sense.

The wide range of magnet school themes makes this point in a powerful way. *There is no one best school for everyone.* As a people, Americans need some common core of cultural literacy, but this core can be achieved in different settings and by differing methods. There are many ways of approaching and appropriating the common culture. Indeed, the reality of the modern American city is different people with differing interests and differing learning styles. And differing teaching styles, we might add.

That last observation is important, because it brings us full circle to the question of the effects of schools. Do schools make a difference—or is the secret simply smart youngsters? At one level, the question is bizarre. Does anyone *really* think that schools *don't* make a difference? Students don't master Advanced Placement calculus by osmosis; they do so because the course is offered and because they work at it. The same can be said for ballet, the French novel, computer programming, and critical reading. These are precisely the kinds of reasons for which schools exist. Street-wise youngsters may learn to run numbers, but they don't learn differential equations on the street corner.

Conclusion

Magnet schools are not a panacea, any more than comprehensive high schools were. Magnet schools are, however, a powerful tool for educational change. They can and do meet the objectives set for them, including higher academic standards and greater integration.

Magnet schools are effective, in large part, because of two ingredients: choice and commitment. Magnet schools also have flexibility with regard to which students are admitted to their programs and encouraged to remain. Not surprisingly, these characteristics of magnet schools produce improved learning, high morale among students and teachers, and a sense of community. There is now sufficient evidence available to support the establishment of magnet schools for youngsters committed to the study of science and mathematics.

The magnet school story has implications both for the culture of schooling and for the federal role in education. With regard to the culture of schooling, magnet schools afford an example of how diversity, choice, and commitment can empower teachers and students to perform more effectively. Schools with strong curricular themes permit students and teachers to form communities that are characterized by shared values—communities that transcend differences in socioeconomic background, race, and ability level.

Allowing schools to be different from one another makes sense pedagogically and organizationally. Learning demands an intellectual engagement between student and teacher that is more easily achieved if both parties know why they are there. Effective teaching thrives in an environment that supports professional growth and collegial interaction. Magnet schools offer just such an environment, and thus they provide a model for changing the culture of U.S. schooling.

Meanwhile, what we now know about magnet schools—beyond anecdotal evidence—has come from federally funded research. The importance of this federal effort cannot be overemphasized. No other unit of government has the financial and the organizational capacity (much less, the incentive) to conduct research of national scope and with national implications.

Too often, policy stems from opinion, only casually informed by fact. Although social science research will never have the precision and the sharp focus of research in the natural sciences, thoughtful analysis of a solid database improves the decision-making process. And so it is with magnet schools. More research on them remains to be done, and the federal government has a continuing role to play in conducting that research and in disseminating the findings.

The federal government could also play a significant role in helping local districts think through the questions related to the design and implementation of magnet programs. A program of federal matching grants for planning and implementation activities could provide such support for a specified number of communities.

For example, a federally funded magnet school demonstration program—deliberately modeled on a major American success story, the land grant college—could be designed today at low cost, at low risk, and with a high probability of substantial payoff. The strength of the land grant model is its decentralization, with funding and control shared among the federal government, the states, and the private sector.

Seed money from the federal government could be catalytic. The preliminary information on cost coming out of the Lowry study of magnet schools indicates that federal grants of about $100,000 per school provide the marginal resources that enable recipients to get a magnet program under way. Clearly, $100,000 is not enough to do more than shake loose local resources, but that is precisely the right strategy to employ in the creation of a reform program that requires local "ownership" for its success.

With such a modest level of funding for individual buildings, the magnet school demonstration program that we are proposing could become a national program of great scope. Since magnet schools are particularly well-suited to urban areas, the federal government might begin by providing funding for magnet schools in each Standard Metropolitan Statistical Area (SMSA). Three magnet schools in each area would permit the communities to launch three thematic schools simultaneously. The logical first candidates would be a math/science magnet school, a humanities magnet school, and an art/performing arts magnet school. But the final decision should be left to the individual communities, which know best their own resources and needs.

Politically, a magnet school demonstration program should have broad appeal, since it would affect a majority of U.S. congressional districts and would reach a substantial majority of the U.S. population. In 1980, for example, there were 318 SMSAs with a total population of 169 million, or 74.6% of the total U.S. population of 227 million.

Logistical and transportation problems may make magnet boarding schools a better choice for rural areas than day schools; thus funding for one or several boarding schools, modeled on the North Carolina School of Science and Mathematics, might be included in the demonstration program. Indeed, federal funds for establishing nonmetropolitan magnet schools could be made available to each state by a formula.

One of the most appealing aspects of the magnet school demonstration program is the fact that it sidesteps old and acrimonious disputes about school boundaries and zones of attendance. By their very nature, magnet schools designed to serve SMSAs (or even larger regions) would cross old boundaries and would involve the various school districts and units of local government within their service areas.

Such a magnet school demonstration program would not involve long-term federal funding. The federal government would simply provide the critical start-up funding to permit local authorities to initiate programs that would best serve local needs.

With more than two decades of federally funded research behind us, we now know one thing with some confidence. Federal funding can stimulate reforms, but these reforms will not last unless the local community appropriates them and makes them its own. The process of schooling goes on in the classroom and in the school building—a complex interaction of teacher and taught, between a given school and the community it serves. But the federal government can strengthen that process, if the role it plays is thoughtfully chosen and carefully delineated.

The class of the year 2001 was born in 1983. Unless we initiate major changes today, that class may face in the space age an educational system designed for the era of the covered wagon. Magnet schools offer a strategy for low-cost, highly visible, incremental change that could conceivably transform American education.

FOOTNOTES

1. James B. Conant, *The American High School Today* (New York: McGraw-Hill, 1959).
2. See Denis P. Doyle and Bruce S. Cooper, "Is Excellence Possible in Urban Public Schools?," *American Education,* November 1983, pp. 16–27.
3. Fred Hechinger, "About Education: Debate on the Role of Elite Schools," *New York Times,* 5 February 1982.
4. Albert O. Hirschman, *Exit, Voice, and Loyalty: Response to Decline in Firms, Organizations, and States* (Cambridge, Mass.: Harvard University Press, 1970).
5. Theodore R. Sizer, "High School Reform: The Need for Engineering," *Phi Delta Kappan,* June 1983, pp. 679–83; and idem, *Horace's Compromise: The Dilemma of the American High School* (Boston: Houghton-Mifflin, 1984).
6. The Office of Program Evaluation of the U.S. Department of Education funded a major study of magnet schools that began in October 1981)USOE Contract No. 300-81-0420). The prime contractor was James H. Lowry & Associates, Washington, D.C. The subcontractor was Abt Associates, Cambridge, Mass. This was the first comprehensive study of U.S. magnet schools—both those that were funded through the Emergency School Aid Act (ESAA) and those that were not. Much of the material in this article has been drawn from *Survey of Magnet Schools, Interim Report* (30 September 1982), the only published document on the study at the time we were writing, and from extensive oral briefings and preliminary materials in draft form. Phase I of the study was completed in September 1982. Phase II is now completed; the final report was released in September 1983.
7. For a more complete review of the recent research on school effects, see Barbara Lerner, "American Education: How Are We Doing?," *Public Interest,* Fall 1982, pp. 59–82; Denis P. Doyle, review of James Coleman et al., *High School Achievement: Public, Catholic, and Private Schools Compared,* in *Teaching Political Science,* Summer 1983, pp. 201–3; Andrew Greeley, *Catholic High Schools and Minority Students* (New Brunswick, N.J.: Transaction Books, 1982); and Michael Rutter et al., *Fifteen Thousand Hours: Secondary Schools and Their Effects on Children* (Cambridge, Mass.: Harvard University Press, 1979).
8. The Gallup Organization has been conducting annual polls of the public's attitudes toward the public schools for 16 years; the results appear in the *Phi Delta Kappan* each fall. The first 10 polls have been reprinted in Stanley M. Elam, ed., *A Decade of Gallup Polls of Attitudes Toward Education, 1969-1978* (Bloomington, Ind.: Phi Delta Kappa, 1978).

Chapter 15
A Collaborative School Dropout Prevention Program: College Students as Mentors

Natalie A. Silverstein, Hope B. Richardson, and Patricia R. Lanier*

Introduction

Mentoring is not new. The word mentor comes to us from Greek mythology. Mentor in Greek legends was an Ithacan and the friend of the Greek hero Odysseus. Odysseus made him the guardian of his household. Mentor played a prominent part in giving Odysseus' son, the hero Telemachus, good advice. History is replete with examples of such relationships: Socrates and Plato, Freud and Jung, Lorenze de Medicia and Michelangelo, Haydn and Beethoven, Sartre and de Beauvoir. Hence the modern adoption for the name for a sage advisor and the concept of a mentor, a friend and good advisor—and hence the legacy of mentoring as a powerful emotional interaction. This concept of a mentor to shape the growth and development of the protege is now being recognized and accepted by major businesses corporations; colleges, universities, and schools; and various agencies, career and human resource development centers. But what does a mentor really do and how important can a mentor be in a person's life? Researchers report that there are many benefits from mentor-mentee relationships (Edlind & Haensly 1985). These investigators state that there are many benefits derived both for the mentor and the mentee.

For the mentee, the benefits include: advancement of career; increase in knowledge and skills; development of a personal ethic; friendship; and enhancement of creativity. Among the benefits for the mentor are: getting work done; having ideations stimulated; establishing a long-term friendship; and receiving personal satisfaction.

Mentoring Models

There are many different kinds of mentoring models which illustrate this kind of intense interpersonal relationship. Basically mentorship falls into five categories: (1) sponsorship for beginning teachers; (2) an aspect of adult development; (3) people in the business world; (4) on the college campus; (5) involvement with youth.

An interesting approach to mentorships for new teachers may be found in the reports from many local education agencies as well as school districts which are designing induction programs for beginning teachers. One feature of these programs is the appointment of a mentor or sponsor teacher. A review of the literature concerning this kind of mentoring phenomenon substantiates the fact that education professionals are interested in initiating a ''mentor teacher'' concept. Many programs underscore the need for assistance for the beginning teacher, and that mentoring is equally prevalent among elementary and secondary teachers (Galver-Hjornevik 1986). Programs from Communication Services, Research & Development Center for Teacher Education at The University of Texas at Austin, have summarized the salient elements of the teacher mentoring relationship.

Their focus is on the characteristics and functions of the mentor; selecting and attracting a mentor; the interpersonal relationship; the character of the mentor-protege relationship; precautions in engaging in the mentor-protege relationship; what and how proteges

*Dr. Natalie A. Silverstein is an Assistant Professor, as are Dr. Hope B. Richardson and Dr. Patricia R. Lanier, in the Department of Special Educational Services at Bronx Community College of the City University of New York.

learn from mentors; and the guidelines for formal and informal mentor programs. The role of the mentor is traced in the literature of adult developmental psychology. Four primary motifs throughout the literature illustrate this second category. Basically, programs which speak to adult development point the way at a developmental crossroad, offer material and/or emotional support and challenge (Daloz, 1983). Programs that foster the growth of the managerial woman are excellent examples of adult developmental mentoring programs. These programs offer fertile opportunities for both mentor and mentee to offer advice for each other and other career-minded women. Other developmental adult projects focus on attitude and goal achievement. Life cycle programs emphasize the differences in male and female development, thereby recognizing the need for sponsorship during periods when adults strive to renew the direction of life and work.

People in the business world have recognized the need to establish a mentoring partnership. The Ysleta Schools Vocational Equity Project conducted in El Paso, Texas, exemplifies a program that was implemented to develop and test methods to link education and industry in a mentoring project. Students were paired with successful role models to provide first-hand experience and encouragement in nontraditional jobs. The mentors provided strategies or accessibility to the industry and made industry aware of qualified students.

The business community's efforts to enhance students' aspirations and opportunities for employment in nontraditional jobs provided a valuable link between education and industry. Other mentoring programs involving this protege concept attest to the fact that the mentoring experience offers the mentee motivation, support for coping with failure, and opportunity to make learning tasks meaningful. Interviews that were collected in 15 programs to examine 30 mentors revealed that what occurred in the mentorship was related to employability and the value of the mentorship experience. Mentees reported that they felt the mentorship had been the most important influence. Both mentor and mentee saw the mentorship as positively and significantly helpful in preparing for the world of work.

Building a mentoring relationship is a time-honored tradition in the academic community. The domain of faculty growth is often measured by a mentor and mentee partnership in academic activities. Programs such as the Florida Council of Educational Management provide mentorships for future educational administrators. This organization focuses on the mentor/coach role, thus affording potential school administrators the opportunity to dialogue behaviors in

leadership, authority, and power in management in professional fields. Additionally, several approaches to support students in distance education have been reported in the United Kingdom. Britain's Open University support services are offered through a mentor. The mentor initially helps each student develop an individual study program and is then involved in the student's progress.

In the U.S. University Without Walls, a teacher-mentor helps students develop a learning contract that serves as a basis for evaluating each student's performance. Various types of educational technologies, such as telementoring via an electronic bulletin, are also sources in distance education (King et al, 1982).

Literature on mentoring programs (Kramer & White, 1982) involving youth supports the notion that a mentor-mentee relationship is an immensely enriching experience for both. Numerous studies (Gaskins & Baron 1985, Keating 1984; Edlind and Haenlsy 1985) report the effectiveness and benefits of mentorships. Studies of gifted youngsters' experiences report that their mentee experience enabled them to deal with motivation, cope with failure, and provided opportunities for self-expression. This experience aided them in expression in the arts and in developing social skills (Short 1985). Other studies reported findings of mentee growth in personal appearance, performance skills, and career assets (Bryan & Wierick). A "mentor approach" has demonstrated that students can make significant gains in achievement, increase student knowledge/skill in specific areas, and change attitudes. Perhaps this aspect of the mentoring concept holds the most promising area of study for educators today. Therefore, the purpose of this paper is to describe the growth and development of a unique New York City mentoring program to aid today's youth.

The Student Mentor in The City University

The Board of Education of the City of New York and The City University of New York (CUNY) recently entered into a collaborative agreement in which CUNY college students serve as mentors for students. The Student-Mentor program, as this special collaborative effort is called, is one of the ways in which New York City educators are attempting to ameliorate the problem of the City's 45% drop out rate.

Chronology of the Program. Joseph Murphy, Chancellor of The City University of New York, and Nathan Quinones, Chancellor, Board of Education of City of New York, have joined hands to address the problem of retention and achievement of high school students. In initiating the Student-Mentor Program, Dr. Joyce

Brown, (1984) and Dean for Urban Affairs, The City University of New York stated:

> It is clear that we have an obligation to create conditions sufficiently motivating that students will complete high school so that they might read, write, critically analyze, and communicate; that they might become contenders in the job market with proper skills and attitudes to be gainfully employed,[1] that they might set goals for themselves and expect to reach them; that they might think beyond survival and be challenged to achieve; avoiding failure, but rather that they might know the joy of excellence; that they might have options to choose a life path for themselves and pursue it.

The design of the student mentor program includes the following goals:

1. To improve student performance at the secondary level.
2. To increase retention in the secondary schools.
3. To help students set realistic life-goals while providing opportunities for reaching those goals.
4. To expand the number of students prepared for college study.

One of the more significant means to achieve these goals is through the use of a student mentoring program. This program is viewed as a means of critical intervention in the lives of "at risk" high school students, by utilizing high achieving City University students in the role of peer tutors and role models. It is the belief of the City University that through this proposed method of critical intervention on the part of high achieving college students who share backgrounds and experiences that are similar to those of the low achieving high school students, the latter can be motivated to succeed.

The Structure of the Program

The student mentor program matches students from The City University of New York with students in local New York City high schools.* Mentees are recruited on a one-to-one basis by the mentee coordinator at the high school. The youngsters are selected on the basis of need, academic achievement and a willingness to participate in the program. The mentor's role is to help the mentee realize the importance of school and the tragic consequences of working in today's society without a high school diploma.

Selection of Participants. College students who are succeeding in school are selected to serve as mentors

*The District 10 Prep School, located on the campus of Bronx Community College, also participates in this project. This school is the only Junior High School currently participating in the program.

for the program. In some instances, they come from the same communities as the mentees. These college students are matched with high school students who are really struggling with many of the same kinds of pressures that the college students faced and overcame.

In seeing the college students overcome these problems, and come from the point where the high school students find themselves, the youngsters are encouraged to strive for success. The fact that the college students are achieving, have plans for themselves, and goals for the future, does impact on the high school students. This model does indeed cause these youngsters to think about their own future. The genuine interest and concern conveyed to the mentee by the mentor can be enough to motivate the mentee to be successful in academic life.

Once the college students have been selected and made a commitment to the program, they attend mentoring training workshops held by specialists from The City University of New York and the New York City Board of Education. The workshops assist prospective mentors in developing skills they will need to build a successful helping relationship. Additional criteria for mentors and mentees are:

Mentor	Mentee
Indication of sound academic standing.	Expressed interest in improving his or her academic standing.
Participated in the training program	Expressed interest in having a mentor.
Indicated a willingness to be a role model for high school students.	
Indicated an interest in working with under-achieving students†	

Student Mentoring at Bronx Community College

The Student-Mentor Program at Bronx Community College of The City University of New York is coordinated by the three professors who provide mentors for public schools. Mentoring is a special field experience within the education curriculum. This three-credit course stresses interpersonal skills needed for a helping relationship. Although the professors work in tandem and are indeed a tightly woven team, each professors adds an idiographic dimension to the mentoring experience.

Clearly, it has been demonstrated at Bronx Community College that mentors as well as mentees have profited from their mentor/mentee relationship. Mentors report that they have begun to think very seriously

†Students taking part in the program are carefully screened to make sure that they possess good character and possess the necessary characteristics of good role models.

about the system of education in New York City, and about community service in general. They have begun to think seriously about their own younger brothers and sisters, and also about the education of their own children. The mentees state that they have begun to think deeply about making a contribution to society instead of standing back, merely being passive participants. Similarly, a growing body of evidence indicates that the personal qualities of the mentors are as significant for positive growth of mentees as are the methods they use. High school mentees who work with Bronx Community College mentors report that they perceive their mentors as able to solve their own problems and manage their own lives. Mentors are perceived also as dependable, friendly, and worthy people. Mentees view the mentor as an individual who has the capacity to cope with problems, a person with whom they feel comfortable, and someone whose opinions are valued.

The compatibility of the mentors' and mentees' personalities has been a key factor in the successful mentoring process. Throughout the mentoring relationship, mentors encourage mentees: to ask questions in class; to become aware of high school resources that are available to them, i.e., the library and homework helpers; to become aware of the requisites to reach goals, and to seek information by talking to teachers and counselors.

Bronx Community College has had a successful student mentoring experience. Probably the element most crucial to that success has been the very strong commitment on both sides of the relationship. Both the mentor and the mentee have had to believe in the program, keep appointments, attend all training sessions, and trust one another. Student mentoring is about college students helping high school students to grow toward their personal goals and strengthen their capacities for coping within the educational system. Few of us achieve our growth goals or solve our personal problems alone. Student-mentors are the helpers in this relationship. Helping and mentoring is a function of all concerned human beings.

Summary and Conclusions

Several important points may be gleaned from this discussion. First, we can recognize a life theme in the mentoring concept. An examination of the literature indicates that since its appearance in Greek mythology (*Telemaque,* by Francois Fenelon, describes the advisor-friend relationship between Ithacan and Odysseus), the mentoring relationship has been a recognized, acceptable, and invaluable means of contributing to individual growth and development.

This intense interpersonal relationship is indeed an ongoing motif throughout history. Currently, successful mentoring programs are reported in a variety of organizations: in education, business, and human services. Specifically in education, successful mentoring programs include: on-the-job training programs for beginning teachers; teacher internships; adult career education programs; programs linking education and industry; mentor-counselors in universities; mentoring-coaching relationships for future educational administrators; and mentor programs which help youths negotiate and handle life's challenges. These previously mentioned programs aid youngsters in handling more and coping with failure, motivation, and attitudes. All of the programs, however, do have salient characteristics which contribute to the growth and development of both parties in the mentoring relationship.

A second important point to note is that a mentoring relationship has proven to be an enriching experience for both the mentor and the mentee. Research indicates that the benefits for the mentor include: (1) advancement in career; (2) increase in knowledge and skill; (3) development of a personal ethic; (4) establishment of friendships; and (5) enhancement of creativity. The benefits for the mentee include: (1) assistance in completing various projects; (2) having ideas stimulated; (3) establishing long-term friendships; and (4) receiving personal satisfaction.

A third important point to be remembered is that a joint effort on the part of two great institutions has been made to ameliorate the pressing problem of school dropouts. Administrators at both the New York City Board of Education and the City University of New York have demonstrated their desire to impact on the lives of youngsters in New York City. In creating a collaborative relationship and knitting together professors and high school teachers, college students and high school students, they have shown a level of commitment to today's youth and recognition of the positive aspects of mentoring.

Pressures which cause youngsters to drop out of school cannot be easily solved. One organization cannot care for the ills in today's atomic society. The significant fact is that two important educational institutions have joined hands and reached out to one another in recognition of the problem. These educators have marshalled their forces and committed their resources to a collaborative effort. Another important point to note is that mentoring is a potent force. The growth of the mentoring corps of professors and student mentors at Bronx Community College clearly indicates the significance of this concept.

Implications

Our experience at Bronx Community College has shown that mentoring, a beneficial educational tool, has been underutilized. One of the major assets of mentoring is its universality, flexibility, and adaptability to a variety of settings.

The success and growth of the program at Bronx Community College and the fact that a mentoring unit now exists at almost every City University campus in New York today provides evidence of the versatility of mentoring as a learning experience. A corps of college mentors now interacts with youngsters in high schools in each of the five boroughs. Mentoring partnerships are equally successful in comprehensive and alternative high schools. A mentoring partnership has proven to be successful for youngsters of junior high school age as well. Future mentoring programs could be designed to include partnerships between any two groups of learners such as high school youngsters and elementary school children; secondary school teachers and elementary school educators; parenting support partnerships and peer mentors and tutors. As we strive to meet the challenge of teaching and learning in the 21st century, mentoring can be a vital resource!

SELECTED BIBLIOGRAPHY

Brammer, L. (1985). *The Helping Relationship. Process and Skills.* New Jersey: Prentice Hall.

Brown, J. (1984, Dec.). The mentor program is a critical intervention. *Student Mentor Program Newsletter of The City University of New York and the New York Board of Education.*

Burke, J. (Ed.). (1984, Summer/Fall). *Linkages. A High School Consortium.*

Daloz, L.A. (1983, Sept.). Mentors: Teachers who make a difference. *Change.* 15. (6). pp. 24–27.

Edlind, E.P. & Haensly, P.A. (1985, Spring). Gifts for mentorships. *Gifted Child Quarterly.* 29. (2). pp. 55–60.

Galvez-Hjornevik, C. (1985). *Mentoring: A review of the literature with a focus on teaching.* National Institute of Education, Washington, D.C.

Gerstein, M. (1985, Oct.). Mentoring: An age old practice in a knowledge-based society. *Journal of Counselling and Development.* 64. (2). pp. 156–157.

Gray, W. A. & Gray, M.E. (1982). Utilizing preservice teachers as mentors to provide enrichment experiences for gifted talented E. S.L. students. *Educational Research Institute of British Columbia,* Vancouver, Canada.

King, B. et al. (1980, Dec.). Support systems in distance education. *Open Campus Occasional Paper. (3). Deakin University. Geelong Centre for Educational Services.* Australia.

Kramer, G.L. & White, M.T. (1982). Developing a faculty mentoring program: An experiment. *NACADA Journal,* 2. (2). pp. 47–58.

Merriam, S. (1983, Spring). Mentors and proteges: A critical review of the literature. *Adult Education Quarterly.* 33. (3). pp. 161–173.

Sample, J.A. (1984). *Exploring Management Development Roles Educational Administrators: Coach, Mentor and Sponsor.* Prepared for the Florida Council on Educational Management.

Solitis, J. F. (1985, Jan.). Imagine a school. *Phi Delta Kappan.* 66. (5). pp. 321–22.

Student Mentor Newsletter Program Newsletter (1984). The City University of New York and The New York City Board of Education.

Chapter 16
The Bilingual Controversy
Teresa A. Trimarco*

One issue that always seems to generate controversy among educators at all levels is that minority students are associated with lower achievement in schools in the United States. These students fare poorly in public school settings (Cardoza & Rueda, 1986). A variety of factors contribute to this relatively poor academic performance. Language proficiency certainly is one of these factors (Laosa, 1977; Cummins, 1980). How can minority students work up to their potential and be prepared for the college scene? Is bilingual education in America's schools the answer? Therein is the controversy over how schools should go about educating students with limited English proficiency.

The concept of "bilingual" education—that is, teaching in two languages—emerged out of civil rights and anti-poverty movements. Using bilingual teachers to provide instruction in other languages as well as English was seen as a way to help students whose progress and achievement was limited due to lack of knowledge of English during the 1960s and 1970s (Fiske, 1985). In 1968 Congress passed the Bilingual Education Act, Title VII of the Elementary and Secondary Education Act. This insured federal support for students with limited English proficiency. In 1974, Congress specified that federal funds could be spent only on programs that made use of native language instruction. Approaches in which the primary language of instruction was English could no longer be utilized. In 1984, Congress softened bilingual requirements. 1986 is a year which will see a national debate over proposed regulation and statute changes sought by Secretary of Education, William Bennett (Melendez, 1986). An issue that will undoubtedly emerge concerns teachers and teacher-aides who are often forced to teach on bilingual waivers because of the difficulty recruiting bilingual teachers in rural areas. Another controversy is centered around the length of time a student remains in a bilingual classroom. Will changes in procedures take place concerning the reclassification of these students?

To date, research has not given the answer to the question of "How long is long enough?"

Some educators and politicians feel that we need a common language. English is the language in the United States. Our history is written in English and our forefathers spoke in English. Not everyone is in agreement with this concept. For example, "The first university in this hemisphere was in Mexico in the 1400's," said Gene T. Chavez, president of the bilingual education association. "My ancestry goes back 400 years in the Southwest. My sense of history predates the landing on Plymouth Rock." The proponents of bilingual education say that educational needs of children with mother tongues other than English requires that they be taught in their native languages–until they have a chance to learn English, thus bolstering self-esteem and hopefully academic performance will improve. And, teaching children in their native language does not undermine their self-concepts (Cardenas, 1986). In fact, placement of a language-minority child into an all-English curriculum before the child has achieved sufficient mastery of the English language could be a disaster. The eager and voracious learner has had the power of language removed and he is sentenced to an animal-like existence until such time he acquires sufficient fluency in a different language! Negative concepts through the use of native language instruction *can* be prevented; the child's whole future capability for learning can be effectively enhanced.

Criticisms of bilingual education come from every type of person and for a myriad of reasons. Perhaps opponents do not use an accurate definition of bilingual education. They often do not present a fair description of it. Sometimes, factual information is absent; emotionalism takes over, overshadowing any rational considerations. Misinformation about bilin-

*Dr. Teresa A. Trimarco is an Associate Professor and Chairperson of the Division of Education, Notre Dame College, St. John's University, New York.

gual education is created by emotional critics. The news media is also responsible for consistently failing to give fair coverage to the topic of bilingual education. Articles concerning shortcomings of bilingual education are controversial and get good coverage; those dealing with the positive side are short and played down. Thus, criticism of bilingual programs stems from emotional responses, misinformation and often racist attitudes (Cardenas, 1986).

Bilingual education must be valued as an asset, not considered as a liability. It should not be viewed as a remedial program. In fact, it should eliminate the necessity of remedial instruction by providing the student with educational concepts in both the native language and the acquired second language (Ballesteros, 1978).

A Pro-Con Look at Bilingual Education (Melendez, 1986):

Pros

- Bilingual education offers English instruction to the pupil while not letting him/her lose ground in academic subjects.
- Bilingual education fosters multicultural awareness and cooperation among students of different cultures.
- Bilingualism is an asset vital to our nation's economy and our nation's security.
- All children have a right to equal access and equal benefit from the educational system.
- Bilingual programs have been criticized unfairly for failure when they have not even been fully or adequately implemented.
- Limited English students are often moved out of bilingual classrooms before they have attained adequate levels of proficiency in English.

Cons

- Bilingual education is un-American. English should be our official language.
- It is impossible to find qualified bilingual teachers for our classrooms, so it is unrealistic to require them.
- Bilingual education is a separatist notion and encourages ethnic isolation.
- Bilingual education is an inflexible state mandate requiring large amounts of school resources, but without large amounts of accompanying state or federal funds.
- Other immigrant groups have "made it" without bilingual education, so why should we provide it for Hispanics?

- Asian and Indochinese parents want their children to speak English—they do not want them in bilingual classrooms.

Not only does bilingual education stir controversy in education circles but it "excites political passions" (Rohter, 1985). Thousands of jobs and several billion dollars in federal and state funds are in question. As a result, the issues concerning bilingual education have produced likely alliances and have raised fundamental social issues. For example, it is said that bilingual education is responsible for opening doors of the schools to parents who have been locked out. Dependence on the home language tended to isolate making parents more manipulable. A minority parent or student who learns English automatically becomes involved culturally with society, making political control difficult. At the same time, bilingual education has disrupted traditional political coalitions, such as between blacks and Hispanics. Many blacks believe that a bilingual program in the school diverts funds (that are always scarce) away from needed compensatory programs designed specifically for black children. Also teachers' unions around the nation see bilingual programs as a threat to their jobs because the vast majority of teachers in our country speak only English.

With the possible exception of desegregation, no subject has aroused as much passion over schools as educating students with limited English proficiency. The controversy over bilingual education continues—possibly because educational researchers have not demonstrated, to the satisfaction of the public, the effects of various methods. In fact, the existing research is contradictory (Fiske, 1985). Perhaps this stems from conflicting terminology used by the researchers. Perhaps the research on bilingual education has too narrow a focus; there are no long-term studies that examine and compare different approaches (Reed, 1985). So, the intensity of the debate over bilingual education goes on.

BIBLIOGRAPHY

Ballesteros, D. (1978). Bilingual/bicultural education: Beyond the seventies. *Bilingual Education for the Latinos,* 98.

Cardenas, J. (January 1986). The role of native-language instruction in bilingual education. *Phi Delta Kappan,* 359, 362.

Cardoza, D. & Rueda, R. (1986). Educational and occupational outcomes of hispanic learning-disabled high school students. *The Journal of Special Education,* 20 (1), 111.

Cummings, J. (1980). The entry and exit fallacy in bilingual education. *National Association for Bilingual Education Journal,* (4), 3.

Fiske, E. (1985). One language or two? *The New York Times Education Fall Survey,* p. 46.

Laosa, I.M. (1977). Inequality in the classroom: Observational research on teacher–student interactions. *Aztlan International Journal of Chicano Studies Research,* (8), 2–3.

Melendez, M. (January 1986). Bilingual education: Legislative prospects in 1986. *Thrust,* 12–13.

Reed, S. (1985). What the research shows. *The New York Times Education Fall Survey,* p. 98.

Rohter, L. (1985). The politics of bilingualism. *The New York Times Education Fall,* p. 46.

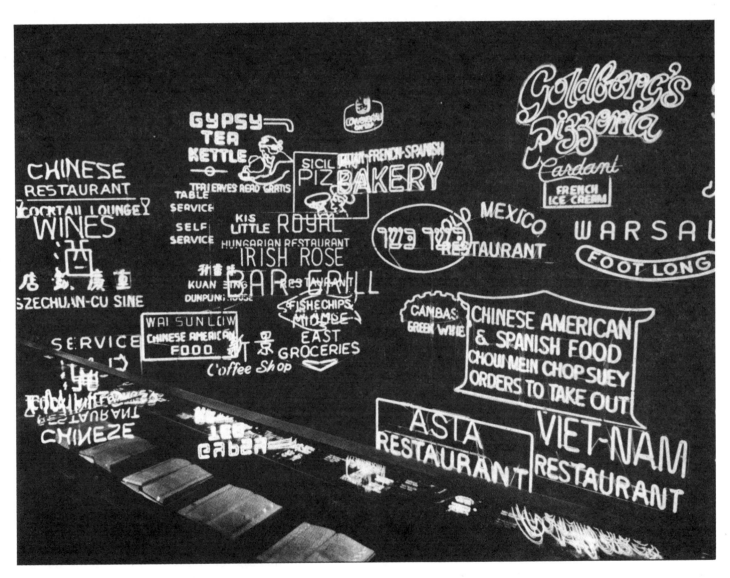

Peter Garfield

Chapter 17
Reflections on Child Abuse
Jean Bethke Elshtain*

Few topics are as guaranteed to create alarm and a demand to "do something" than the abuse and exploitation of children. Visions of beaten, abducted, and sexually traumatized children exert a terrifying and even morbid fascination. At the moment we cannot seem to get enough of it.

"Missing," proclaims the milk carton. As I eat my breakfast cereal I stare at rather indistinct photos of two children, a "White Female" and a "White Male." Additional data includes "date missing," "from," "DOB," height, weight, eye color and hair color. I am asked to report these children, if I identify them or "any other missing child," to "The National Center for Missing and Exploited Children." An "800" number is provided. Sorting through bulk mail, I find a card, addressed to "Resident" and advertising a carpet-cleaning service, that asks in bold print: *"Have you seen me?"* A photo of a single missing or exploited child appears with the pertinent data and the same "800" number. Missing children pop up on Cable News Network and on the screen of my local movie theater just before previews of coming attractions.

Glancing through a local publication consisting of advertisements placed by individuals to hawk no-longer-wanted household items, to sell cars, or to publicize tag sales, I run across a full page ad placed by "Child Seekers." The logo above the headline is a drawing of a human eye. A single tear drop tumbles down, partially covering the letter "d" in the word "child" below. Six children, with data, are pictured. In addition to the "800" call number, I am informed of the scope of the problem in bold capitals:

1.5 MILLION CHILDREN ARE REPORTED MISSING EACH YEAR.

SOME 20,000 TO 50,000 CHILDREN DISAPPEAR EACH YEAR AND THEIR CASES REMAIN UNSOLVED, SOME FOREVER.

3,000 UNIDENTIFIED BODIES ARE FOUND IN THE UNITED STATES EACH YEAR AND HUNDREDS OF THOSE ARE CHILDREN.

This is the stuff of nightmares. One's imagination is given free rein and there are just enough real horror stories to lend credence to every individual's worst-case scenario: young Adam Walsh, abducted from a shopping mall and beheaded; Lori, a Denver three-year old, lured into a car from the street outside her home, sexually abused, then dumped in a sewage pit. (She lived to tell the tale.)

In addition to the terror of child abduction and molestation outside the home, we are bombarded with statistics and stories of abuse by parents, ranging from neglect to incest, repeated beatings, and even murder. *Newsweek* for May, 1984 (the year we discovered child abuse in a big way) headlined: "The Hidden Epidemic," The magazine painted a picture of incestuous families and child sex rings in day-care and the community-at-large, and featured a "Letter from a Pedophile" which concluded with the words: "Have you hugged your kids today? If not, a child molester will!"

Every possible location for the child—his or her own home, foster care, and child care, is now suspect, *Newsweek* declared, providing reports on each situation. A world of apparent Dickensian dimensions begins to take shape as one reads that 1984 saw investigations and arrests at day care centers in California, New York, New Jersey, Illinois, Alabama and Tennessee.

Proposed solutions range from individual therapy—bringing everything out into the open and talking about it, to films and puppet shows teaching children as young as three or four that they can't trust anybody, including mommies and daddies, to fingerprinting children and establishing a national computerized file under FBI auspices, to harsh punishment for child molesters (including treatment with Depo-Provera, a

*Dr. Jean Bethke Elshtain is Professor of Political Science, University of Massachusetts, Amherst, MA.

synthetic hormone used experimentally with male sex offenders), to stricter laws and regulations governing day-care centers.

Clearly we are in the midst of a socially constructed crisis concerning this society's treatment of its children. By that I mean that the way particular issues gain public attention—in the case of child abuse even hysterical attention—is a complex coming together of political, economic and cultural forces. Americans seem unusually prone to dramatic lurchings on a whole range of questions: from prohibition to almost unlimited access to alcohol to attempts to partially restrict; from almost no legal abortion to almost no legal limits to abortion; from attempts to proscribe sexually explicit material to a pornographic free-for-all.

Surely, as in the case of rape and battering, the problem of child abuse has long been with us. Why, then, the "discovery" of the issue at this time? How do social realities become political problems? Who identifies and names these problems and to what ends? Have incidents of abuse really risen dramatically? Are parents, child-care providers, and the average man-on-the-street more venal, less trustworthy, than in the past? Such questions are probably unanswerable in any definitive sense. But there are a few things to be said.

Several years ago when I researched the 'violence against women' question, I learned that the rate of forcible rapes showed little overall change as compared with the crime rate in general. Appalling as rape is, it accounts for about 6 percent of violent crimes. Yet, as a result of public awareness largely inspired by the women's movement, we are not only *rightly* concerned about the crime of rape, and its punishment, but we *wrongly* believe that rape is skyrocketing and that women are special targets of violent crime. Yet the figures on this score have been remarkably consistent for years: Most perpetrators of violent crimes are males; most victims of violent crimes are males.

Child abuse taps even deeper fears and rouses even stronger visceral reactions than rape because children are the most vulnerable members of any human population. I understand these reactions very well. My own opposition to capital punishment has been challenged on more than one occasion when I proclaimed to myself or in private conversations with family or friends that death, perhaps even lingering torture, was the only fit punishment for some brutal crime against a child. As a parent, my concern for the well-being of my own children plays directly into my reflections on child abuse as a social concern and a public policy question.

About a year ago I began to gather, or to attempt to gather, data and found it was very difficult. *If* we agree with most "experts" that reported incidents notoriously underestimate the problem, we enter a shadowy realm that *presumes* some form of child abuse or neglect as the norm rather than the deviation from one. For example, under the headline "Reports of Child Molestation Increase by 35%, Study Finds," the *New York Times* for February 18, 1985, Anne H. Cohn, executive director of the National Committee for the Prevention of Child Abuse, proclaims that the soaring figures represent only "the tip of the iceberg." Her Chicago-based committee's report estimates instances of sexual molestation as 123,000 per year and over-all abuse at 1,273,000 per year—again with the proviso that we can let those numbers rise as high as our Hobbesian inclinations take us. The National Committee report goes on to say that "the more we work to uncover the problem of child abuse, the more we are able to find."

True, no doubt, but what are "we" finding? I found that it is impossible to get any clear definition of what constitutes "abuse" in the first place. Richard Wexler has (in his recent essay) showed us how sloppy notions of child "neglect" often wind up indicting parents, particularly single-parent households headed by women, simply because they are poor. The burden of "neglect" falls upon those who are themselves victims of the injustices of our political economy.

Similarly, what counts as "abuse" is a contested notion. Dr. Joyce Brothers, television's favorite pop-psychologist, insists she was abused because society told her that there were some things little boys were better at than little girls. Public figures and comic figures (e.g., "Spiderman") rush to confess that they were abused as children although some also note that they did not know it was abuse at the time. We seem most obsessed with sexual abuse. Senator Christopher Dodd, a founder of the Children's Caucus, clearly accepts the upper-range figures when he insists that, "A child is sexually abused within the United States every two minutes." *Parade* magazine (July 29, 1984), tells us that "only about 2 percent of sexual molestation against preschool-age children is ever reported"; hence, "the vast majority of guilty adults are never even identified."

If we focus only on sexual molestation or battering, leaving aside the question of whether slapping a child's hand if she is about to stick her finger into an electric socket is abuse or parental responsibility, who are these "guilty adults"? In the case of sexual molestation, the image that pops into mind is either father/daughter incest or a degenerate male pervert out to snatch children off the streets or abuse them in some hidden place.

It is more difficult to capture the prevailing picture of non-sexual abuse, though I have a hunch we *prefer* to see an out-of-control (perhaps drunken) father who hits the wife and kids and kicks the dog rather than a mother driven to maim or destroy a child to whom she has given birth.

To these we must now add newly hatched fears that those to whom we entrust the care of our children, particularly day-care workers, may be molesters. Although the most sensationalistic case of alleged sexual abuse in child-care, the Manhattan Beach, California affair, focuses on six female and one male perpetrator, our popular images are of (male) pedophiles. This image is reinforced by experts.

"Pedophiles are naturally drawn to jobs where they have close contact with children," says Suzanne Danilson, described by the New York Times (April 3, 1984), as "an expert in the care of children in institutions." In addition to parents and other relatives, "bus driver, camp counselors, coaches, pediatricians and ministers" are singled out. Pamela Klein, director of the Rape and Sexual Abuse Care Center at Southern Illinois University, proclaims "abuse in school systems" to be "pervasive." She cites the case of a "popular and respected teacher" who was "suspected of molesting at least 20 girls," a "not atypical case" which "can happen in your town, too," according to a local attorney. A play put on by the Illusion Theater of Minneapolis, designed to help children "recognize the perils of sexual abuse," includes a scene of sexual abuse in which "a grandfather's good-night kiss" turns into "fondling of the breasts," reports Newsweek. Thus far, this theater company has taken "Touch" to 35 states, primarily playing in elementary schools.

Trying to come up with empirical evidence on this question is like attempting to eat jello with a table knife. The most interesting question, perhaps, is our current societal-wide inclination to believe the most overblown figures. In part, no doubt, we are dealing with a justifiable reaction against those who said, over the years, that children were "making the whole thing up." Just as we once placed the onus of rape on the woman, we also placed the onus of "abuse" on the child.

No more. Now we have lurched to a situation in which those accused of abuse are presumed guilty until proven innocent. We have moved from doubting the veracity of children in constructing out of the often-wrenching stories of children a scenario that initially placed all parents under suspicion and has since added nursery school workers and child-care providers to the growing list of probable offenders.

Into the breach come the "experts"—psychologists, bureaucrats of various agencies, researchers, criminologists, and legislators—out to save us, once again, from ourselves or, in this instance, our children from those who care for them. I do not mean to belittle the

problem: it is real. But why are we so willing to trust individuals with a vested interest in constructing this issue as a social question over which they have effective say or power? Going through the Annual Sourcebook of Criminal Justice Statistics, and in light of recent challenges concerning statistics on missing and abused children, I tried to get some handle on the problem. What emerged was rather interesting and it threw many of our popular images out of focus.

First, the vast majority of missing children are runaways, not abductees. For example, according to a June 14, 1985, article in the Boston Globe, of the 1,080 children currently listed as missing in Massachusetts, 75% are runaways and most of the remaining 25% are cases of parental abduction. All told, Massachusetts has about "26 unsolved cases of child abductions by non-family members, many going back several years." Maine has one 10-year old case of child abduction on the books. Nationally, the current number of unsolved cases of missing children is about 32,000—of whom 95 percent are runaways. The figure of 50,000 missing children, used by Child Find and featured in literature from the Adam Walsh Child Resource Center, the one staring out at me from all those ads, is now declared to be "erroneous." Challenged on its figures, Child Find currently estimates that there are fewer than 600 cases a year.

A wrenching feature of the problem of abducted children in those instances in which children have indeed disappeared and presumably been snatched by strangers with evil motives, is that parents become the first suspects. In line with the anti-family ideology of official child-protectors, parents find this insult added to their injury. According to Newsweek, "Many are made to submit to lie-detector tests and intensive investigation of their past." Mothers and fathers are put on unofficial trial—even in cases where the missing child is from an intact family rather than from those fragmented families with disputed custody cases in which abduction is a desperate act of last resort, or a dire way for estranged spouses to wound one another.

We find, then, a double-whammy when the problem is missing children: a nearly paranoid over-inflation of the problem coupled with a tendency to revert to notions of the "enemy within"—either parents did it or they are responsible because they did not care adequately for their children. Another load of guilt, or potential guilt, is layered onto the already enormously difficult and sensitive task of child-rearing in a society that has little real respect for child-rearers, especially mothers.

Second, in the matter of child-abuse, the findings are bound to be somewhat murky. But two important pieces of data emerged. According to Criminal Justice

Statistic sources, females are the prime perpetrators of abuse through all age brackets up to 40—by about 3–1 through age 34. At that point the statistics reverse themselves and males take over. The answer to this apparent riddle is probably demographic: by the age of 40 most women are past child-bearing years and the vast majority are no longer mothers of very young children. The population available for abuse is just not there. But males dominate in other non-parental roles that open up possibilities for abuse. (A cautionary note: "abuse" is not defined in the Sourcebook, so it is not at all clear what gets subsumed under this rubric.)

In the incendiary matter of "father-daughter" incest, in fully two-thirds of all cases the offender is not a biological parent but a step-father or live-in roommate of the mother. The popular image, then, is only partially correct: about 90% of all accused molesters are male. But incest and sexual abuse are not everyday affairs in the overwhelming number of intact homes. The at-risk population is most likely to be children in socially isolated and unstable domestic situations, with alcoholism and drug-abuse major factors. This parallels the findings of the most credible research on battering, for at least "half the American women battered each year have no blood or legal ties to the men who assault them," found Evan Stark, Anne Flitcraft and William Frazier in an essay on domestic violence for the *International Journal of Health Services*. Violence and sexual abuse are major symptoms of familial breakup and domestic stress in a time of widespread social dislocation, rather than probable features of stable relationships.

As more and more women emerge as alleged offenders in sex-ring and day-care cases, we are also prompted to reflect upon the social double-standard that comes into play in how we evaluate sex between a fifteen-year old girl, say, and a 40 year old male, on the one hand, and a teen-age boy and the mythic "older woman," on the other. The former conjures up perversity and exploitation—the "dirty old man" and the despoiled maiden. But the latter has long been the stuff of pulp fantasies, B-movies, and serious romances, sometimes with a French accent. In other words, social expectations gear us to expect male offenders, perhaps seeing many more than there are, and to be blind to possible female abusers, perhaps seeing fewer than there are.

Overall, the thrust of current awareness programs designed to root-out and to prevent sexual abuse of children aims to instill in children mistrust of family members and the placing of confidence instead in helping professionals, those who presumably have nothing to cover up. The results are not in on what this sort of awareness training does in terms of actually preventing child abuse. Surely it enhances the fears of children, perhaps even prematurely sexualizing their relations with adults, implanting in the child's mind notions that were not previously there in the form of vague fears, apprehensions and sensations. Many would insist that we cannot protect children unless we make them fearful and suspicious, so that they know when something wrong is being done. Maybe. But stories are also accumulating from divorced or separated fathers who say they are afraid to hold or to hug their children, or even change soiled clothing, for fear a vindictive or suspicious ex-spouse may conjure a tale of sexual abuse out of it.

Families in general and individual family members in particular have long been almost powerless against the ministrations of various agencies in terms of a warrant to pry, probe, and harrass. One friend of mine reported an incident that became part of her own move to feminism. Separated from her husband, living with her two young children in a communal household (the time, you may have guessed, was the mid-60s), she found herself being investigated by the local child welfare agency on a report lodged by her estranged mate and mother-in-law. The charge was that the children were being "twisted" and "perverted" by living in a non-nuclear household consisting of unmarried political radicals. Although this was clearly a power-play on the man's part, with a divorce and possible child-support pending, the woman had no choice but to submit to a demeaning investigation, including several unannounced visits by bureau sleuths out to assess whether a household of friends, who were also political dissidents, by definition constituted a situation of child abuse and neglect.

A new twist, however, has been added to the tale over the past year. Families that neglect and abuse children, under notoriously loose definitions, have been joined by foster-case homes and day-care institutions as dangerous, or potentially so, places. Foster case has been problematic as a "solution" to family "neglect" for a long time. In some instances, children have been placed at risk by being removed from homes where they were "neglected" into foster-care situations where they were abused—either by foster parents or boyfriends of foster mothers. Yet foster care is the preferred non-institutional prescription for poor or economically marginal families who fall into the net of official child protection. (My intent is not to indict all foster-care homes but to take the measure of our approaches to the problem under review. I know there are many loving and secure foster home situations.)

In a large public hospital north of Amherst, Massachusetts, a ward devoted to "psychiatric" treatment includes among its numbers of voluntary admittees together with a sizeable population of involuntary patients, mostly "troubled" teenagers. These young people are institutionalized by police, social agencies, doctors, and sometimes families for "de-tox," drug, or alcohol problems. Sometimes "behavioral" problems are at issue. Sometimes attempted suicide is the reason for admittance. According to my informants, an interesting pattern can be found in terms of prescribed treatment once the teenager is allowed to leave the hospital. For poor or lower-middle class families, the "solution" is invariably to remove the child from the home: off to foster-care. For upper-middle class families, the "solution" is invariably to remove the child from the home: off to private school. In this single instance, and there are no doubt many more like it, already economically marginalized children are taken away from "neglectful" parents and resituated in a way that may leave them at even greater risk. Apparently, nearly any situation is preferable to the child's own family in the view of many official child protectors. As a society, we have become adept at coercing and "disciplining" families that fail to meet certain norms, but we are notoriously inept at providing a supportive surround in which parents might rear their children.

The day-care situation is the latest and most troubling wrinkle. Current fears about day-care speak in part to parental guilt, especially that of mothers, at leaving their children, sometimes in less than optimal day-care situations. Fears about day care have come into focus at a time when more and more women, driven either by economic need, personal desire, or the sanctioned insistence that women should get out of the home and into the real world of economic society, are in the labor force. Although the vast majority of working mothers are not employed full-time, those with children under school age require day-care. The high divorce rate further promotes a need for out of the home day care.

We have made of day-care an economic function, best performed by specialized providers. But we don't really respect those who care for children very much, so day-care workers receive lousy salaries, have few long-term prospects, and often labor under difficult conditions. Child-care is severed altogether from the home. Mutual suspicions between day-care providers and parents are aroused. Shunting our children off to their own ghettoes, for they are not yet of "productive" age, we feel in our bones something is wrong. What is wrong must be with the day-care situation, frightened parents conclude, not with the overarching ordering of a political economy geared towards a bureaucratic industrial structure in which *all* those who cannot work do not fit—including our children.

The truly horrific tales coming out of various day-care scandals tap already extant guilt and promote a new climate of fear and suspicion. Eileen W. Lindner, director of the Child Advocacy Office of the National Council of Churches, reports that the hysteria accompanying sexual abuse in child-care centers prompted 100 staff members in nine church-housed child-care centers in the mid-West, to issue an ultimatum to their director: "Fearing they would be falsely accused of sexual abuse," Lindner writes in *The Christian Century,* May 13, 1985, "they [child-care staffers] refused to return to work until the board of directors issued precise guidelines for physical contact with their young charges."

In principle this may seem reasonable, Lindner continues, but in practice such precision is impossible to implement. Moreover, good child care "demands physical contact. Touching is a part of caring for and affirming young children." The upshot of all this is that children, some of whom are in day-care from 7 a.m. to 5:30 p.m., hence literally out-of-touch with parents and other family members all day long, may find precious little hugging, holding, and caressing among their frightened day care-takers.

If day-care workers are frightened, and parents are paranoid, politicians and professionals are up-in-arms, prepared to do various things. One garden variety proposal is to beef up staffs in already extant bureaucracies. In the Northeast, for example, budget increases in the six New England states would "add a total of 221 child protective workers," according to *The Boston Globe,* June 12, 1985. In January of this year, the Department of Health and Human Services urged states to pass stricter laws and regulations governing day-care. The Department's "Model Child Care Standards Act" proposed screening all potential employees, doing background checks for criminal records or past abuses, requiring probationary periods for all employees "until background checks are completed" and "training staff members" to detect and report abuse. In order to implement such proposals, a whole new level of bureaucracy must be set up.

Fortunately, a few voices are being raised against what Rebecca Shannon Shipman, an associate professor of human services at Massasoit Community College, Brockton, Massachusetts, calls the leap to a "Big Daddy" approach to the day-care/abuse problem. For the "Model Child Care Standards Act" as well as the National Child Protection Act, introduced in the Senate, Fall, 1984, by Sens. Alfonse D'Amato (R, NY) and Paula Hawkins (R, FL), offers a mega-institutional "solution" that requires a national child-care system. This legislation is primarily coercive (withdrawal of federal funds from states that do not adhere to prescribed monitoring programs) and policing (a national hot-line for reporting allegations of child sexual abuse by day-care workers and a criminal-records check of all employees of licensed day-care facilities).

But there is no evidence whatever that criminal records checks will prevent child abuse. The scandal at the Bronx day care center in 1984 showed that none of those charged with abuse had criminal records. "Furthermore," writes Diana R. Gordon in the *New York Times* (March 2, 1984), "among the more than 6,000 day care workers fingerprinted and reviewed in the wake" of the Bronx scandal, "not a single one" had a record of sexual or any other abuse of a child. The finger-printing review, however, likely turns up very old misdemeanor charges that do not necessarily ill-suit a person for his or her present responsibilities but may nevertheless haunt an individual by becoming knowledge available to current and prospective employers.

The likely result of the rush to tighten-up the order, gain control, and attain a homogenous national day-care system, is the loss of diversity in day-care, whether in churches or private homes, and to frighten many decent people away from day-care work entirely. Shipman makes a good point: experts cannot agree on whether out-of-home or in-home child care is most helpful to child development. Why should they be trusted to determine "the type and amount of day care that is best for millions of different children?"

She proposes a Big Sister approach that emphasizes "security, trust and love . . . personal involvement and responsibility." This sounds good, to be sure, but how would it play itself out institutionally? For starters, if we are to have day care, and surely it is here to stay, it should be more closely controlled by parents, more integrated into work and home. We need more rather than less "slack" in the order. This, in turn, requires important political initiatives that soften some of the most harsh features of our political economy, including our relentless demands or productivity that constitute people as "wage-earners," leaving them precious little time to be family and community men and women, parents, friends, activists, sharers in a way of life.

Admitting that our children are at risk, we need not leap into the arms of Big Daddy. (Interestingly, many conservatives who fret so much about government control are behind the initiatives I here criticize.) Different community standards should prevail, diversity must be acknowledged, both in families and in day-care. Were we to alter the surround in which child care, both familial and institutional, takes place, were we to remove some of the hot-house pressures that are more likely to explode into abuse, this problem would take on more appropriate proportions and colorations. This is a project for the long haul.

In the meantime, we need far less media hype that frightens us all out of our wits and freezes our responses to children in our care, and more emphasis on the fact that genuine love and concern between adults and children remain, however fragile this nexus has become. One now withered bond that we must find ways to restore is that between the young and the old, between children and grandparents or grandparent surrogates. Surely the present crisis of confidence concerning our treatment of the young cannot be severed from a second national scandal, our treatment of the old.

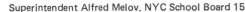

Superintendent Alfred Melov, NYC School Board 15

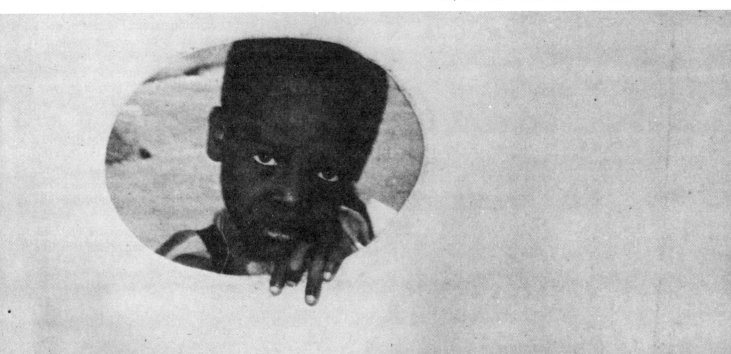

Chapter 18
The Great Self-Care Issue
E. Riley Holman*

"Hurry home, Dad! Clay made soup and set fire to the tablecloth."

—Older sibling in child care

"Fires and other emergencies pose a very real threat to children in self-care" (Rhodes & Long, 1983, p. 7).

"Jenny, be sure to call me as soon as you get home."

—Working single mother

"In factories and offices throughout our country, parents wait anxiously for their children to call and confirm their safe arrival home." (Riegle, cited in "School Facilities," 1984, p. 10).

"Sam, don't you think you should put your key away before you lose it again?"

—Primary teacher

"I was constantly reminding students who wore their keys displayed to place them inside their shirts or blouses" (Long & Long, 1983, p. i).

"Hey, Tommy, are you coming over to smoke with me again after school?"

—Adolescent latchkey friend

"Many others argue that lack of supervision can encourage experimentation with sex and drugs" (Rooney, 1983, p. 10).

These actual recorded statements are illustrative of a gigantic social phenomenon and some of the accompanying problems that have occurred with pressing suddenness during the past two decades. More and more children now and into the next century are likely to spend their childhood in families with a single working parent or with two parents, both of whom are working. Many of these children will be involved in self-care or sibling care.

Often, children involved in self-care are referred to as "latchkey children," a term used to "describe a child who is regularly left without direct adult supervision before or after school" (Strother, 1984). There is no agreement as to exactly when or how the term originated. Strother indicates that it was coined during World War II, but McCurdy (1985) attributes its origin to the 19th Century. It was, however, derived from the observation that "many young school-age children of working parents are carrying housekeys to gain entrance to their homes" after school closes (Clifford, 1980, p. 14).

Estimates as to how many children are involved in self-care are enormously conflicting. In order to clarify the reasons for the conflict, reference is made here to the first hearing of the House of Representatives Select Committee on Children, Youth, and Families ("Child Care," 1984) where a number of interested people testified in order to raise the level of national debate on child care. Dr. Kamerman of Columbia University testified that "there are no national data on where children are cared for after school or when school is closed . . . just as there are no national data on who is doing the caring or what kinds of care are available. What is known is that the demand for after-school care is growing as is the supply, but the supply is in no way able to meet the demand." (p. 11)

It is also known that the demand will increase as we move into the next century. Dr. Zigler, Director of the Bush Center in Child Development and Social Policy of Yale University (cited in "Child Care," 1984), testified that "currently more than half of the mothers whose children are too young to care for themselves are working outside the home." By the end of the century, this figure will top 75%. (p. 24)

Because there are no national data on how children are being cared for and by whom, Kamerman (cited in

*Dr. E. Riley Holman is Professor of Childhood Studies and Reading, Education Department, West Chester University, PA.

"Child Care," 1984) estimates that the number of children in self-care range from between 1.8 and 7 million. The disparity relates to who is doing the counting, how self-care is being defined, and the ages of the children involved. For example, the most often mentioned ages of children in self-care appear to be between 6 and 13 years (Long, 1983 and Hall, 1985). However, sources often report ages as low as 5 and as high as 14 years. The Center for Early Adolescence ("Setting Policy," 1984) is most concerned about the increasing number of young adolescents in the 10 to 15-year-old age range who do not have adult supervision after school.

Social Trends

The reasons for the tremendous increase in the number of children involved in self-care are ingrained in the social conditions of the times. So many dramatic changes have impacted either indirectly or directly upon the family in general, and children in particular, that the problem of self-care is one of national concern. Pell (cited in "School Facilities," 1984) and Rooney (1983) present a number of social and demographic trends that are at the root of the problem. Some of the trends affecting children indirectly include:

1. Economic realities that force many families to depend on two incomes and demand that single parents (especially women) join the work force.
2. The heightened mobility of modern society that encourages families to move often and makes immediate neighbors strangers.
3. Age-segregation housing that separates young families from older family members thereby reducing the number of adults available to care for children as was one of the trends in the past.

Changes that are directly family related include:

1. The increased divorce rate that impacts in part on the growing number of families headed by single parents (mostly women).
2. The gradual decline in the size of the average family resulting in fewer teenage siblings to care for younger brothers and sisters.
3. The decline of the extended family resulting in fewer live-in adults to care for children.
4. The strong and ever-building number of women entering the labor force resulting in acute child-care needs.

These social conditions are among those that have created an unprecedented demand for child care as well as have caused a disruption in many sources of traditional child-care arrangements. According to Kuchak (1983), the traditional care providers such as friends, neighbors, and relatives are now less available. In addition, women who might once have stayed home to care for their own and/or another's child are themselves needing child-care arrangements. Often, self-care appears to be the best answer to child care and, in many cases, the only financially feasible solution.

Issues

Self-care is not a new issue. Selligson, Genser, Gannett, and Gray (1983) indicate that as a nation, we have been grappling with the problem for a long time. What is new, according to McCurdy (1985) is the staggering numbers of children in self-care in America. Indications are that more and more school-age children will be caring for themselves as our society moves into the future.

Any great social concern is accompanied by a number of issues. The self-care issue is very complex; just as there is no one reason for the emergence of the problem, there is no one correct view regarding the issues involved. Most discussion has centered around the following:

Are Children in Self-Care at Risk?

Whether children involved in self-care are at risk and if so, how extensively, is a question that is not settled. According to Wellborn (1981), there is evidence to indicate that unsupervised children are at risk to a greater or lesser extent, depending on the context of their care arrangements. Selligson et al. (1983) maintain that research in this area rarely has focused on the cumulative effects of self-care. The research is far from definitive and has been "either cross-sectional or based on local studies which are not generalizable." (p. 15) Galambos and Garbarino (1983) concur that the results from a number of studies show that there is insufficient evidence to point to clear-cut, positive or negative consequences of self-care.

Lipsitz ("Setting Policy," 1985) indicates that whether a young adolescent is at personal risk depends on where he or she lives, the safety of the neighborhood, and the quality and character of the family. Garbarino (1984) adds to the list by suggesting that risk depends on the age and maturity of the child.

Burtman (1984) surveyed suburban children who felt safe in their homes and positive about the self-care arrangement. These children reported a sense of independence, self-sufficiency, responsibility, and capability. Galambos and Garbarino (1983) investigated the effects of the self-care experiences on rural children. The children in self-care performed no differently in school than did their peers, nor were they more fearful of going outside alone. Long and Long (1983) found that children in self-care in an urban setting experienced more fear and nightmares than did their peers who were not in a self-care arrangement. McCurdy (1985) emphasizes that common sense indicates that many children are in jeopardy. He feels that many children are too young and vulnerable to care for themselves in "this modern and dangerous society." (p. 11)

However, Lipsitz ("Setting Policy," 1985) does not see the matter of risk as the main issue. She reminds us that:

> the larger issue goes beyond preventing risk and harm to preventing lost opportunities for helping. Young adolescents explore their personal potential, their community, and the larger world. Let us not forget the vulnerability of young adolescents to positive experiences with caring and respectful adults. Let us not forget that we can act positively to enrich young people's lives, to enhance their opportunities, not just to avoid them. . . . (p. 14)

What Should Be the Role of Government?

Kuchak (1983) summarizes the role of government in day-care policy traditionally as being conceived at the state levels and implemented by state and local agencies. The federal government has provided support for day-care services chiefly in periods of war and primarily targeted to low-income families. Generally, the federal rule has been "one of a crisis mediator during times of natural, social, political, and economic change." (p. 1.1)

The involvement of the federal government under the Reagan administration has drastically affected all types of child care. Major cuts in existing programs were sustained until centers servicing low-income children have drastically curtailed services or eliminated them altogether.

Edelman ("A Children's," 1986) reports that the impact of reduced child-care help on families has been severe. She explains that while the dearth of adequate care is taking its toll on most working families, it is hurting the poor the most. The situation is causing parents to settle for makeshift child-care arrangements and/or leaving children alone to care for themselves. Edelman claims that "despite the complex child-care problems many Americans now face, the federal government has virtually abdicated any leadership role in helping to meet the need." (p. 292)

Many child-care advocates are convinced that the whole society has a stake in the kinds of adults children become and therefore the kind of care children receive when they are young. Kamerman (cited in "Child Care," 1984) contends that if many people become convinced of the need, support for more administrative investment in child care may take place. However, if present trends continue and the high cost of good child care is ignored and inadequate funding appropriated, the quantity may increase somewhat but the quality will remain an "unaddressed issue." Kamerman concludes that: "This is a very strange outcome for a rich society allegedly concerned with children and said to lead the world in child-development research." (p. 23) She points out that the only significant federal development is the expansion of the child-care tax credit in 1982. This expansion made it available to those who do not itemize deductions on their income taxes. However, she feels that the credit must be increased and be made refundable or it will have very little or no value to low and moderate-income families.

Child-care advocates visualize some federal help with the problems of school-age child care through two bills that appear to include some financial relief and encouragement from the federal government, that is, Senate Bill #1531 entitled "The School Facilities Child Care Act" and HR 2242 entitled "The Child Care Information and Referral Act." In the final analysis, the bills were combined and less than $5 million was authorized for problems related to school-age child care ("Latchkey Aid," 1986). The money was authorized to set up new programs. No money was allocated to help existing programs and no money was authorized for administrative costs in operating programs. Apparently, the federal government does not see school-age child care as much of a problem or it is willing to abdicate its leadership role in such a gigantic social issue.

State governments, according to Kuchak et al. (1983), traditionally have been responsible for licensing requirements, creating standards, distributing federal and state funds, giving professional help, and patronizing research. Some states have responded to the need for increased and more adequate after-school care by sponsoring legislation. Other states are considering legislation or are offering special incentives to schools and community groups to start school-age care programs (Selligson, 1986). According to Tompkins (cited in "Child Care," 1984), however, many states have reduced standards in child care as a result of cutbacks in Title XX and the elimination of federal requirements.

A few states have been successful in initiating gubernatorial and legislative programs where federal effects have failed despite creative legislation introduced in Congress. Gannett (1985) reports that successful state proposals range from instituting legislation encouraging the use of public school space for before-and-after-school programs to full-scale funding programs for school-age child care. Successful programs in 11 states, i.e., Arizona, California, Florida, Indiana, Maine, Massachusetts, Missouri, New Jersey, New York, Pennsylvania, and Wisconsin, are summarized in Gannett.

Arizona and Massachusetts, for example, have legislated monies to encourage using public school space. New York, the first state to appropriate funding programs for school-age child care, and California, the state appropriating the largest amount of money for school-age child care, both have full-scale funding programs.

Pennsylvania recently approved $1.5 million for care for school-age children. Indiana passed a pilot school-age child-care bill that includes $270,000 for operating costs. New Jersey approved $1 million, targeting a portion for school-age child care; Wisconsin earmarked $77,800 for 2-1/2 years to fund three different types of school-age child-care programs in three areas of the state. Other states are beginning to react to the need. For example, Kansas made a tiny contribution by allocating $15,000 for school-age child care. Where federal effects have failed to provide leadership, the need for states to offer help is considered paramount.

Communities have generally participated in conducting assessments of local needs for day-care services and in developing their own programs. The private sector has also been involved in meeting the needs and demands of families and their children (Kuchak et al., 1983). A community can address school-age child care needs in a variety of ways. There are many before-school and after-school programs sponsored by family day-care centers, religious groups, community organizations, and public schools. However, Stroman and Duff (1982) report that efforts have been scanty when compared to the need.

Scherer (1982) suggests that some of the most highly successful community programs are those housed in public school buildings and sponsored by parent and/or community groups. Many of these models involve schools contracting with community groups to provide care in a school setting. Local governments sometimes have made funds directly available to community groups. Often, arrangements have been made for parents to pay on a sliding scale with free care for the poor, thus guaranteeing low-income children access to school-age child care.

An example of a community attempt to research the problems and issues related to care of school-age children is provided by Adams and Strupp (1984) and involves the City of Madison, Wisconsin. In 1983, the city of Madison Day Care Advisory Board established a task force "to examine information regarding school-age self-care needs and problems related to lack of supervision and to make recommendations which could help decision makers address the problems." (p. 3) Parents served by the school district were surveyed to gather information on a number of self-care issues. Findings characterized the self-care needs of Madison in a number of ways. They also indicated that many parents are willing to offer support for more and better services.

What Role Should Public Schools Play?

The use of public schools as the most efficient and effective solution is supported by a number of groups interested in finding answers to the school-age child-care crisis. Many believe that schools have the best facilities and that school personnel have the expertise and the experience to provide leadership to answer many of the problems associated with self-care. Some feel that present attempts to fill the need through a variety of programs are piecemeal approaches and lack a rational priority (McCurdy, 1985). Hawkins (1984) states that the use of schools would be an inexpensive and efficient way to provide federal leadership to this growing national problem. He sees partnerships being built between schools, parents, and nonprofit day-care providers.

Selligson et al. (1983) see the possibility of a school program providing continuity and dependability that may not be available in more informal care arrangements. That is, the program of the school has the possibility of always being available. They suggest that current problems of enrollment and image may be alleviated through the school's participation in child care.

In spite of the growing surge to use schools for before and after-school programs, there are a number of concerns from both the public and educators. McCurdy (1985) reports that those outside the school system may have difficulty accepting the fact that a school is entering into the "day-care business." Private day-care operators might perceive the school's involvement as unfair competition and could pursue legal channels to prevent the school from what they see as an encroachment on their territory. Others view the problem as a family responsibility and feel that schools should not have a role in its solution. The involvement of schools could be seen as an intrusion by government into family matters. In addition, Campbell and Flake (1985) point out that some community groups may be reluctant to contact the schools because of the difficulties in negotiating school-community partnerships. Also, many groups may not understand how to approach school personnel or who to contact first in order to initiate school involvement. Still others worry about who is going to pay the bill for public-run programs. Will school taxes be raised?

Educators have several concerns regarding the use of schools in after-school care. Many of these concerns are legitimate and involve accountability and liability, preparation of personnel, budgetary matters, and philosophical objections. Selligson (1986) and McCurdy (1984) both refer to the concerns of educators. Some of the most-often-asked questions include: Who will pay the liability costs if a child is injured on school grounds before or after the regular school day? Do school personnel have sufficient knowledge about day care? Is it babysitting or is it remediation? How will additional programs be financed? Who will pay additional costs for janitorial services, electricity, heat, etc.? Will there be a tendency to siphon money away from regular school programs to meet costs of an after-school program? How can education continually attempt to relieve all of society's ills? Will school programs develop as recreational programs or more of the same?

Regardless of the mixed reactions to public school involvement with school-age child-care programs, many schools have initiated programs with varying degrees of success. Campbell and Flake (1985) report that the most successful programs have a broad base of community support. Generally, the type of program desired has been decided by a community group before meeting with the superintendent. Often, the school assists in helping the interested group survey community needs and form a viable proposal.

Levine (1979) suggests that communities are so diverse that it would not be wise to assume categorically that the school is the "best possible sponsor or provider of day care." He also contends that it would not be in the national interest to exclude the schools. Local values and planning must be considered in any approach to after-school care. A school might be used fully, partially, or not at all depending on the circumstances and needs of a given community.

Seltzer (1981) summarizes the various forms of involvement public schools may take. Often a school teams up with a community group to offer programs. The programs may be housed in an empty classroom, a part of the school such as the cafeteria, or the entire school. Often there is an understanding that if the school needs space, the program will move. Many programs use the space and services at no cost, others pay rent and/or others defray costs of additional energy and custodial services. Still other schools may develop their own programs.

How Do Parents Respond to Self-Care Conditions?

Today's working parents are forging a new course which is drastically different from the traditional definition of "parenting" where a homemaker was available when children left for school and returned home from school. Many parents begin their days very early to attend to household chores and manage the daily destinations of family members. Modern parents wear a lot of hats, and often they need help to make it all work.

Long and Long (1983) found that most parents using the self-care arrangement began on an occasional experimental basis. When nothing serious happened and their children appeared to be able to manage, the parents increased the duration and frequency of self-care. Other parents started self-care as a result of some traumatic family problem such as a divorce, and self-care began one day and may never cease.

Thomas and Makris (1983) report that parents are more likely to use the resources available to the family for child care no matter what the family income. As households with the least resources for child care are headed by single parents, children in these families will likely be left alone more often.

McMuray and Kazanjian (1982) summarize a follow-up study of a 1979 survey of families involved in New York City's public day-care programs. This study revealed that despite parents' expressions of confidence in the fact that their children involved in self-care were old enough and responsible enough to be left alone, it was clear that there was a great deal of ambivalence, concern, and dissatisfaction with the arrangement. A number of parents worried about safety matters and their children being confined to the house. Parents generally believed that the children would do better in an organized program. Even some parents who expressed satisfaction registered concern regarding the adequacy of the arrangement. Almost all parents wanted some alternatives. Most wanted a structured program where supervision, help with homework, and recreation with other children was provided.

Pecoraro, Theriot, and LaFont (1984) feel that while self-care may appear to be free, it is not entirely without cost. Many parents suffer guilt feelings which are generated by a conflict between their belief system and their actions in leaving their child alone. Their traditional concept of roles and parenting responsibilities causes stress. Parents of children in self-care worry about a multitude of possible problems. This is substantiated by employers who are well aware of what is now referred to as "the three o'clock syndrome" where parents wait for their self-care child to call on the telephone to check in and let the parents know that he or she has arrived home safely.

Many parents suffer from guilt feelings as a result of the self-care arrangement. Long and Long (1983) report that "there is a kind of conspiracy that causes the latchkey phenomenon to maintain a low profile in day-to-day society." (p. 18) This occurs because of the guilt parents feel, even though in many instances the self-care arrangement may be the only alternative.

Grier and Grier (cited in Emlen, 1982) report that employees' on-the-job absenteeism rate is related to child-care arrangements. In their study conducted in the greater Washington D.C. area, employees who needed to make out-of-home child-care arrangements reported missing twice as may days as those without parental responsibilities. They also found a relationship between absenteeism and the kind of child-care arrangements parents used. Parents who used family day-care arrangements had the highest absenteeism rates. Somewhat higher rates than other parents were reported for "those using day-care centers, those relying on older brothers and sisters, and by those whose children look after themselves." (p. 14)

How Do Children Respond to Self-Care?

Most studies, whether they have concentrated on self-care or after-school supervised activities, have failed to consider the impact of the child-care situation on the child's development. Research has not seriously probed the long-term effects of self-care on various aspects of the child's personality. No longitudinal studies have been conducted to compare the effects of self-care with various other child-care provisions (Strother, 1984). Much more needs to be done in this realm.

Below are two statements gleaned from adult women who, as children, were involved in self-care. The differences in the way each perceived the situation is illustrative of the varying ways in which children perceive self-care.

Beginning in fourth grade, I came home to an empty house. My parents owned their own business, therefore, they needed to work. As a young adult, I am now terrified of the dark, and I can't stand to be by myself in a house at night. I feel that these fears originated because I was a "latchkey" child.
                                        —College Sophomore, 1986

As the only child of professional parents (both in the teaching profession), I was met at the school gate by our housekeeper every school day until the beginning of eighth grade. I hated it and often felt embarrassed. For me, having my own key from that time on was the

biggest and grandest step to adulthood. This was my opportunity to be independent, responsible—a chance to meet aloneness head-on and master satisfying the use of that time alone.
                                        —College Professor, 40 years old, 1986

The effects of self-care on children depend on a number of variables. There is no consensus among child-care advocates and professionals as to the positive or negative effects of self-care on children. Factors generally considered include the maturity, age, attitude, neighborhood, structure of the self-care situation, family income, and presence of other siblings or peers. The maturity, planning, and attitudes of the parents are also considered important factors (Pecoraro et al., 1984 and Toenniessen et al., 1985).

The statement from the college sophomore indicates that certain adult fears started from being alone in an "empty house" after school. Indeed, some research does indicate that children often experience fear. Zill (1983) studied boys and girls from ages 7 through 11. They were asked if they worried when they had to stay at home without adults. Thirty-two percent of the boys and 40% of the girls said, "Yes." The most frequent fear expressed was that somebody bad might get into their house.

The statement from the college professor indicates that she thrived on the experience of self-care. Research also indicates that some children mature through the experience; and that, for some, it is indeed a way for gaining independence (Burtman, 1984).

Some research has focused on the age and maturity of the child when he/she enters the self-care arrangement. Generally speaking, the older the child is when beginning self-care, the more likely it is that the experience will be positive. In the statements presented, the college sophomore was approximately 10 years old when self-care began; the college professor was about 14 years old when she received her own key.

Sibling care is another alternative parents have used. Stroman and Duff (1982) indicate that although the presence of siblings may reduce loneliness, sibling care also increases tension and responsibility for children in self-care. Older children who stay at home with siblings report problems (Rhodes & Long, 1983). Older siblings often resent the responsibility. Their freedom is restricted when caring for younger siblings. In addition, peer interaction is often limited by time and restrictions of parents. Older siblings may also experience difficulty in controlling younger siblings, and often younger siblings may not respond to their requests. Younger siblings often have trouble coping with older siblings who are in charge of them. Most older siblings are not equipped to handle many of the problems associated with caring for a younger brother or sister.

The three worst problems for many children in self-care appear to be fear, loneliness, and boredom. While this is true for many average children in self-care, it is even more true for special children such as the learning disabled. Learning disabled children, as reported by Rhodes and Long (1983), are more likely to be less mature, less socially adept, and more in need of structured experiences. They are more likely to be fearful, unable to structure time, and have fewer problem-solving skills and emergency strategies than average children. Rhodes and Long conclude that learning disabled children are not likely to have a successful self-care experience.

Some child-care advocates are concerned that the responsibilities given to children in self-care are often more than they are capable of handling. This granting of increased adult responsibility has caused many scholars to react to what they see as a disappearance of childhood. For example, Meyorwitz (1982) reports that the children he sees around him manifest interests, experiences, and language that seem more adolescent and adult-like than child-like. Others have written similar themes questioning whether forces are at work to deprive children of the full experience of childhood.

Garbarino (1984) contends that children should be sheltered from the direct demands of economic, political, and sexual forces. Children have a right to receive support from their families and communities. They should not be fair game for political activity, and they are not supposed to be sex objects. She suggests that childhood is about creating social space to lay the foundation for optimal human development. There are two important aspects of childhood which go together, that is, play and the development of basic competence.

Many observers feel that the premature granting of responsibility for self-care to younger children and "the extensive involvement of children in formal activities that mimic adult work, play, and sexuality and make extensive maturity demands" (Garbarino, 1984, pp. 9-10) indicate a disappearance of childhood. These maturity demands are not only evident in families but in the academic, social, and socioeconomic world as well. Some researchers feel that the current maturity demands involve risks that outweigh the benefits found in the socioeconomic context.

Solutions

Just as there is no one answer to other social problems we face as a nation, there is no one answer to how the problems regarding self-care can be solved. Most child-care advocates dealing with these problems feel that the solutions will need to be addressed jointly; that is, by the federal government, state governments, industries, various social groups, parents, schools, and communities.

Communities across the United Sates are working out ways to respond to the needs of children in self-care. Many communities have recognized and are sensitive to the problems, but attempts to offer help to solve them have been both modest and dramatic. Long and Long (1983) emphasize the importance for all concerned parties to pay attention to the "care arrangements parents make for children among which self-care is rapidly becoming paramount." (p. 209) They maintain that not only are the needs of children more adequately met, but the national economy is also affected by finding better ways to solve the problems associated with self-care.

Long (1983) stresses the importance of parents, schools, and community groups cooperating as a result of the increased needs of families for self-care choices. He believes that cooperation is the key to improved services for children (p. 15) and that each community will need to require a number of approaches to adequately respond to family needs for child care.

Hawkins (cited in "School Facilities," 1984) indicates that in many communities concerned groups are working together to develop programs to meet self-care needs. He cites Pineless County, Florida, as having an exemplary program achieved through a "unique spirit of cooperation and community service." (p. 5)

While the ideal way to meet the needs of children in self-care may be a concentrated community effort, in actuality it appears that most services to provide before and after-school care have been initiated by separate organizations such as private day-care centers, the YMCA/YWCA, schools, etc. In pockets of communities all over this country, individual groups and organizations have made responses to the self-care problem without the benefit of a planned community effort.

Examples of a number of self-care programs and a brief description of each are provided below. They illustrate the many alternative forms of assistance established to help solve the problem.

Telephone Hotlines

Various organizations in many communities have initiated telephone hotlines for children. Generally, the hotlines are established to help children in self-care find ways to deal with boredom, loneliness, fear, worry, and/or emergency.

One such service is provided in Lancaster County, Pennsylvania. It is sponsored locally by the Lancaster County Council of Churches but is affiliated nationally with Contact Teleministries USA and Life Line International. It is managed by a director and a staff of volunteers. Advertisement for the kids-line is promoted through newspapers, television, and in elementary schools. The director for the program sees the service as a supportive one, not an intervening mechanism to assume the responsibility of parents. The philosophy is to talk the caller through the problem. The kids-line also offers a service to parents and guardians who wish to list their names and where they may be reached in case of emergency. The staff has been surprised at the number of calls received from teenagers, as the service is advertised to younger children. They have also been surprised at the dramatic increase in calls on snow days and teachers inservice days when children are at home alone all day (Thomas, 1986).

Check-In Programs

A check-in program is a flexible care and supervision arrangement that allows a child to report to a trained, neighborhood-based family care provider after school and during times when school is not in session. It is designed for older elementary and junior high school children who are not yet ready to completely take care of themselves.

An example of a check-in program can be found in Fairfax County, Virginia, where it has been designed and tested under a grant from the Department of Health and Human Services (Administration for Children, Youth, and Families). McKnight and Shelsby (1984) explain that parents designate exactly how much freedom and responsibility they want their children to have by writing and signing a special contract. The contract also defines the role and responsibilities the parents assume when they enroll their children in the program. Each child's day is planned differently. After check-in, and with parental permission, children can visit friends, play in their neighborhoods, attend after-school and community activities, and/or spend time in their own homes.

Before-School and After-School Programs

There are may programs sponsored by family day-care centers, religious groups, various community organizations, and public schools. Stroman and Duff (1984) report that the efforts to establish programs has been scanty when compared to the need. Nevertheless, more and more organizations are responding to the problem by offering before-school and/or after-school programs. Stickney (1981) indicates that there are programs funded by universities, governmental bodies, private industries, philanthropic organizations, and

profit-making businesses. Some are custodial; some help prepare children for school; while others supplement school experiences. Many are nothing more than babysitting services while others are remedial and some are developmental.

One unique after-school recreational program described by Hamilton (1985) was developed for children in self-care in the Winnebago School District #323, Winnebago, Illinois, under a grant from the Illinois Board of Education. The focus of the program uses high school students enrolled in a child development class as "teachers" in a laboratory experience that allows them to work closely with children. They prepare daily lesson plans for after-school activities and help children with homework. High school students in food service classes have also joined in this project to prepare nutritional snacks. Students are paid for their work. The program is held in a middle school and supervised by a director and an instructor. There has been an enthusiastic response to the program from school administrators as well as from the high school students and the children involved.

There are several sources available for helping interested parties establish programs. Wellesley College houses an exemplary School-Age Child Care Project where staff members provide information and technical assistance on the design and implementation of programs. The project has been conducting research since 1979 under the direction of Selligson (1983) on the type of school-age child-care services available nationally.

Hamilton (1985) offers help on steps in setting up a "latchkey" program; Morlock (1984) gives information on "A Model School-Age Child Care Program Operated in the Public Schools;" and Stickney (1981) offers a manual geared to starting, operating, and maintaining a successful after-school program with a focus on child development.

Mass Media

Mass media in many areas of the country has contributed to raising the consciousness of the people toward self-care issues. Generally, the thrust of the media has been toward providing information and encouragement to elements of the community to aggressively consider the problem as serious.

A good example of the contributions that television has made is demonstrated by a series of programs aired by CBS's Channel 10 in Philadelphia entitled "Latchkey Families." The project (Cohen, 1986) was produced in consultation with the National Television Workshop, Inc., New York. The comprehensive project included four broadcasted programs that focused on informing viewers about the state of working parents, the problems associated with self-care, and some of the ways the problems are being solved. Some of the programs were distributed for use in schools and youth agencies as a public service of Channel 10.

Survival Training

One solution to the child-care issue has been to provide support to children in self-care by training them in coping skills designed to improve their safety and well-being. Strother (1984) refers to business groups which have arranged with educators, social workers, and private organizations to present programs that parents and children on developing coping skills. However, Fosarelli (1985) believes that it is the parents' responsibility to impart self-survival skills. She feels that others may impart information with which a parent may disagree, and that in some cases a person other that the parent cannot possibly impart accurate information because of the uniqueness of the child's home. She advises that other interested adults should counsel parents, recommend courses for them, and be prepared to recommend books on the topic for both parents and children.

Long (1985) recommends that teachers include self-care skills in their curricula to help children with emergency situations because most parents give their children only rudimentary preparation for staying at home alone. She suggests nine topics as a fairly complete curriculum for preparing children to function safely on their own, that is: key care, safe travel, being safe at home from strangers, telephone skills, fire safety, handling household emergencies, first aid, safe snacks, and facing fears. She also suggests that teachers incorporate these skills into regular curriculum subjects such as reading and mathematics. An example is given of how Baltimore teachers have found ways to do so.

Flex-time

Some industrial leaders have developed flex-time arrangements that permit workers to adapt their hours to their needs as parents. Bell (cited in Kameran & Hayes, 1982) reports that many small businesses have informal flexibility in work scheduling for some employees but do not have a formal policy or even a consistent practice. Garbarino (1981) explains that there are limits to this solution in that many parents cannot expect to be at home both before their children leave for school and when they return from school.

Informational and Referral Services

Child-care information and referral (I&R) services provide an important tool for helping parents learn about what kind of care is available. It also helps parents choose an adequate child-care service to meet their needs and the needs of their children. Kamerman ("Child Care," 1984) sees the expansion of I&R services by employers as probably the most significant development on the part of employer-sponsored child-care services. However, Thompkins ("Child Care," 1984) explains that while this is a very worthwhile endeavor, it certainly is not the solution to existing child-care needs. He reports that the most extensive service is in California where public subsidy is provided for these services.

The Future

The problems associated with self-care will not disappear. In fact, everything we know leads to the conclusion that the numbers of children left alone will increase as we move into the future. Naisbitt (1984) contends that there are specific states where most of the social invention occurs in this country. He suggests that, in the future, we should keep an eye on these areas for answers to some of society's most pressing problems. There are key programs, researchers, and ideas that may help provide answers to some of the self-care issues and problems as we approach the next century. Below are several possibilities that may prove to be beacons on which to focus attention.

1. Metropolitan Washington, D.C., is said to lead the nation in trends regarding new lifestyles such as greater diversity in types of households, fewer children per household, increased number of working women, etc. (Grier & Grier, 1982). Just as Naisbitt (1984) suggests that in the future we watch Florida (the state with the greatest elderly population) for answers to problems related to the age-youth ratio, so we might also watch the greater Washington, D.C., area for answers regarding school-age child care.

2. Long and Long, through the School of Education at Catholic University in Washington, D.C., have been active writers and researchers concerning the issues, and their work will undoubtedly make important future contributions.

3. The Wellesley College Center for Research on Women, in Wellesley, Massachusetts, through the School-Age Child-Care Project, has demonstrated genuine interest in the problem and has made important contributions in finding solutions. As a result of demonstrated interest, we can expect that future contributions will be significant. The center currently offers information and technical assistance regarding school-age child care. It also provides several publications regarding the issues involved.

4. National organizations which exist to provide a strong and effective voice for children might also be beacons for future efforts. One such organization is The Children's Defense Fund which pays particular attention to the needs of poor, minority, and handicapped children. The organization focuses on programs and policies that affect large numbers of children. It gathers data and disseminates information on key issues affecting children and monitors the development and implementation of federal and state policies. The Children's Defense Fund is a national organization with roots in communities all over America. The main office is in Washington, D.C. It has developed cooperative projects with groups in many states. It is supported by foundations, corporate grants, and individual donations.

5. Prominent states such as New York and California, where interest and initiative have resulted in legislative action, are key states to watch in providing help to others in the future.

6. Efforts of key communities where cooperative efforts of several groups have come together to focus on the problems may also be key places to watch in the future.

Currently, school-age child-care programs are popping up all over. Community organizations such as the YMCA and private day-care centers are responding to the need. However, many of these programs for before-school, after-school, and school holiday care are rather expensive and unaffordable for many parents. The sponsoring organizations can certainly not be blamed. Good child care is expensive, and society should not expect child-care professionals to carry the financial brunt of the problem. Until various levels of government realize the need and assume a great deal more responsibility, many child-care advocates are worried that the problem will just continue to grow.

Finally, Kamerman and Hayes (1982) and other child-care advocates recommend a research agenda to help solve the self-care problems of the future. However, they explain that as there is no defined body of knowledge "of child-family-work-community, there is no agreed-on field of research." Each issue requires a different view and raises new questions. They plead for not "more studies but different studies," that is:

studies which focus more directly on children, what happens to them and why; and studies that acknowledge the complexity of the environment in which children are reared. . . . They (children) must be studied in their living environment, an environment that increasingly includes working parents (p. ix).

REFERENCES

Adams, D. & Strupp, R., *School-Age Child Care Parent Survey, Final Report.* Wisconsin: Research Report. (ERIC Document Reproduction Service No. ED 251180) 1984.

Burtman, A., The new latchkey kids. *Working Mother, 7*(2), 1984, pp. 78–86.

Campbell, L. & Flake, A., Latchkey children—What is the answer? *Clearing House, 58*(9). May 1985, pp. 381–383.

Child Care: Beginning a National Initiative. Washington, DC: Select Committee on Children, Youth, & Families. House of Representatives. U.S. Government Printing Office (Stack No. 052-070-059-66-4), April 4, 1984.

A Children's Defense Budget. Washington, DC: Children's Defense Fund, 1986.

Clifford, H., *Status of Day Care in Canada, 1980: A Review of the Major Findings of the National Day Care Study.* Ottawa, Canada: National Day Care Information Centre, 1980.

Cohen, S., *Latchkey families.* Philadelphia: Channel 10 (CBS), 1986.

Emlen, A., *When Parents are at Work: A Three-Company Survey of How Employed Parents Arrange Child Care.* Washington, DC: Greater Washington Research Center, December 1982.

Fosarelli, P., *Children Left Alone: Latchkey Problems—Future Research Questions and Interventions.* Paper presented at the Annual Conference of the National Education Association, Washington, DC, February 22, 1985.

Galambos, N. & Garbarino, J., *Identifying the Missing Links in the Study of Latchkey Children.* Paper presented at the Annual Meeting of the American Psychological Association, Washington, DC, August 1982.

Gannett, E., *State Initiatives on School-Age Child Care.* Wellesley, MA: School-Age Child Care Project, Wellesley College Center for Research on Women, October 1985.

Garbarino, J., *Can American Families Afford the Luxury of Childhood?* Paper presented at the National Conference on Latchkey Children, Boston, MA, May 1984.

Garbarino, J., Latchkey children: How much of a problem? *Education Digest, 46*(6), February 1981, pp. 14–16.

Grier, G. & Grier, E., *Metropolitan Washington: Leader in Changing Lifestyles.* Washington, DC: Greater Washington Research Center, 1982.

Hall, Janet M., Latchkey children: Is anybody home?

Our responsibility. *Illinois Teacher of Home Economics, 28*(3), January-February 1985, pp. 117–118.

Hamilton, T., *Vocational Recreational Programs for Latchkey Kids.* Springfield, IL: State Board of Education, Department of Adult, Vocational and Technical Education, June 1985.

Kamerman, S. & Hayes, C., Eds., *Families that work: Children in a changing world.* Washington, DC: National Academic Press, 1982.

Kuchak, J., *School-Age Day Care Study.* Final Report. Research Report. (ERIC Document Reproduction Service No. ED 242411) 1983.

Latchkey aid to states available, *Education Week, V*(33), May 7, 1986.

Levine, J., Day care and the public schools: Current models and future directions. *The Urban and Social Change Review,* 12(1), 1976, pp. 17–21.

Long, L., Safe at home, *Instruction,* February 1985, pp. 64–69.

Long, L. & Long, T. *The handbook for latchkey children and their parents: A complete guide for latchkey kids and their working parents.* New York: Arbor House Publishing Co., 1983.

Long, T., *Working Parents, Schools and Children in Self-Care.* MD: Position Paper. (ERIC Document Reproduction Service No. 238552).

McCurdy, J., Schools respond to latchkey children. *The School Administrator, 42*(3), 1984, pp. 16–18.

McKnight, J. & Shelsby, B., Checking in: An alternative for latchkey kids. *Children Today,* May/June 1984, pp. 23–25.

McMurray, G. & Kazanjian, D., *Day care and the working poor: The struggle for self-sufficiency.* New York: Community Service of New York, April 1982.

Meyorwitz, J., Where have all the children gone? *Newsweek,* 1982.

Morlock, L., *Latchkey, a model school-age child care program operating in the public schools.* Largo, FL: Latchkey Services for Children, Inc., 1984.

Naisbitt, J., *Megatrends.* New York: Warner Books, Inc., 1984.

Pecoraro, A., Theriot, J., & Lafont, P., What home economists should know about latchkey children. *Journal of Home Economics, 76*(4), Winter 1984, pp. 20–22.

Rhodes, S. & Long, L., *Latchkey and Learning Disabled: Some Problems to Consider.* MD: Position Paper (ERIC Document Reproduction Service No. ED 253982) July 1985.

Rooney, T., *Who is Watching our Children? The Latchkey Child Phenomenon.* Sacramento, CA: Senate Office of Research, 1983.

Scherer, M., Loneliness of the latchkey child. *Instructor, 91,* May 1982, pp. 38–41.

School Facilities Child Care Act. Washington, DC: U.S. Senate Subcommittee on Education, Arts, and Humanities, Committee on Labor and Human Resources. Congress of the United States, April 27, 1984.

Selligson, M., Child care for the school-age child. *Phi Delta Kappan, 67*(9), May 1986.

Selligson, M., Genser, A., Gannett, E., & Gray, W., *School-Age Child Care: A Policy Report.* Wellesley, MA: School-Age Child Care Project, Wellesley College Center for Research on Women, December 1983.

Seltzer, M., Planning school-age child care in public schools. *Education Digest, 46*(6), February 1981, pp. 17–18.

Setting Policy for Young Adolescents in the After-School Hours. Proceedings of conference, Chapel Hill, NC: Center for Early Adolescence, November1984.

Stickney, F.,*Latchkey Cares for Kids: A Guide for a Successful Child Development Program.* California: Non-classroom material. (ERIC Document Reproduction Service No. ED 225689) 1981.

Stroman, H. & Duff, R., The latchkey child: Whose responsibility? *Childhood Education, 59*(2), November-December 1982, pp. 76–79.

Strother, D.,Latchkey children: The fastest-growing special interest group in the schools. *Phi Delta Kappan,* December 1984, pp. 290–293.

Thomas, N., Hotline helps troubled kids. *Intelligencer Journal,* Lancaster, PA, March 18, 1986.

Thomas, N., & Makris, B., *Child Care Consumer Education: A Curriculum for Working Parents.* Washington, DC: Wider Opportunities for Women, Inc., 1983.

Toenniessen, C., Little, L., & Rosen, K., Anybody home? Evaluation and intervention techniques with latchkey children. *Elementary School Guidance and Counselling,* December 1985, pp. 105–115.

Wellborn, S., When school kids come home to an empty house. *U.S. News and World Report,* September 14, 1981, pp. 42–47.

Zill, N., *American children: Happy, healthy and insecure.* New York: Doubleday-Anchor, 1983.

Chapter 19
Preventing Adolescent Suicide
Richard A. Schere*

Despite the popular belief that adolescence is a wonderful, exciting, and enthusiastic time of life, the research has always indicated that, in fact, adolescence is one of the most difficult stages of development. Classic studies (Erikson, 1950 and 1963) as well as more recent studies (Hiam, 1974) clearly describe the conflicts and ordeals adolescents must confront. In essence, adolescence is a transition between childhood and adulthood during which a sense of personal identity must be established and role confusion must be overcome. Independence must replace dependence. Conflicts regarding career, sexuality, and meaningful relationship must be explored and resolved–all this, at a time when body growth, physiological change, and the pull of new cultural and subcultural demands create agonizing pressure on the teenager.

The suicide rate of youngsters from ages 15 to 24 has increased 150% in the last twenty years and is now near the average for the population as a whole *(Harvard Medical Health Letter,* 1986, No. 8). This increase may well reflect the many social tremors that have shaken modern American society. The teenagers' traditional support system has been devastated by the high level of divorce and remarriage that has caused typical adult supporters to be unavailable and preoccupied with therere own new difficult adjustments. In addition, the erosion of traditional standards of morality and custom has caused an inability to be certain of right and wrong. Finally, the rocketing rate of general change in the current era has made it nearly impossible to be rooted, stable, and secure.

It is no wonder, then, that a study of 5,600 high school youngsters (Freese, 1979) found that depression was second only to colds, sore throats, and coughs in frequency. Researchers clearly established the relationship between depression and suicide, but a lesser known fact is that 95% of people come out of depression unless suicide intervenes (Maggie Scarf, 1980). It is therefore very important to establish a sharper focus on the nature of the depression the suicidal adolescent manifests. To begin with, suicidal adolescents often keep their depression concealed (Hyde and Forsyth, 1978). Because of their lack of experience and perspective, adolescents tend to overreact to problems that later in time are apt to be perceived as less significant. The depression of teenagers has also been traced to the loss of parent by death, divorce, separation or extended absence. This results in the removal or displacement of a developing youngster's important role model (Miller, 1975 and McAnarney, 1979), alienation from family (Wenz, 1979 and McAnarney, 1979), and failure to achieve in our highly competitive society (de Catenzaro, 1981 and Grueling and De Blassie, 1980). Additional causatives are parents who neglect, severely punish, or perceive their adolescent as unworthy (Frederick and Resnick, 1971), confusion about sex roles in a period of very strong sexual stimulation (Miller, 1975 and Finch and Poznanski, 1971), and a magical concept of death as a way of producing a problem-free life (Miller, 1975).

Research efforts to measure an adolescent's potential for suicide has yielded important information about the quality of reaction a teenager, seriously at risk, takes to these causatives as compared to peers who are much less at risk. A feeling of hopelessness, defined by Beck (1975) as negative expectation of the future has been found to be a critical quality linking depression to suicidal behavior. Teenagers with external locus of control (believing that their circumstances are caused by outside forces, not themselves) have been found to feel more hopeless than teenagers with internal locus of control (believing that their circumstances are caused by their own behavior or personality) (Kohant and Gagton, 1977 and Topol and Reznikoff,

*Dr. Richard A. Schere is Professor of School Psychology, Brooklyn College, CUNY, and Director of the Kennedy Learning Clinic. The author wishes to acknowledge the contribution made by Roseanne Moreno in the preparation of this chapter.

1982). Suicidal adolescents tend to feel they have more total problems, more serious problems and more family problems than adolescents less at risk. Finally, suicidal adolescents manifest a progressive isolation from meaningful relationships which seems to develop after maladaptive behaviors like withdrawal or running away prove ineffective (Topol and Reznikoff, 1982). In light of these critical qualities, one seeking to screen adolescents for suicidal potential ought to consider such measures as (1) The Hopelessness Scale (Beck, Weissman, and Lester, 1974), (2) The Mooney Problem Checklist Revised High School Form (Mooney and Gordon, 1950), and (3) The Locus of Control Scale for Children (Norvicki and Strickland, 1973), (4) The Family Concept Test (van der Veen, 1965), and (5) The Social Desirability Scale (Marlowe and Cowne, 1969).

Indeed, it would seem that in this era of computer technology, it would be prudent to employ a sample of these five measures to identify adolescents in the public high schools who need to be monitored more closely than their peers. Furthermore, it would appear that if a prevention program is to prove effective, these specific dynamics must be addressed. They represent a check list of criteria by which a proposed intervention can be evaluated.

1. Does the program include strategies that attempt to help adolescents feel more positive and optimistic about their future?
2. Does the program include strategies that attempt to help adolescents feel more in control of their circumstances?
3. Does the program address the personal problems perceived as serious by each participating adolescent?
4. Does the program provide adults who can serve as supports, role models, and liaison to the families of the adolescents involved?
5. Does the program include strategies that encourage reluctant adolescents into meaningful relationships and active participation?
6. Does the program educate its participating adolescents about the realities of suicide and death, the nature of the developmental stage through which they are going, and the specifics of themes that are particularly important and confusing to them (sexuality, vocational trends and preparation, and social myths—e.g. what boys look for in girls and vice versa)?

Too many programs seem more concerned with form than content. There are many valid approaches to preventing adolescent suicide as long as the content of the approach attends to the critical issues research indicates press upon the teenager who is most vulnerable.

Certainly programs should be initiated in the schools. Charlotte Ross (1980) presents the argument for schools being a focal point for prevention programs. In addition to computer screening, teachers trained to see the vital signals given by teenagers at risk could be crucially valuable–but they must be trained. Discussion of the problem is far more preferable than the silence that presumably protects youngsters, especially in light of research that indicates that adolescent suicide, despite the myth, is not contagious (Lester, 1972 and Ross, 1980). Peer group programs are also recommended as valuable. Adolescents feel an especial need for peer confidence (Mishara, 1979) and so teenagers can be perceived being both potential victims and potential rescuers. Furthermore the peer group can be a valuable aspect of the total support system. However, in light of the needs of at-risk teenagers we have discussed, peer group programs should be sub parts of a more comprehensive approach. Hotline programs seem generally ineffective. Severely suicidal people are usually too isolated, fearful and despairing to call a stranger. Studies indicate that cities with hotline programs do not have a lower suicide rate than cities without them. (*The Harvard Medical School Mental Health Letter,* March, 1986, No. 9). The only group found to benefit from hotlines is that of white women under twenty-five, who are the most frequent callers to hotlines. However, hotlines are impersonal and are limited as to what effective strategies they can employ. Bargaining for delay is one hotline strategy that has proven somewhat useful. Callers can be urged to postpone action until after coming to a prevention center to discuss problems and alternatives more fully.

There is no greater tragedy than the self-caused loss of a young person who has only just begun to live. Parents, siblings, and peers are affected in ways that are unlike the trauma of most other death experiences (Cantor, 1974). Usually, the suicide of a teenager has more to do with his internal depression and confusion than with any of the events in his reality. Prevention programs that contain strategies that deal with the important dynamics underlying the vulnerable teenager's depression and confusion can effectively reduce the alarming increase in suicide and can contribute calm to this restless concern held for that which most of us care most about—the welfare and future of our children.

REFERENCES

Beck, A.F., Weissman, A., Lester, D., and Lester, L. "The Measurement of Prevention: The Hopelessness Scale." *Journal of Clinical and Counselling Psychology,* 1974, 42, 861–865.

Cantor, P. "The Effects of Youthful Suicide on the Family." *Psychiatric Opinion,* 1974, 6–11.

Cowne, D.P. and Marlowe, D. "A New Scale of Social Desirability Independent of Psychopathology." *Journal of Consulting Psychology,* 1960, 24, 349–354.

de Catanzano, D. *Suicide and Self-Damaging Behavior,* New York: Academic Press, 1981.

Erikson, Erik H. *Childhood and Society.* New York, W.W. Morton and Co., 1950 and 1963.

Finch, S. and Poznanski, E. *Adolescent Suicide.* Illinois: Charles E. Thomas, 1971.

Frederick, C. and Resnick, H. "How Suicidal Behaviors are Learned." *American Journal of Psychotherapy,* 1971, 25, 37–55.

Freese, A.I. *Adolescent Suicide: Mental Health Challenge, (Public Affairs Pamphlet No. 569).* New York: Public Affairs Committee, 1979.

Grinspoon, Lester (Editor), *The Harvard Medical School Mental Health Letter),* volume 2, numbers 8 & 9, February and March, 1986.

Grob, Mollie, Klein, Arthur and Eisen, Sue "Role of the High School in Identifying and Manning Suicidal Behavior." *J. of Youth and Adolescence*—1983 (Apr., Vol. 12(2) 163–173.

Grueling J. and De Blassie, R. "Adolescent Suicide" *Adolescence,* 1980, 15, 601, 1980.

Hiam, A. *Adolescent Suicide*—New York International Universities Press, 1974.

Hyde, M. & Forsyth, E. *Suicide,* New York: Franklin Watts, 1978.

Lester, D. *Why People Kill Themselves.* Illinois: Charles E. Thomas, 1972.

McAnarney, E. "Adolescent and Young Adult Suicide in the United States—a defection of Societal Unrest." *Adolescence,* 1979–Vol. 13, p. 209–213, 1979

McBrien, Robert—"Counselling Student *School Counselor,* 1983 (see) Vol. 31 (1) 75 & 82.

Miller, J. "Suicide and Adolescence" *Adolescence* 1975, Vol. 10, pp. 13–23, 1975.

Mishara, B.L. "Suicidal Verbalizations and Attempts in Collect Students: A Multivariate Log—Linear Analysis of the perceived Helplessness of Peer Reactions." In: Proceedings of the 10th International Congress for Suicide Prevention, Ottawa, 1979.

Mooney, R.L. and Gordon, L.V. *The Mooney Problem Checklist: Manual, 1950* Revised. New York: Psychological Corporation, 1950.

Nowicki, Jr., S. and Strickland, B.R. "A Loss of Control Scale for Children." *Journal of Counselling and Clinical Psychology,* 1973, 40, 148–154.

Ray, Lydia & Johnson, "Adolescent Suicide," *Personnel and Guidance Journal.* 1983, Nov., Vol. 62 (3), 131–135.

Ross, C.P. "Mobilizing Schools for Suicide Prevention." *Suicidal and Life Threatening Behavior,* 1980, 10(4), 239–243.

Ross, C.P. "Teaching Children the Facts of Life and Death." In: Peck M. Litman, P., and Farberoza, N. (Eds.) Youth Suicide, New York: Springs Publishing, 1982.

San Francisco Chronicle, September 29, 1980, p. 17 (Interviews with M. Scharf).

Selkin, James "The Legacy of Emile Durkheim." *Suicide and Life Threatening Behavior.* 1983 (SPR) Vol. 13(1) 3–14.

Stone, M. "The Parental Factor in Adolescent Suicide." *Int. J. of Child Psychotherapy* 1973, 2: 163–201.

Topol, P. and Reznikoff, M. "Perceived Fear and Family Relationships Hopelessness and Locus of Control Adolescent in Suicide Attempts." *Suicide Life Threatening Behavior,* 1982, 12, 141–150.

van der Veen, F. "The Parents Concept of the Family Unit and Child Adjustment." *Journal of Counselling Psychology,* 1968, 12, 196–200.

Wenz, F. "Self-injury Behavior, Economic Status, and the "Family Anomie Syndrome Among Adolescents." *Adolescence,* 1979, p. 387–397.

Chapter 20
School Finance's Future: Addressing the Adequacy
Margaret Godfrey*

Education will not occur unless there is money available to finance it. In the post World War II period American education has been grappling with court decisions and legislative mandates which address inequities and special needs of children. Financial crises were a continual problem as inflation and rising costs eroded school budgets. But it was the onset of reports like "A Nation at Risk" that caused the public to place a greater priority on the adequacy of funds which were available to education.

Anyone involved in running a school system doesn't really need to wait for results of a Gallup poll to find that lack of financial support is one of education's most persistent problems. School systems are financed through local property taxes which are also supplemented by state and federal funding. The local real estate taxes used to support schools necessarily couple the number of students with the total assessed property value of a community with their potential for tax revenue. Assessed property can be private homes or commercial development. A community with a high ratio of total assessed property value to student population could be labelled a wealthy district, and a low ratio of total assessed property value to student population could be labelled a low wealth district. These ratios are not absolute because communities vary considerably.

The property wealth of a district can strongly influence the amount of money that can be spent to educate each child in it. The obvious result is that districts with low property wealth are often unable to compete with higher property wealth districts on their education budgets. Indeed some districts may strain to their financial limits as federal and state mandates are placed on them with no provision to supply the money needed to implement the mandates. A good example of this was the U.S. district Court in 1972 in the Pennsylvania Association of Retarded Children ruling that schools must provide for education of mentally retarded children regardless of cost. It was not until 1975 with the passage of Public Law 94–142 that some funds were provided by Washington for handicapped children. (Soares, 1982).

Some communities undoubtedly find themselves serving more students with special needs which predictably cost more. But another aspect of local real estate taxes is that they are also used by communities to support municipal services. A community may find it has to supply needed services to a greater number of citizens, such as handicapped or elderly. One outcome of this disparity is the use of "municipal overburden" aid where a state such as New York can give more money to school districts which have a greater need to supply special services to their citizens through the principle of "municipal overburden."

In the early 1970s it was apparent that the financing of schools by local property taxes had inequities which were to be corrected by court order. In 1971 in the Serrano v. Priest case the Supreme Court of California found substantial dependence on property taxes discriminated against the poor. To remedy this, the state's wealth as a whole rather than local property taxes were to be used to determine educational expenditures for children. The quality of the schools was too dependent upon the real estate wealth of a community and the inequities produced, per pupil, did not give equal protection under the state constitution (Reutter & Hamilton, 1976).

The California State legislature had been given until September 1980 to establish a plan to equalize the expenditures throughout the state. AB 65 (Assembly Bill 65) was passed in 1977 to improve the funding and the quality and public schooling. State assistance was to be administered on a more equitable basis to provide funds for school districts, especially by increasing per pupil expenditures in low wealth districts.

*Dr. Margaret Godfrey is a Math Teacher Trainer, PS 75, Bronx, New York City Board of Education.

School budgets are the concern of local school boards and community members, but their source of funding can be a constant problem which inevitably must be solved through a political process. The way school budgets have emerged in recent years has been shaped by the turmoil of the legal and societal changes taking place. A dramatic example of this emerged in California's implementation of Serrano.

The Foreword to "California Schools Beyond Serrano" (1979) had to look backward to the Serrano court decision and its projected impact on the schools. This report on Assembly Bill 65, which was passed in 1977 to implement Serrano, was written before June 6, 1978 when the voters of California decided upon Proposition 13 which limited local property taxes to one percent of market value. The ominous conclusion stated, "Obviously this limitation prevents full implementation of these school finance provisions of AB 65 that requires certain levels of local property tax revenue."

In 1973 another Supreme Court decision citing the Fourteenth Amendment addressed another aspect of financing the schools by maintaining poor districts did not have to provide children with the same education as wealthy districts (Sherman, 1976). A ruling in the Rodriquez v. San Antonio case found the use of local taxation for schools does not provide full freedom of expenditure for all districts because the real question was that education was not "explicitly or implicitly guaranteed by the Constitution." (Reutter & Hamilton, 1976). This decision left to the states decisions about how to equalize educational opportunity based on clauses of their state constitution. (Fiske, 1982).

Appropriately, the Robinson v. Cahill case in New Jersey was being watched closely by school boards and administrators (Canfield, 1976). A more equitable finance plan had been sought in this decision. The shift in local financing was traced by Goertz (1979) from 1975-1976 to 1978-1979 when the state's share of total expenditures increased from 23.5% to 31.3%. Expenditures of the wealthiest districts rose 40% per pupil while in the poorest districts they increased a mere 15%. State aid could not overcome the expenditure potential of high wealth districts. The conclusion was that the court mandate had produced a very small amount of change.

One of New Jersey's poorest municipalities which has an extremely high total net property valuation and an extremely low equalized valuation of property value per pupil has not improved its financial base despite the court decisions and passage of the New Jersey Public School Act of 1979 (Thomas, 1979).

The Levittown court case in New York also tested whether additional state funding should be used to equalize educational expenditures to low property wealth districts through additional state funding. The New York State Court of Appeals found that the state's methods of financing its schools was constitutional (Dionne, Jr., 1982). The majority opinion called New York's financing system "rational" and emphasized that forcing uniformity of educational opportunities throughout the several hundred school districts would contribute to the dismantling of local control of education.

The value of the local school district and control by boards of education was reasserted through this decision. Differences based on decisions made in local communities were maintained. Municipalities that want to use zoning laws to increase commercial or residential ratables are encouraged to create the type of tax base they want. State and federal aid can be sought and applied for as the priorities are determined (Sobel, 1982). Most important, however, is the sentiment that local school districts that choose to spend large amounts of their tax money on schools are free to do so without being concerned that they are providing unequal, though superior, educational opportunities for the children in their community.

The public views financial issues as important. Perennial issues that attract their attention include tax rates, school budgets, bond issues and salaries (Iannaccone & Cistone, 1974). Expenditures according to Zeigler and Johnson (1972) were related to economic variables while other types of outcomes were related to political variables.

Gittell and Hollander's analysis (1972) of six large urban school districts lead them to conclude school systems are a part of the political culture of a city and that school board political independence is not assured by fiscal independence.

In a small town a board of education's actions are watched more closely. The businessmen, mostly farmers, are organized and exert pressure to promote a "low-tax, low expenditure ideology." The five-member board exerts power in the educational hierarchy by their control of the "purse strings" (Vidich & Bensman, 1968).

A study in Ohio highlights the financial plight of the schools in the cities. According to Murphy (1978) municipal overburden is increasing and large cities do not place as much of their budget into education. Per pupil expenditures prior to 1950 were greater in the cities, by 1957 a certain equality was reached, but in the next decade, cities declined to the lowest point. During the 1970-1978 period state and federal aid revived per pupil spending in the cities to the levels of the suburbs.

According to the National Center for Education Statistics (1984) it was during the 1970s that state revenues became a more frequent source of funds for the public schools. In 1970-1971 the states' share of public school revenues was 39%. But by 1980-1981, the state provided 47% and two years later 48%. Federal revenues also increased from 8% to 9% during the period from 1970-1971 and 1980-1981, but in 1982-1983 they decreased to 7%. Federal funds, however, are particularly important in Southern states because they contribute to a much higher proportion of their education funds.

State revenue is derived primarily from sales and income taxes, both of which are influenced by the general business conditions in the state. These conditions can also be a controlling factor in determining the amount of state aid that local school districts will receive. Enrollment figures of a district usually are another method of determining how much state aid a district receives.

The local revenues which are collected through property taxes and their stability make school budgets less subject to changes in business conditions or enrollment changes. However, state revenues can be used to reduce differences in how much districts spend per pupil even if they are not mandated to do this by court order.

Tax revolts such as Proposition 13 in California also produce changes in the finance patterns of schools. California had the largest shift from local property taxes to state taxes. California was one of four states where per pupil expenditures dropped in comparison to the United States average despite an increase of 15 percentage points of the state's share of educational expenses. Hartley (1981) alluded to several trends based on his analysis of California where after Proposition 13 the state's share of education expenses grew from 45 percent to 70 percent in 1978-1979. He predicted a shift of financing away from property tax to a state tax and equity of per pupil expenditures.

Another view of these changes in school finance was given by Adams (1982) who found that between 1959-1976 states had created over 41 new taxes and passed 586 tax increases. This was a necessary step to reduce property taxes which were regarded as regressive for education. Throughout the seventies until 1978 a greater amount of federal aid was given to local communities. During the period, educational spending continued at a pace that was higher than the economy in general. But from 1977-1980 the states began to lower tax rates. In what Adams calls a "tax revolt" many states lowered sales and income taxes.

Politics and public opinion can exert influence. Just (1980) notes that education is now finding itself in greater competition with other public services for the limited amount of resources available. Iannaccone (1972) also reinforces that one way that public power can manifest itself is through limiting the resources available to the schools.

A look at the years 1980-1981 and 1982-1983 shows that expenditures per pupil were far from consistent when adjustment for inflation was considered. Sometimes this was caused by increases or decreases in enrollments. Utah's increase of 8 percent in average daily attendance had a per pupil spending increase of only 3 percent which was below the national average. In Massachusetts which had passed Proposition 2-1/2 to limit taxes to 2-1/2 percent of a city's property base (Collins & Lucove, 1982) school attendance fell 13 percent but expenditures managed to stay on a par with inflation. High spending states between 1980-1981 and 1982-1983 tended to have greater increases in expenditures. The top five states in 1981-1982 averaged 118 percent more than the bottom five, but by 1982-1983 the top five spent 140 percent more. Thus the disparity in spending became more pronounced.

This pattern or ability of high spending districts or states to increase their budgets and per pupil expenditures more than their lower spending counterparts may be the tell-tale sign that signals the commitment to the educational system. According to Collins and Lucove (1982) Massachusetts was one of 17 states that had passed laws to ease their communities' tax burden. In Massachusetts a prioritized list of budget cuts was followed starting with non-personnel items non-academic program services. Academic programs and teachers were the last to be cut. In California with Proposition 13 there were cut-backs in high school offerings and summer school (Savage, 1982). Another consequence was that SAT's dropped from 1976-1980. In general education did not suffer severely because of the powerful state lobby in the state capital.

As education moves into the last half of the 1980s much attention has been focused on the need to improve education. In this climate of change, a proliferation of reports have come forth to admonish the public that schools must receive greater support. But even with this climate, localities will necessarily adjust their financial support of schools as they perceive the needs of their communities. School boards and superintendents will set policies and present budgets that their constituents demand. Communities have a wide range of ability to finance education because of tax bases that are vastly different. Complicating this is the needs of the children. A greater number of children requiring compensatory education will often come from a district which, because of poor socio-economic status, cannot afford to spend the extra tax dollars that are needed to educate these children properly. For instance, mandates for remedial education may be dictated by state or federal laws but the full amount of financing needed may not have been provided.

Conclusion

There is no invisible hand which will keep educational finance in a state of equilibrium. School boards, superintendents and their staffs and the citizens in local communities along with state and federal money are needed to assure that schools will be adequately funded. Without this support, the children of today will not be prepared for the future. The public must be continually apprised to address the sufficiency of school finance. Educators must not hesitate to shake loose the bureaucratic mold and find new paths which will lead them to the sources of funding for their schools.

The federal mandates which are frequently insufficiently funded were addressed by *American Education* magazine (1983). States can be placed in a position where they must direct localities to divert their tax dollars to comply with these regularions. To remedy this, it was recommended that autonomy be returned to the state and local levels with support through block grants, vouchers, and tuition tax credits. However, what is needed with this viewpoint is a statement on how the inequities of state and local finance are addressed. Poorer districts and states may have no feasible method of raising enough money to adequately finance their schools. Richer districts and states can continually enjoy paying for the luxury of excellent schools. This is a great injustice to children in our democracy which all fair minded educators should seek to correct.

The children of our nation are its most precious resource. Regardless of philosophy or ideology—conservative, moderate or liberal—the inequities of school finance are everyone's problem.

BIBLIOGRAPHY

Adams, E.K. "The Fiscal Conditions of the States." *Phi Delta Kappan* 1982, 63(9).

American Education "Toward More Local Control: Financial Reform for Public Education." May 1983, 19(4).

California Schools Beyond Serrano Sacramento: California State Department of Education, 1979.

Canfield, J. in Golubchick, L. & Persky, B., editors. *Urban, Social and Educational Issues.* Dubuque: Kendall/Hunt Publishing Co., 1976.

Collins, J. & Lucove, J.S. "Proposition 2-1/2: Lessons from Massachusetts." *Educational Leadership,* 1982, 39(4).

Dionne, Jr. E.J. "Financing Method of Schools Ruled Valid in New York." *The New York Times,* 1982, CXXXI (45,354).

Fiske, E.B. "A Setback for the Move to Alter School Financing." *The New York Times,* 1982, CXXXI (45, 354).

Gittell, M. et al. *School Boards and School Policy. An Evaluation of Decentralization in New York City.* New York: Praeger Publishers, 1973.

Goertz, M.E. *Money and Education: How Far Have We Come? Financing New Jersey Education in 1979.* Princeton, N.J.: Educational Testing Service, 1979. (ERIC Document Reproduction Service No. 172 436)

Hartley, H.J. 1980's Education Scenario: From Tax Revolt to Governance Reform. *Music Educators Journal,* 1981, 67(5).

Iannaccone, L. & Cistone, P. *The Politics of Education.* Eugene, Ore: National Institute of Education, Oregon University, 1974. (ERIC Document Reproduction Service No. ED 091 803).

Murphy, J.F. "Fiscal Problems of Big City School Systems: Changing Patterns of State and Federal Aid. *Urban Review,* 1978, 10(4).

National Center for Educational Statistics. Source: U.S. Department of Education.

Reutter, Jr. E.E., & Hamilton, R.R. *The Law of Public Education.* Mineola: The Foundation Press, 1976.

Savage, D. "The Unanticipated Impact of Proposition 13." *Educational Leadership,* 1982, 39(4).

Sherman, J.D. *Educational Research in the Courtroom: The Analysis of Inequities in School Finance Suits, 1976.* San Francisco: American Educational Research Association, 1976. (ERIC Document reproduction Service No. ED 122 447)

Soares, L.M. "The Impact of American Jurisprudence on American Education." New York: American Educational Research Association, 1972. (unpublished paper)

Sobol, T. "After Levittown: Looking Ahead." *The New York Times,* July 4, 1982.

Thomas, E.P. *Education in Jersey City: An Assessment of the Impact of Robinson V. Cahill.* New Jersey: Greater Newark Urban Coalition, 1979. (ERIC Document Reproduction Service No. ED 174 725)

Vidich, A. J. & Benson, J. *Small Town in Mass Society.* Princeton: Princeton University Press, 1968.

Zeigler, L.H. & Johnson, K.F. *The Politics of Education in the States.* Indianapolis: The Bobbs-Merrill Co., Inc., 1972.

Chapter 21
Should We Lengthen the School Term?

Nancy Karweit*

Time-on-task is generally regarded as an important element for student achievement. One indication for the consensus concerning the importance of time-on-task is the number of recent legislative actions aimed at increasing time in school or at modifying how schools use their existing time. About two-thirds of the states are considering legislative actions or committee task force reports to change the amount or scheduling of school time.

These proposals, especially the ones aimed at extending the amount of school time, have far-reaching implications for schools, teachers, students, and their families. Given the potential costs and significance of increases in the amount of school time, we need to know how likely it is that such changes will produce the desired result-sizeable increases in student achievement. This paper examines selected research on time and learning to judge how useful increases in school time might be for increasing student achievement.

Time and Learning

Carroll's (1963) model of learning as a function of time is the usual starting point for most recent studies of time and learning. Although Carroll's model expresses learning as a function of time needed and time spent, most empirical studies of school time have only measured time spent.

Time spent has been measured by a variety of indicators. Days in the school year, hours per day, attendance, and minutes of instruction have been used as well as proximate measures of time use such as student attention or engagement. Perhaps because of the diversity of time and achievement measures used, the zero order-correlation found across these studies shows an appreciable range, from .09 to .70 (Walberg & Frederick, 1983). When controls for beginning achievement or ability are introduced, the partial correlations between achievement and time are in the range .10 to .60. Walberg (1984), summarizing the various studies of time and learning,

reports the average effect size for time to be .38. Collectively, these studies suggest that time spent is positively and moderately related to student achievement.

For understanding the potential of school time as an agent for school reform, these global indications of the effect of time tell us very little. An average effect size encapsulates information about factors that we can directly manipulate—such as days in the school year—and factors that we cannot directly manipulate—such as student engagement with learning. Thus, for gauging the impact of increasing time in school, such aggregated measures are not very informative. Instead, we need to disaggregate time into its separable components. To gauge the power of time as an educationally relevant variable, studies that accurately measure the link between student engagement and learning are useful. To gauge the potential of engaged time, studies that document how engaged time is related to allocated time, such as length of school term or day, are useful. Engaged time, which is the educational variable of interest, is not directly manipulable by legislative or other actions, whereas allocated time, from which it is derived, is. As a result, to determine the potential effect of allocation changes we need to examine how engagement is related to both allocation and achievement.

Allocated and Engaged Time

The amount of time a particular student spends actively engaged in appropriate learning—time-on-task—is the result of decisions and actions made at many different locations and by many different persons. Legislative actions governing days in the school year, hours in the school day, and minutes allocated to particular topics prescribe the amount of opportunity time. Opportunity

* Dr. Nancy Karweit is a research scientist at the Center for Social Organization of Schools, Johns Hopkins University, Baltimore, MD. Her areas of interest are the sociology of education and research methodology. Reprinted with permission of *The Educational Researcher*, June/July, 1985.

Figure 1. Time use in 12 classrooms showing variations in student engagement, time-off-task, and classroom management time.

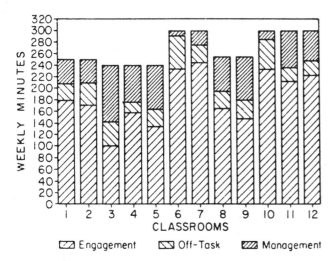

Variability in these use of allocated time in classrooms and schools implies that studies of the effect of allocated time are of limited value for understanding the likely effect of increasing the school term or day. Allocated time measures are too far removed from the variable of interest—time engaged with instruction—to unambiguously tell us about their impact.

Cross-national comparisons of achievement and time illustrate these points. The 180-day school term in the United Sates is significantly shorter than the 240-day term in Japan or Taiwan. Achievement of first graders in the U.S. also is behind that of similar students in Japan and Taiwan (Stevenson, 1983). The interpretation is directly made or implied that if we increase the U.S. time allotments, student achievement in the U.S. will become comparable to that of Japanese or Taiwanese students. Such interpretations clearly ignore the necessary cautions for attributing causality in correlational studies. First, there is the need to separate selection and time effects in the studies that compare elite and mass educating systems. Second, there is the need to convincingly argue that time effects are in fact due to time differences and not to some other effects masquerading as time. Although differences in time allocations may vary with achievement differences, manipulating the time allocations may not drastically alter achievement because time per se may not be the cause of achievement differences. For example, nations that allocate more time to schooling probably do not have longer school terms by accident; school terms are longer because their societies attach greater importance to education. If greater support for education is the primary reason for greater achievement, manipulating a manifestation of this emphasis—the amount of school time—will not necessarily alter achievement. Stevenson's (1983) finding that between-nation achievement differences existed at the first grade prior to possible impact of time allocation differences suggests that societal and cultural differences in education, not time differences, are largely responsible for achievement differences.

Studies examining the effect of differences in the length of the school term or school day within the U.S. have these same interpretive difficulties. For example, Wiley and Harnischfeger (1974) documented impressive effects for quantity of schooling (number of days X attendance X hours in the day) in an analysis of time effects on achievement in a 40-school subsample of the Equality of Educational Opportunity Survey (EEOS). That these results failed to generalize in an extension of these analyses to additional settings in the EEOS data (Karweit, 1976) should hardly be surprising, given the problems with using global time measures as proxies for student engagement measures. More important, even had the results been significant in every instance, interpretation

time, in turn, is scheduled for academic and nonacademic times by school and teacher decisions. The actual use of scheduled time depends on many other factors, including the student's school attendance and the erosion of instructional time by nonacademic activities and events. Finally, given that instruction is taking place, the instruction may or may not be needed and the student may or may not be paying attention.

The number of minutes engaged with appropriate instruction is the amount of time we wish to increase. But because engaged time is the end product of many influences, the same engaged time may be produced by very different allocated times. Likewise, the same allocated times may produce quite different engaged times. The chain from allocation of time to actual use of time may follow different paths, depending on student, classroom, school, and community influences.

In Figure 1, data from 12 classrooms (Karweit & Slavin, 1981) within the same school district illustrate the diversity of classroom time use. Three aspects of time use are shown in the figure: scheduled minutes, instructional minutes, and engaged minutes. Scheduled minutes are the weekly minutes each teacher allots for mathematics instruction. Instructional time is the time left in scheduled time after classroom management time and interruptions are deducted. Classroom engaged time is the time left from instructional time once student inattention is deducted. Figure 1 demonstrates that losses in scheduled time follow different patterns across the 12 classrooms and therefore that different strategies to recover lost time are appropriate in different classrooms. For example, classroom 3 clearly uses more classroom management time, whereas classrooms 6 and 10 appear to have relatively high amounts of student off-task times.

of these "effects" to imply that time was the cause would still be an issue. Recent comparisons (Harnischfeger and Wiley, 1984) of time allocated and achievement in New York and California have again been interpreted to imply that more allocated time is the cause for more achievement. Allocating more time, however, may or may not be a reasonable strategy for increasing achievement. The wisdom of this strategy depends on how much of the additional time can actually be used for instruction and how engagement during instruction is related to learning.

Of the existing time that schools have available for instruction, there is evidence that an appreciable portion for the day is not spent by students actively engaged in learning. For example, in the Beginning Teacher Evaluation Study (BTES), observation of elementary school classrooms indicate that of the 360 minutes in the school day, 171 minutes were allocated for math, language arts, and science instruction and 65 minutes were used for nonacademic instruction, with the remaining time going to lunch, breaks, and classroom management activities. Given that students pay attention to instruction about 80% of the time, these time allocations suggest that students spend about 190 minutes per day engaged with academic and nonacademic instruction. Of these 190 minutes, about 135 minutes per day would be engaged with academic instruction, or about 38% of the school day.

In many classrooms, these estimates may be too high as instructional time is eroded by student and teacher absence, by interruptions for nonacademic purposes, by discipline and classroom management, by lack of coordination of pull-out programs, and by early dismissal from school for non-academic reasons. There is an increased awareness of these "thieves of teaching time" and implementation of interesting scheduling changes to minimize such time loss (Hawkinson, 1984).

It is important to recognize that in actuality we know very little about reasonable goals for how much of the school day can be expected to be used for instruction. How long can teachers be expected to productively interact with their students? How long can students be expected to be on-task? We have little systematic evidence to suggest time performance guidelines for teachers and students under different settings and for different types of tasks.

Not only do we have few guidelines for how to create a desirable balance between instructional and noninstructional activities, we also lack guidelines about expectations for the efficiency of instruction once instruction is taking place. The assumption is usually made that the major problem is one of getting enough time for students to be on-task. But another problem, at least as difficult, concerns making the time-on-task appropriate, given the usual range of student abilities in the classroom, the usual class size, and the usual arrangement for one teacher per 25 or more students. We need to examine the evidence that indicates how well usual classroom arrangements solve this problem of making instruction appropriate to diverse students. The relationship between engaged time and achievement provides an important indication for the appropriateness of instruction as usually practiced. If time spent and achievement are highly related, then instruction as practiced is probably efficient and adding more time may be a reasonable strategy. If time spent and learning are not so strongly related, then a strategy of improving the quality and appropriateness of instruction may be more beneficial. To address these issues, we need to examine the relationship between time and learning in studies that have measured time as engagement with learning. In these examinations, we use studies that have frequently been cited as indicating the importance of student attention for achievement (see, e.g., those cited in Bloom, 1976). The studies examined here are not intended to be an exhaustive review of the effects of time-on-task, but are intended to cover frequently cited or methodologically suited studies.

Engagement and Achievement

The Beginning Teacher Evaluation Study or BTES (Denham & Lieberman, 1980) is one of the most widely known studies to examine the effects of time on learning. During the 6-year project, four separate samples were studied (known as Phase II, Phase III-A, Phase III-A Continuation, and Phase III-B). The last of these field studies is the one to be considered here. From a set of volunteer teachers, classrooms were selected that fell into the 30th to 60th percentile range on reading and mathematics tests that were designed specifically for this study. Within these classrooms, six students (three males, three females) were selected for observation, producing a final sample of 139 second-grade students in 25 classrooms and 122 fifth-grade students in 21 classrooms. Observations of selected students within classrooms took place for a complete day. In most instances, each classroom was observed about 15 times. Targeted students were observed once every four minutes to gauge the activity, the content area, engagement rate, and level of success.

Achievement data were collected in October 1976, December 1976, May 1977, and September 1977. The intertest period, October to December, is referred to as the A-B period. From December to May is referred to as the B-C period. The results from the B-C period are of primary interest here. During this 17-week period, time allocated to reading and mathematics instruction was documented in teachers' logs. Specific content categories within subject matters were coded (e.g., mathematics speed test, decoding consonant blends). The teachers recorded the allocated time per content and per student for each school day during the 85-day inter-test period.

The post- and pretests were designed especially for this study to test what was taught during the inter-test period. The allocated minutes are the number of minutes, from teachers' logs, during which instruction occurred in the particular subtests. To convert these minutes into the number of minutes per day it is necessary to divide by the number of data days covered in the study. Although there were 85 possible data days during the B-C period, the actual number of days with data is appreciably smaller. For grade 2 reading, there were 71.5 data days, for grade 2 mathematics there were 65.6, for grade 5 reading there were 55.7 data days, and or grade 5 mathematics there were 52.8 data days (from Dishaw, 1977, and Fisher et al., 1978). This loss of days came about either because scheduled instruction did not take place due to field trips or other events, or because observation did not take place.

Separate regression analyses at the individual level for grades 2 and 5 for reading/language arts and mathematics subtests were carried out using matched pretest, time, and posttest measures. Academic Learning Time (ALT) was entered into the regression as four separate variables: allocated time, engaged rate, percent of low-difficulty questions, and percent of high-difficulty questions. Borg (1980) summarizes the results of 29 of these subtests and reports that the individual ALT variables were significant ($p < .10$) in 41 of the 4×29 (116) possible cases, or 35% of the time. If we use the criterion of $p < .05$, we find that there are 29 significant effects for the individual ALT variables, or 25%. Engagement rate and allocated time accounted for 9 of these 29 significant effects. This information is important because most of the discussions about improving learning time center on allocating more time or improving student attention. These data do not support this strategy.

Of these significant time effects, there may be overestimates of the true effects for several reasons. Pre-achievement, engagement, and post-achievement are all highly correlated. Controlling for pre-achievement is critical to remove ability effects from the correlation between engagement and post-achievement. However, partialling out the effect of a third variable from the correlation between two other variables does not completely remove the effect of the third variable when the intercorrelations are high and the reliability of the control variable is less than perfect (see Lord, 1960). In other words, because students who tend to be highly engaged are usually significantly higher in ability than minimally engaged classmates, controlling for ability will only partially remove ability effects from the engagement-post-achievement correlation. In fact, the use in the BTES of

short, criterion-references pretests as control variables may exacerbate this problem, as such scales would likely be less reliable than longer norm-referenced measures such as IQ or standardized test scores. Further, use of "percent easy" and "percent hard" as part of ALT almost certainly inflates the uncontrolled effect of student ability on student achievement. These measures are derived from student responses to instruction. More able students will obviously answer correctly more often than less able students.

The problem of under-controlling for prior achievement would be largely solved by analysis of class means rather than individual scores on all variables. Use of class means would focus the analysis on classroom practices rather than on student-to-student ability differences. "Percent easy" and "percent hard" for the whole class might be influenced by the overall class ability level, but less so than individual students' "percent of correct answers" would be influenced by their own abilities. Class-level analyses were conducted in the BTES (Fisher, Berliner, Filbey, Marliave, Cahen, & Dishaw, 1980). Across the 29 subtests for grades 2 and 5 for mathematics and reading, of the 9 "percent easy" effects that were significant at the individual level, only one was significant at the class level. For percent hard, of the 11 that were significant at the individual level, again only one was significant at the class level.

Of course, the BTES is not the only study that has examined how time-on-task is related to student learning, net of ability. Lahaderne (1967) examined the effect of student attention on sixth grade reading and arithmetic achievement across eight subtests. Attention, measured by observer rating over a 3-month inter-test period had correlations of .37 to .53 with achievement. However, the partial correlations between attention and posttest score, controlling for IQ, were significant in only three of the eight subtests, with a range of .26 to .31.

Cobb (1976) examined the relationship between concurrent achievement and a composite measure termed survival skills in which attention was included. In this data on fourth graders in two schools, the correlations between arithmetic achievement and attention were .40 in school A and .48 in school B. Attention and reading were related .25 in school A and .24 in school B. Without controls for initial ability, IQ, or readiness for instruction, it is impossible to know what these correlations imply for the importance of attending to instruction. For this purpose, we estimate a partial correlation had a "pretest" been given, using estimates of correlations of .70 between posttest and pretest and a correlation of .45 between pretest and attention. Using these hypothetical, but realistic, figures produces estimates ranging from .22 to .40 for the partial correlations of attention with achievement.

Edminston and Rhoades (1969) reported the zero-order correlation between CAT general achievement and attention for 12th graders to be .58. Again, this study is difficult to interpret because it did not include a pretest measure, so that only estimates of the partial correlations can be made. Using typical values for these missing correlations of .7 with the posttest and .45 with attention, the partial correlation between attention and posttest is reduced from .58 to .40.

The independent effect of time-on-task on the achievement of 462 students in 23 classes was assessed in a study by Bell and Davidson (1976). The achievement tests were teacher-made and were specific to the content of instruction. Bell and Davidson used observational indices of time-on-task and additionally employed measures of IQ as a control variable. Analyses were carried out separately for the 23 classes. They report the partials between time and achievement for each class, controlling for IQ. In only three of the 23 classes were these partials correlations statistically significant.

Everston, Emmer, and Clements (1980) provide data on the importance of time-on-task for achievement for junior high school students. Using content-specific English and math tests and controlling for CAT scores, the partial correlation of time-on-task and English score was computed to be .20 and laws .34 for mathematics. The unit of analysis here was the class ($n = 150$).

Karweit and Slavin (1981) report the effects of student engaged time from a pretest-observation-posttest design where the observation interval was about 3 months. Six mixed second and third grade classes and 12 mixed fourth and fifth grade classes comprised the sample. Within each class, the attentive behavior of six students was observed for a period of at least 10 consecutive school days. Achievement was measured by the mathematics subtest of the CTBS and by chapter-specific tests. In regressions examining the effects of engaged minutes, inconsistent results were obtained. Significant engagement effects were found in grade 2/3 for the standardized tests, but not the chapter tests, Grade 4/5 had significant effects for the chapter tests but not the standardized tests.

Summarizing the results of these studies of time-on-task and achievement, we found the engagement measures to be related to achievement in the range of .25 to .58. Once initial ability was controlled, the partial correlation between achievement and engagement was found to be between .09 and .43. In terms of the proportion of variance explained, the engagement variables were found to explain between 1 and 10% of the unique variance in achievement outcomes.

What conclusions can one reach about the importance of time-on-task for achievement from these studies? In light of this evidence, is increasing the school term a reasonable strategy for policymakers to pursue in an ef-

fort to increase student achievement? We note that very few negative effects of time-on-task on achievement are found, and we would agree that it would probably be helpful (and certainly not harmful) to encourage teachers to minimize time wasted and to try to increase student engagement. However, as researchers attempting to discover the critical elements of classroom practice, we must be clear about where the strong effects really lie. For a theory of classroom organization, it is of considerable consequence that time-on-task is not so strongly associated with learning after ability is partialled out. We would argue that these findings point toward an explanation of classroom learning based more on accommodating student diversity in readiness for instruction and rate of learning and on quality of instruction than on the gross quantity of instruction delivered to or consumed by students. In other words, if time-on-task is not a strong factor influencing achievement, then we must consider how quality and level of instruction might influence learning. In addition, if time-on-task in and of itself is not a strong predictor of achievement, we need to seriously question the wisdom of enacting policies aimed at school improvement by sheer increases in instructional time. A wiser policy would aim first at increasing the use of available opportunity time and second at increasing the appropriateness of instructional time.

Summary and Discussion

Recent commission reports and studies of time and learning have focused our attention on the importance of school time. Numerous states are presently considering lengthening the school day and/or the school term. On the surface such action may seem worthwhile, but a closer look at the research results on which these proposals are based reveals weak and inconsistent effects for allocated time and engagement rate.

Even had the effects been significant in every subtest across all grades, the results could not be interpreted to mean that all the variance accounted for could be actually manipulated were time allocations changed. It is not clear how much of the variation in time-on-task is actually open to manipulation. Students differ in their willingness and tendencies to stay on task. Some of this variation can probably be altered, but certainly not all of it can be. Similarly, teachers use time well or poorly. Some teaching practices may use time more efficiently, but even with the same teaching techniques some teachers will simply be more efficient in their time use and more aware of what is going on in their classroom than are other teachers. Thus, like student variation in engaged time, teacher variation in the use of time is not entirely open to manipulation.

Sources of differences in time-on-task may not be uniform, making alteration of time-on-task a less general enterprise than it first appears. The factors responsible for loss of learning time in one classroom or school may not be problematic on another setting. Student absence, for example, continues to comprise a major loss of instructional time for thousands of students in urban schools. But in many other schools, student absenteeism is not a problem of the same magnitude.

The inconsistencies of the research results, the often weak effects for time, the concentration of studies on elementary school populations, and the diversity of sources and problem with school time all suggest that blanket increases of time for schooling are at best likely to have an uncertain outcome. The addition of raw number of hours obviously does don't guarantee that the additional time will be used to any better purpose than the present time is used. Because resources for school and for school improvement are limited, decisions to act in one direction often foreclose pursuit of other actions. In this case, other options—such as implementing what we already know about effective instruction and classroom management—seem to have a much greater potential payoff than simply keeping the school doors open for a longer period of time.

REFERENCES

Bell, M.L., & Davidson, C.W. (1976). Relationship between pupil-on-task performance and pupil achievement. *The Journal of Educational Research, 69,* 172–176.

Bloom, B.S. (1976). *Human characteristics and school learning.* New York: McGraw-Hill.

Borg, W. (1980). Time and school learning. In C. Denham & A. Lieberman (Eds.), *Time to learn.* Washington, DC: National Institute of Education.

Carroll, J. (1963). A model for school learning. *Teacher's College Record, 64.* 723-733.

Cobb, J.A. (1976). Relationships of discrete classroom behaviors to 4th grade academic growth. *Journal of Educational Psychology, 63,* 74–80.

Denham, C., & Lieberman, A. (1980). *Time to learn.* Washington, DC: National institute of Education.

Dishaw, M.M. (1977). Descriptions of allocated time to content areas for B-C period. In *Beginning teacher evaluation study* (Technical Note IV-2b). San Francisco: Far West Laboratory for Educational Research and Development.

Edmindston, R.W., & Rhoades, B.J. (1969). Predicting achievement. *Journal of Educational Research, 51,* 177–180.

Everston, C.M., Emmer, E.T., & Clements, B.S. (1980). *The junior high classroom organizational study: Summary of training procedures and methodology* (R&D Report 6101). Austin: University of Texas, R&D Center for Teacher Education.

Fisher, C.W., Berliner, D., Filbey, N., Marliave, R., Cahen, L.S., & Dishaw, M. (1980). Teaching behaviors, academic learning time, and student achievement: An Overview. In C. Denham & A. Lieberman (Eds.), *Time to learn.* Washington, DC: National Institute of Education.

Harnischfeger, A., & Wiley, D.E. (1984, April). *Time and learning: A statewide policy analysis.* Paper presented at the Annual Meeting of the American Educational Research Association, New Orleans.

Hawkinson, H. (1984). Hatch school-not at risk. *Phi Delta Kappan, 66* (3), 181-182.

Karweit, N. (1976). A reanalysis of the effect of quantity of schooling on achievement. *Sociology of Education, 49,* 236-246.

Karweit, N., & Slavin, R.E. (1981). Measurement and modeling choices in studies of time and learning. *American Educational Research Journal, 18* (2), 157–171.

Lahaderne, H.M. (1967, February). *Attitudinal and intellectual correlates of attention: A study of four sixth grade classrooms.* Paper presented at the Annual Meeting of the American Educational Research Association, New York.

Lord, F.M. (1960). Large-sample covariance analysis when the control variable is fallible. *Journal of American Statistical Association, 55,* 307–321.

Stevenson, H. (1983). Comparison of Japanese, Taiwanese and American mathematics achievement. Stanford, CA: Center for advanced study in the Behavioral Sciences.

Walberg, H. (1984). Improving the productivity of America's schools. *Educational Leadership, 41* (8), 19–27.

Walberg, H., & Frederick, W.C. (1983). Instructional time and learning. *Encyclopedia of Educational Research,* 917–924.

Wiley, D.E., & Harnischfeger, A. (1974). *Explosion of a myth: Quantity of schooling and exposure to instruction, major educational vehicles.* Studies of educative processes (Report 8). Chicago: University of Chicago.

Section IV
Teaching as a Profession
Introduction by Thomas A. Mulkeen*

There was a time when society seemed to change very slowly. Institutions and value systems were relatively stable, clearly understood, and generally supported throughout the community. This is no longer the case. Pervasive forces are now reshaping American society. We are now in the process of shifting away from a traditional mass production economy to one stressing high technology, service, information, and communication. The new electronic, biological, nuclear, and solar technologies are transforming the lives of Americans at home and in the workplace. In the coming decades we will see an increased information flow, rapid change and impermanence in the workplace, a new family structure, the decentralization of institutions and systems, people-centered organizations, and major demographic shifts.

The American education system, designed in the early part of this century for a mass production economy, is ill prepared to respond to the pervasive forces that are now reshaping American society. The reshaping of the occupational structure, the technological revolution and the internationalization of the economy requires a basic restructuring of an educational system designed for an industrial economy. With the shift to an information economy comes the need for new learning skills. Mastery of the curricula can no longer be the prime educational goal. Schools must strengthen the analytical and communicative skills of students who need to acquire critical thinking skills. Students must become active learners, busily engaged in the process of bringing new knowledge and new ways of knowing to bear on a widening range of increasingly difficult problems. The focus of schooling must shift from teaching to learning, from passive acquisition of facts and routines to the active application of ideas to problems. Education must teach us how to learn, how to cope with change, how to build a body of knowledge that endures throughout life, and how to adapt to a changing work environment. That transition changes the role of the teacher.

The likelihood of continuing change in society has profound implications for teachers. Clearly, the increasing information flow negates the traditional notion of teaching content for mastery. Students will, in the coming years, need to acquire critical thinking, decision making, and communication skills with an emphasis on the cognitive processes of inquisitiveness, sequential thinking and problem solving. This suggests that the role of the teacher as the source of information and as disseminator of knowledge will have to change to one in which teachers become facilitators of learning. This also implies that teachers must become lifelong learners as the knowledge required to do their work changes with new challenges and the progress of science and technology. Teachers will not come to school knowing all they have to know, but knowing how to figure out what they need to know, where to get it, and how to help others make meaning of it.

In a world where knowledge can no longer be acquired once and for all, where technology will play an increasing role in the educational process, where the forces of change in the social fabric have overcome the forces of continuity, teachers' initial preparation cannot be expected to sustain them throughout their professional life. It is clear that professional educators cannot acquire in their initial preparation all the knowledge and competencies that will be helpful during future years because some of the skills that will be needed are not now recognized or have yet to be developed. The increasing information flow suggests that the distinction between preservice education as a period of intensive training followed by an in-service period when training is less extensive or even haphazard is no longer valid. Education for teaching in the modern

*Dr. Thomas A. Mulkeen is an Associate Professor at Fordham University.

world must be a lifelong process, and there must be an institutional framework that reinforces and directs the continuing education of school personnel. This requires a basic reassessment of how teachers are prepared and promotes thinking about the whole character of the profession.

New policies are needed for teacher education that recognize its pivotal role in strengthening the teaching profession. Sweeping changes are required both in the institutional structure of teacher education and in the continuing education of the practicing professional. Taking into account the emerging economic trends and gleaning the best elements from current research, our authors offer a series of interesting commentaries on the reform movements attempting to transform the teaching profession.

In the first article, Dal Lawrence presents a discussion of the Toledo Plan. He offers peer evaluation as a way to transform schools from the traditional factory model to the professional model so desperately needed and envisioned by many of the current critics of public education. In the second article, Gregory Anrig discusses the pros and cons of state-required testing of teachers, a movement that is spreading to nearly every state.

The third article is N.L. Gage's update of his seminal work, "The Scientific Basis of Teaching," which discusses current research about teaching and its effects on student achievement. The next two articles discuss preservice teacher education programs and examine models designed to promote teacher effectiveness.

The article by Edwin M. Bridges shifts attention to methods of coping with incompetent teachers, while Paula E. Lester writes about teacher job satisfaction. Edward A. Wynne examines the central role that philosophic issues play in teaching, and Brian R. Metke discusses how a "quality circle" can become a valuable human resource in our schools.

Each of our authors is presently active in the movement to transform the teaching profession, and their commentary highlights key issues that educators must contend with today.

New York Teacher's Staff

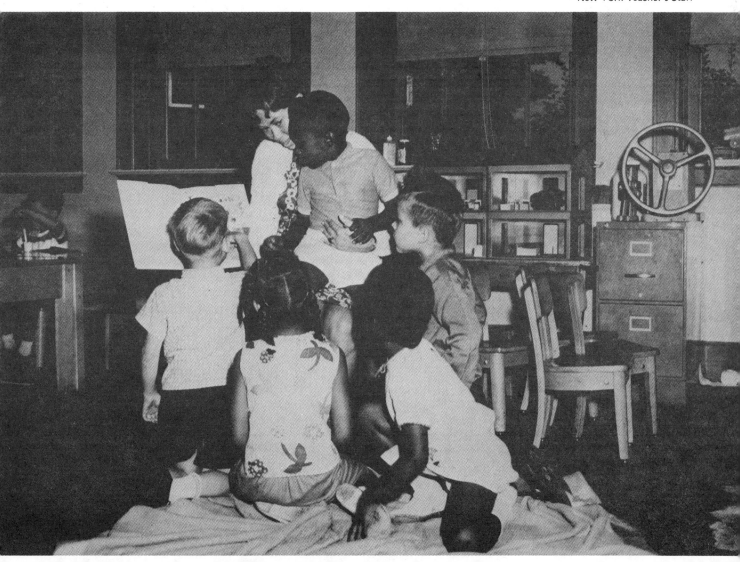

Chapter 22
The Toledo Plan: A Five Year Perspective
Dal Lawrence*

Ask teachers if they want peer review as the American Federation of Teachers has and forty percent answer "no"; another thirty percent only slightly favor it.[1] In Toledo, our twenty-five hundred AFT members are ready to start their sixth year of a tough peer review process that has attracted a remarkable amount of attention nationwide, as well as interest from Australians and Canadians.

It is not surprising that teachers, like other employees, would reject the notion that one's next-door neighbor should evaluate his or her work. Yet, when we asked our members at the end of the third year of our intern-intervention program who they felt should be responsible for removing from the profession those colleagues with severely deficient performance, by an eleven-to-one margin they said "the union." The survey received 1,315 responses, and out of the one hundred questions asked, the "peer review" question garnered the greatest consensus.

Are teachers in Toledo different from teachers elsewhere? Of course not, but teacher ownership of peer programs is uncommon. For most teachers peer review is untraditional and frequently threatening. "Review" implies evaluation. The form it takes and the context in which it is explained is crucial to the process of getting teachers to accept peer evaluation at the elementary and secondary levels. Personnel evaluation in public schools has not been performed with distinction which further complicates acceptance. Quite often peer review amounts to little more than administrators asking teachers to snoop on their colleagues for all the wrong reasons. Little wonder teachers are suspicious.

Teacher evaluation performed by colleagues does not have to be threatening or disgusting. A system of peer mentoring and evaluation, however, that is not seen by teachers as a process they own most certainly will continue to be viewed with suspicion. Typically, peer review is a process where management selected teachers join principals and/or college professors in rating another teacher. The teacher participant in the team makes one-

third of the rating decision while management arbitrarily decides any subsequent termination question. The rest of the teachers feel no responsibility at all because they have no more at stake in the outcome than if the review had been carried out traditionally by a principal or supervisor. Ownership is missing.

How one confronts the peer review issue is critical. Have you ever met a teacher who enjoyed working next door to a hopelessly incompetent colleague? I never have, and I take the time to ask this question everywhere I go. Have you ever met a teacher who didn't want to participate in a profession where dignity, respect and reasonable wages were the result of high standards? A rare find. There is an overwhelming consensus among teachers that building such a profession is desirable for teacher and student alike. Peer review considered within the context of profession building evokes an entirely different response from the peer review that is absent this larger purpose.

Peer review must be considered a basic building block in all efforts to create a real teaching profession with serious professional responsibilities. Building a profession for teachers means reshaping the governance of public schools and reallocating many competence judgments to those who actively practice the profession. Peer review without the responsibility of policing competence standards makes no more sense than calling for professional teachers in one breath and then defending school management's inalienable right to make all important decisions in the next.

That is one of the most significant lessons we learned in Toledo. We did not set out to establish a peer review program; rather, we wanted to build a profession for teachers where none existed. We wanted to shift the traditional administrative responsibility for deciding who was good enough to teach school to the new profession we envisioned. Internships and self-policing of clearly de-

*Dal Lawrence is President of the Toledo Federation of Teachers, AFT.

fined performance standards were two obvious starting points. If we had asked our members in 1973 if they would support "peer review," there probably would not be a Toledo Plan today. But our peer evaluation was always part of a process to build a profession for teachers, and where better to start than to decide who was acceptable as a colleague? Indeed, where else would one start?

A detailed explanation of the mechanics of the intern and intervention programs has been presented elsewhere.[2] A brief description of the plan is presented here as background. An internship of one year is served by all new Toledo teachers, many long-term substitutes, and a few experienced teachers returning to the district after a prolonged absence. Carefully selected, excellent, experienced teachers—we call them consultants—are released full time to devote all their energies and talent to the eight to ten interns assigned to them. These consultants participate as active mentor-evaluators for three years and then are returned to their regular teaching duties. The consultants perform this task in behalf of all their colleagues. Consultants devote twenty to thirty hours each semester to each intern and then in March recommend renewal or nonrenewal of the intern's contract. It is through their deliberations that the fate of each intern is determined.

A board of review hears the recommendations and supporting documentation and decides to accept or reject the consultant's judgment. Five of the review panelists are union members; four are from top management positions. As the union president, I appoint four other teachers to the panel and, on alternate years, chair the board. The district's assistant superintendent for personnel shares that responsibility with me and appoints three management representatives. As alternate chairpersons, we jointly make intern assignments, decide which consultants to use, and determine which consultant applicants will be accepted into the program. The panel must achieve six votes to reject a consultant's recommendation no matter what the recommendation is, thereby avoiding five-to-four splits. Our decisions are passed on to the superintendent, who, in turn, delivers them to the school board as required by Ohio law. All of our decisions have been accepted by the superintendent and the board.

The board of review does not rubber stamp consultant recommendations. Questions from the panel are sharp and to the point. We want to know just how firm the consultant's belief is in what is being recommended. Does the documentation support the conclusion? Do the evaluations show uniformity when similar circumstances exist? Are occasional charges of personality conflict valid? Has the consultant followed the procedures and observed the standards for performance accurately? It is a tense and demanding experience for consultants.

During the second year of Toledo's two-year probationary period, principals evaluate beginning teachers by using the same criteria that is used during the intern year. During the first year they have no responsibility for interns, although a report of compliance with school and district rules is given to the consultant to be used at his or her discretion. It should be noted that we have yet to see a negative evaluation during the second year. Interns who fail to meet district standards do not get a second chance. Our internship, we feel, successfully "weeds out" those who can't handle the job.

In five years we have worked with 314 interns. Twelve have been nonrenewed—about 4 percent. One intern was terminated because of concern for student safety. Others not awarded a second contract are allowed to finish their intern year. By way of comparison, Toledo fired only one new teacher in the five years prior to the intern program.

In the strictest sense, the internship is not an example of peer review. Interns are not thought of as peers. The union charges each intern half the regular dues and does not represent them in terminations or nonrenewals, although other representational services are provided. Dr. Philip Schlecty of the University of Louisville has pointed out that there is nothing wrong with considering beginning teachers inferior as long as there is a procedure in place to overcome the condition.[3] We agree.

Mentoring coupled with evaluation best describes our approach to initiating beginners to the profession we are building. If after seven months of intensive mentoring an intern shows little aptitude for the classroom, he or she will not be practicing in Toledo. Teachers have a vested interest in competence, and here we have made a commitment to screen out of our profession, and our union, those who do not measure up.

The internship represents a shared governance arrangement, but with clearly defined responsibilities. This shared governance is unique to the Toledo Plan, but we feel it must be duplicated if reform efforts are to succeed elsewhere. The internship represents a basic governance reform. The benefit is the recognition Toledo teachers have that competence is important to each of them, and that each of them bears that responsibility. They have ownership.

Intervention is peer review in its purest sense. Experienced teachers who are conspicuously dysfunctional, once identified, must accept peer assistance or face termination. Consulting teachers typically are assigned one or two intervention cases in addition to their intern load. Consultants are not told what to do or how long they may take to bring the intervenee back to acceptable performance levels. It should be stressed that the career of the teacher in trouble is completely in the hands of the consulting teacher.

Identification of troubled teachers requires agreement between the principal and the elected union school committee chaired by an elected building representative. Authorization to meet and cast the two votes is granted only if the president of the union and the assistant superintendent for personnel agree to proceed. (There are other programs of assistance available to such an employee, i.e. the Employee Assistance Program and voluntary confidential mentoring.) The dysfunctional teacher is permitted to appear before his school committee and the principal and can formally protest placement in intervention. Of interest is the fact that two-thirds of the interventions have been initiated by teachers, not principals, something we did not foresee five years ago.

If a formal protest is filed, an arbitrator from the University of Toledo law school reviews the case and makes a binding decision as to whether we followed our identification procedures properly or whether intervention is the appropriate avenue for correcting the individual's deficiencies. Overall competence is not judged because that is not the arbitrator's area of expertise.

When the consultant has succeeded, or failed, and further work with the dysfunctional colleague is not judged appropriate, a status report is issued—typically fifty to one hundred pages of documentation and discussion. The status report says: "This is what I found"; "This is what I did"; and "This is why the relationship is ending." Consultants do not recommend a future course of action in intervention cases.

A negative report invariably triggers termination proceedings. The union then has its grievance personnel review the status report and interview the teacher, the consultant, and any other persons who might be able to provide information. Those four grievance people next recommend to the seven union officers whether representation should be offered or denied. The officers vote on the final decision. Intervention is not something the union takes lightly. To deny representation is to deny arbitration under our contract. Yet, only once have we decided to represent.

These are the mechanics of the intern-intervention program. The Toledo Plan places total responsibility for insuring competence on the shoulders of teachers, where it belongs. Management's role is a joint regulatory one. In retrospect, we can see just how radical our approach was and how close to failure we came. But the concept was right and the people were committed. The idea worked, but not without trouble.

The 1981 contract of the Toledo Federation of Teachers stated only that there would be an intern-intervention program that could be cancelled by either party with thirty days' notice. It still says that. Guidelines for the program were committed to paper and signed as a sidebar agreement.

Precedents established by the board of review govern

the relationship. No one should try to "bargain" such a detailed agreement. It is task enough just to bargain the commitment; in our case, that took nine years of bargaining. Once the commitment was made, we had precious few moments to argue about who was in charge. Credit and control ceased to be issues. We shook on it and went to work.

Surprisingly, few things went wrong, but those that did presented critical challenges. During the first year, an intern who was nonrenewed went to a school board member whom she knew and asked to be given a second chance. The review panel and superintendent refused to budge; the board member dropped the matter. In the second year, an intern, the husband of one of the union's officers, was nonrenewed. She is still an officer and he is not teaching in Toledo. It was becoming clear that relatives, friendships, sex, and race would not be criteria for success. Competence would.

Early in our experience, one teacher was accused of making inappropriate comments of a sexual nature to some of his female students who were of a different race. Teachers in intervention are not immune from disciplinary proceedings. During the subsequent hearing, parents and activists demonstrated in the hallway while we debated the merits of the charge. The consultant had not yet decided to end the intervention, and the evidence of sexual misconduct was shaky at best. Nevertheless, the district's attorney recommended immediate suspension and termination. We had our first crisis. Interventions were not supposed to end this way.

Short of clear misconduct warranting termination, intervention was to proceed until the consultant terminated the relationship. We had agreed that the consultant would have that jurisdiction, although the review panel retains the right to question the progress of the intervenee. The panel had received oral and written reports indicating that progress in this case had been minimal, but the consultant believed more time was needed.

It was clear that intervention could not work as planned if management felt no constraint in its traditional right to initiate termination proceedings at will. The pressure of the demonstration had interrupted the peer review process. I drafted a letter of notice canceling the entire intern-intervention program.

This occurred late in our third year. The Rand Corporation had studied the Toledo Plan and had given it high marks. Newspapers had picked up the story and we were anything but inconspicuous. Rand had cited a study by Charles Kerchner and Douglas Mitchell in which they had traced the evolution and maturity of collective bargaining relationships in public school systems.[4] According to Rand, "The Toledo approach, however, moves beyond traditional collective bargaining toward a professional conception of teaching."[5] We apparently had reached a kind of labor-management millennium that Kerchner and Mitchell had only speculated about with some degree of skepticism. Telling management the Toledo Plan was over was not one of the few pleasures of running a teachers' union.

A meeting was arranged in the offices of one of Toledo's larger law firms. The attorney who represented the district was a partner in the firm and also represented the *Toledo Blade,* the city's only newspaper. A public relations disaster was imminent, if nothing else. I was furious.

How cold this same lawyer who helped me set intern-intervention in motion just three years earlier now show so little sensitivity to its nuances? The meeting was suitably tense as we each explained our point of view. Charges of caving in to community n'er-do-wells or ignoring the welfare of children were hurled back and forth without result. I presented my letter and left.

An accommodation was reached the next day. The teacher stayed in intervention but at a different school. A few weeks later the consultant issued a status report and it was negative. The teacher was given a termination notice and, against my better judgment, the union officers voted four to three to defend him in arbitration, which we subsequently lost.

We had passed our most serious crisis, however. Henceforth, consultants would determine the length of intervention. That new-found confidence in the judgment of consulting teachers has not been misplaced. Both union and management maintain a respectful distance now and routinely perform their separate functions in the dismissal and representation decisions. The concept of shared responsibility has a much sharper focus.

Does peer review work? In five years there have been twenty-six teachers placed in intervention. Five are still in the program. Eight have successfully completed the transition back to acceptable performance norms—three to an astonishing degree. There have been five terminations, and eight others have either resigned, retired, or, as in one case, transferred to the nonteaching bargaining unit at his own request. Without intervention, most of these teachers would still be in the classroom today; none of them would have received assistance.

During the five years we have worked with several hundred teachers aspiring to full status as a Toledo teacher through the internship. None have turned out to be problem teachers. None have had to be disciplined. Most did not feel threatened after their first encounter with a consultant. Joan Schmitz is typical. "I would characterize the role of my consulting teacher as a 'profession parent,'" she told me. "I felt that my survival in the teaching field was directly attributable to my consult-

ing teacher's years of experience and personality."

Only twice have we found consultant recommendations that were obviously inaccurate. In one instance, the recommendation was for a second one-year contract, but the supporting data and rating indicated the opposite. We suspended the consultant and placed the intern in the program for a second year, the only time this has been necessary. (The intern was nonrenewed at the end of the second year.) Another recommendation called for a new contract, but the panel discovered deficiencies in the intern's work that led to a nine-to-zero vote for nonrenewal. Two obvious errors in 314 presentations, both corrected, is a credible record.

Two interns have had excellent student rapport but were nonrenewed because their knowledge of subject matter was deficient. Without question, those cases would have passed muster in most districts, as they would have in ours five years ago.

Teachers generally have negative feelings about evaluations. Management claims that evaluation, usually on an annual basis, leads to better teaching and higher morale do not stand up under scrutiny. Part of the reason is that the wrong people do the evaluating–people who are no longer teaching. Principals are busy and usually cannot devote the time necessary to improve techniques. Areas of expertise are often impossible to match. Administrators have control over too many working conditions for teachers to feel comfortable with an employer-employee mentoring system. Seventy-five individuals using the same standards and criteria do not produce the same reliability as do ten or twelve evaluators. One-a-year perfunctory reviews are a classic outgrowth of the traditional factory model of school governance, which has produced considerably less than widespread confidence in our nation's schools.

The factory model assumes that teachers are line workers–hired hands–to be supervised not by their peers, but by their superiors. Since the disappearance of the one-room schoolhouse, this boss-worker relationship has dominated the decision-making process in public schools with devastating results. It is peculiar, yet understandable, that teachers feel no responsibility for the woes of public education. Why should they when all of the key decision-making apparatus is in someone else's hands, collective bargaining notwithstanding? And, yet, who is in the best position to improve the quality of instruction? Teachers, of course.

People who have responsibility tend to act responsibly. The Japanese have recognized that simple reality with stunning results. College educated people tend not to be very happy working in routine subordinate roles. That is one big reason we don't see many former teachers working on auto assembly lines even though the money is better. It also accounts for a substantial number of teacher dropouts each year. Teaching is too removed from those responsibilities that can make a difference in the quality of the workplace and in the quality of the product.

Teachers do not think in terms of collegiality. Standards of practice do not enter into many lounge discussions. All that is someone else's business. Career advancement inevitably involves a change of careers—from teaching to administering. Nothing about the factory system encourages competence and responsibility except discipline in the most traditional labor-management sense.

Pride is missing. It must be restored before that elusive "quality education" can be achieved. Teachers need a sense of who they are; pride in belonging to a profession they can call their own; and the need to feel and exercise responsibility for that profession and for the profession's standards and competence. Traditional governance of public education in America effectively blocks these reforms even though they are desperately needed.

Little wonder then that building a profession for classroom practitioners meets with teacher approval when they perceive ownership. That is precisely why our review panel has one more teacher member than does management. It is crucial that consultants not be viewed as management trainees. The three-year rotation cycle is important. (We also found that three years of the kind of pressure the program demands is quite enough for the consultants.) Seven consultants are now back in the classroom—much to the amazement of some of their colleagues. Only one, at the conclusion of this fifth year, has been employed in a management position.

What makes sense is not always easy to bring about. School administrators are not eager to reform themselves out of the special status they hold in the traditional governance model, no matter what problems plague public education. Lower level administrators are particularly sensitive to any reforms that strike at the "boss's" turf. For nine years, principals, more than anyone else, blocked the Toledo Plan; but by the end of the 1981–1982 school year we were getting requests from principals to have consultants evaluate the intern's second year, too. That came as a surprise.

I rejected the idea because teacher evaluators are human: give them a second year to make a decision and most decisions will be made the second year. And what about shared governance? We could not be viewed as totally usurping management's role without discouraging other districts from trying the Toledo Plan. Two years is not needed to screen out those who lack aptitude for teaching, especially after the inordinate amount of time spent in undergraduate pedagological training. One year

was enough to accomplish the goal of deciding who is competent enough to practice and join us as colleagues. Profession building does not have to mean unfettered control of all personnel functions by the union.

Line administrators were won over after vigorous resistance by carefully choosing top-notch people for consultants and then showing the skeptics that the new system worked. Our inservices address the sensitivities principals have when consultants first appear at their doorstep. The turnaround in attitude has been remarkable. Today principals and supervisors have their own intern and intervention programs at their request.

What about the argument over whether mentoring and evaluation should be placed in the hands of the same person? Can a consultant be a "professional parent" and an evaluator, too? Personally, I regard separation of these duties questionable even when traditional governance is assumed. In Toledo, neither management nor the union would consider separating these functions.

The intern concept is designed to develop professional skills and eliminate those who fail to reach our defined standards. Separating evaluation from the professional growth function would make no sense at all. What would happen in a court of law or before an arbitrator if growth is evident (as it almost always is) and a second person judged it insufficient! Why would a teacher union, or any other professional group, consent to an arrangement where its member created a record for a nonpractitioner to use against one of its members? Dividing the growth and competence issues would destroy the unique vested interest teachers have in inducting only competent people into their profession. It is far better to fully accept the decision-making responsibility or avoid peer review altogether. In our experience we have not found that the evaluation function inhibits professional growth. Evaluation judgments in December, and finally in March, are a natural conclusion to the mentoring that has preceded.

As I pointed out earlier, some "peer review" schemes popularized by school management involve teams of evaluators most often comprised of a college person, an administrator, and the teacher peer. There might be merit in such arrangements if profession building is not the context for teacher evaluation. For those wedded to the factory model, it can be said that innovation is apparent but little else: there is no ownership, no profession building, no reform, precious little mentoring, and too many fingers in the stew.

In the final analysis, interns have to feel the extra effort in trying to gain a foothold in the teaching profession was worth the effort. We ask interns to evaluate the work of consultants anonymously after their final evaluation. Each year 94 to 96 percent have rated the program "good" or "excellent" with more excellent ratings than good. Despite some understandable fear about serving an internship, the experience of being an intern is quite positive.

The various commissions and reports calling for the professionalization of teaching and overall educational excellence present the best opportunity we are likely to have to restore the credibility of a public education. A management that is wise will seize this opportunity to transform schools from the traditional factory model to the professional model so desperately needed and envisioned by most thoughtful critics of public education. It is not good enough to lose half of our new teachers by their seventh year in teaching. There is no excuse for mediocrity in a democratic society's public school system. The nation is at risk when we entrust our elementary and secondary classrooms to the least talented high school and college students. It is not a good idea to run schools like factories, especially when the product is too often shoddy.

Happily, the solution is not an either/or proposition: ether give the schools to the teachers or see them doomed to continued mediocrity. The solution is to create for teachers a profession of which they can be proud by clearly delineating those responsibilities that their new profession is best equipped to carry out, while continuing other management roles best left to non-practitioners. That is what Carnegie and the Holmes Group envision;

and that is why I believe the Toledo Plan for peer review and internship has contributed significantly to the reforms on the national agenda today.

FOOTNOTES

1.   An unpublished January, 1985 poll of Florida teachers, conducted for the American Federation of Teachers.

2.   Good explanations can be found in the following publications: Waters, Cheryl M., and Wyatt, Terry L., "Toledo's Internship: The Teacher's Role In Excellence," *Phi Delta Kappan,* January, 1985, pp. 365–367.

McCormick, Kathleen, "Swept Away," *American School Board Journal,* July, 1985, pp. 19–25.

Lawrence, Dal, "The Toledo Plan for Peer Evaluation and Assistance," *Education and Urban Society,* Sage Publications, Beverly Hills, Vol. 17, #13, May, 1985, pp. 345–54.

Lawrence, Dal, "Teacher Excellence: Teachers Take Charge," *American Educator,* Spring, 1984, pp. 22–29.

3.   Schlecty address to the 1985 "Quality Educational Standards in Teaching: (QUEST) conference of the American Federation of Teachers. Transcripts and tapes available from the AFT.

4.   Mitchell, Douglas E., and Kerchner, Charles T., "Labor Relations and Teacher Policy," *Handbook of Teaching and Policy,* Longman, New York, 1983, pp. 220–30.

5.   Wise, Arthur E.; Darling-Hammond, Linda; McLaughlin, Milbrew W.; Bernstein, Harriet T., *Case Studies for Teacher Evaluation: A Study of Effective Practice,* Rand Corporation, Santa Monica, June, 1984, p. 132.

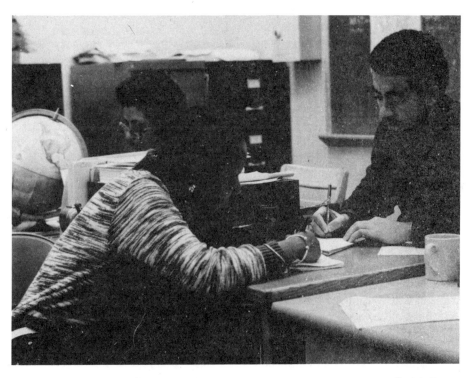

Paul A. Basso

Chapter 23
Teacher Education and Teacher Testing: The Rush to Mandate
Gregory R. Anrig*

Some of the fastest-moving changes in these years of education reform are in the area of teacher testing. In only about five years, state-required testing for those who aspire to enter teacher preparation programs or to become certified has spread from a handful of states—mainly in the Southeast—to become a nationwide trend that now involves 38 states, with seven more currently considering teacher-testing requirements. In 1984 alone, nine states enacted teacher-testing laws or regulations.

The race to begin teacher testing is not only nation-wide but across-the-board. Twenty-one states require students to pass a test before entering a teacher education program. Thirty-two states have (or, by 1988, will have) a testing requirement for certification. A smaller number of states also test at the completion of teacher training, for recertification, or for advanced certification under career ladder/merit pay plans.[1]

The teacher testing movement goes well-beyond the NTE Program, administered by the Educational Testing Service (ETS). Though 25 states currently use one or another of the NTE tests, other tests used by states include the Scholastic Aptitude Test, those of the American College Testing Program, the California Achievement Test, and state-developed tests (used in Alabama, Arizona, California, Connecticut, Florida, Georgia, and Oklahoma). Teacher testing is upon us, and the issues it raises transcend any one of the tests.

What Tests Can Do

There is a place for teacher tests on the American educational scene. National opinion surveys indicate strong public support and strong teacher support for requiring satisfactory test performance as a condition for entering the teaching profession. A 1984 Gallup poll reported that 89% of the public and almost two-thirds of the teachers polled favored state examinations for beginning teachers.[2]

Properly developed and validated, teacher tests can measure the academic knowledge of prospective teachers. Within the limits of any standardized paper-and-pencil examination, teacher tests can demonstrate that a prospective teacher has a basic knowledge of the subject (or grade level) that he or she plans to teach, has the minimum pedagogical knowledge that experienced practitioners and teacher educators deem necessary for beginning teachers, and demonstrates certain basic communication skills necessary to instruct children.

These are reasonable expectations—standards, if you will—for a prospective teacher to meet before being certified by the state. Just as lawyers, physicians, and those in scores of occupations must demonstrate basic knowledge of their fields in order to qualify for state licenses, so too it is reasonable to expect similar competence from teachers. State licenses are a means of consumer protection; school children are the primary consumers of education an are entitled to such protection.

What Tests Cannot Do

No standardized test that I know of can accurately measure such qualities as dedication, motivation, perseverance, caring, sensitivity, or integrity. Yet, when we remember outstanding teachers from our own school days, those are among the qualities that made them excellent. We must admit the limits of tests and the restricted range of qualities that they can measure. Moreover, we should recognize that tests can present and measure only a sample of the knowledge required for teaching.

No test results guarantees that a prospective teacher will succeed and become a really good teacher in the classroom. While no teacher can succeed and be very effective without a strong knowledge of subject matter and of the skills of teaching, professional performance

*Dr. Gregory R. Anrig is president of the Educational Testing Service, Princeton, NJ. Reprinted with permission of *Phi Delta Kappan*, February, 1986.

requires more than academic knowledge. Remember that many of the convicted Watergate defendants were lawyers who had successfully passed the bar exam. Ignorance of the law does not account for their actions.

All of this suggests that policy makers should keep teacher tests in their proper perspective. As in other fields of professional licensure and certification, tests in education are important aids for insuring that new entrants have mastered the basic knowledge relevant to the job. They can also be useful to candidates (and to those who prepare them) as ways to identify strengths and weaknesses in their preparation.

Troubling Signs

As was true in some cases with state competency testing for students in the 1970s, the rush to legislate excellence through teacher testing is raising some troubling questions and leading to some decisions that are educationally unsound.

One such decision, now law in several states, makes continued accreditation of teacher preparation programs dependent on the test performance of the prospective teachers they enroll. The Educational Testing Service has testified against using teacher tests in this way. Such use fails to recognize that from 60% to 80% of the college preparation received by prospective teachers is in academic departments, not in the college or department of education. On the NTE Core Battery, for example, more students seem to have difficulty qualifying on the Test of general Knowledge than on the Test of Professional Knowledge.

Accountability for teacher education should rest with the entire college or university, not solely with the teacher preparation unit. If significant numbers of prospective teachers graduating from a college or university are failing to meet the state's minimum standards for certification, the state certainly has a right and an obligation to question such a trend. The process of review, however, should conform to good accreditation practice, including the opportunity for institutional self-examination and external validation and the allotment of reasonable time in which to improve institutional performance. From the time an institution is placed on probation, some states allow only two years for graduating seniors to meet a predetermined standard of success on state certification tests. I believe that this practice raises some or the same questions of fairness that have been raised in court challenges of testing programs for high school graduation.

A second area of concern regarding teacher testing has arisen in Arkansas and Texas. In the course of enacting comprehensive education reform bills, the legislatures in both states included a requirement that all practicing teachers—regardless of years of service and ratings by their school supervisors—would have to pass a one-time "functional academic skills" or "literacy" test in order to retain their teaching certificates. Such a testing program is unprecedented for any other occupation requiring state licensure or certification.

Certainly no one wants illiterate or otherwise incompetent teachers in the classroom. However, just as with accreditation, there are reasonable and educationally sound procedures for addressing this problem through careful supervision and valuation. Then, in the absence of improvement and with appropriate due process, a teacher's employment may be terminated. To put an experienced teacher's professional career on the line solely on the basis of a mandatory, one-time test is both an injustice to the teacher and a misuse of the test. The Educational Testing Service and the NTE Policy Council, in an unprecedented action for test development organizations, have refused to allow the use of NTE tests for this purpose in either Texas or Arkansas.

A third area that must be of profound concern to all of us in education is the effect of the teacher testing movement on the access of minorities to the teaching profession. ETS has recently published two research reports: one on the general impact of state testing policies on the teaching profession and the other specifically on the impact on teacher selection of the use or the NTE tests by the states.[3] These reports present data that documents the effect of current state testing policies on the access of blacks and Hispanics to the teaching profession.

To understand the dimensions of this problem, let us look at the results of teacher tests in four states. In California, passing rates on the California Basic Educational Skills Tests were 76% for white test-takers, 39% for Hispanic test-takers, and 26% for black test-takers (The California Basic Educational Skills Test is developed by ETS. The Georgia, Oklahoma, and Florida certification tests are not developed by ETS.) In Georgia, 87% of white students passed the Georgia Teacher Certification Test on the first attempt, but only 34% of black students did so. In Oklahoma, the passing rate on the state teacher certification test was 79% for white students, 58% for Hispanic students, and 48% for black students. In Florida, 83% of those who took that state's teacher certification test in 1982 passed each of its four parts. Among black test-takers, however, the pass rate was only 35%. On the Test of Communication Skills in the NTE Core Battery, using national data and the median qualifying score of states that use the test (644), the passing rates would be 94% for whites, 48% for blacks, and 70% for Hispanics.[4]

ETS research reports conclude that, by the year 2000, if there is not significant change in the current status of teacher preparation, the percentage of minorities in the teaching force in the U.S. could be cut almost in half, from its current level of approximately 12%. This decline will be taking place at the same time as the proportion of minority students enrolled in U.S. schools will be increasing dramatically. The growing mismatch between the racial and ethnic composition of the teaching force and that of the student population is a matter with serious social and educational implications for the nation and its schools.

Test Bias or Unequal Opportunity?

A natural and predictable reaction to these differences in the test scores of various ethnic groups is to blame them on racial or ethnic bias in the tests. Similar charges have been leveled against other national tests. Yet something encouraging is happening that counsels against such a reaction. The performance of minority students on the SAT, on the College Board Achievement Tests, on Advanced Placement tests, and on the tests given by the National Assessment of Educational Progress has improved dramatically.[5] Similar patterns of improvement have been reported on state basic skills tests. Minority students are demonstrating that they can and will do better on standardized tests if they are provided better educational opportunities.

Tests certainly can be biased. When they are not, however, they can be useful indicators (used in conjunction with other data) of the quality of education provided to minority and majority students alike. At ETS, we guard against bias in the NTE and other tests we develop. The committees that develop test items are multiracial. Before the new NTE Core Battery was inaugurated in 1982, multiracial panels of experienced classroom teachers, chosen independently by the National Education Association and by the American Federation of Teachers, examined results for every question in the field test of the new Core Battery. (Both teacher organizations are also represented on the NTE Policy Council.) In addition, all ETS test items go through a mandatory sensitivity review process, in which specially trained ETS test development experts examine each item for potential race, sex, or ethnic bias. The NTE and all other tests developed by ETS must conform to the *ETS Standards for Quality and Fairness.*[6]

Even after taking all these precautions, states are required by ETS to conduct their own validity studies before they can use NTE tests. These state validity studies provide an opportunity for an independent review of the tests for potential bias.

It is a regrettable fact that most children from financially poor families—minority or white—attend school in financially poor urban and rural school districts. Working conditions in the schools in such districts are such that the better teachers are more likely to seek em-

ployment in more affluent districts (though many able, dedicated teachers continue to serve in urban and rural districts). As someone whose entire professional career has been committed to the cause of equal educational opportunity, I believe strongly that we do not serve children well or fairly—especially educationally disadvantaged children—when we give them teachers who have not themselves mastered the basic skills that the children must learn before they graduate from high school. If those who aspire to teach can't qualify on state-mandated teacher tests, the solution isn't to do away with the tests. The solution is to improve the education being provided to aspiring teachers. This is what is needed—not permitting poorly prepared teachers, white or minority, to teach children who need and deserve better.

A Challenge for Teacher Education

The combination of a period of reform in education and of the growth of the teacher testing movement provides an opportunity for colleges of teacher education. Up to now the reforms have focused mainly on elementary and secondary schools, but teacher preparation should be at the forefront of reform in higher education.

Teacher preparation is higher education's *primary* responsibility to the schools. Most college and university presidents have by now identified themselves with the drive for school reform in the name of excellence. Their actions and their words, however, have concentrated on what the *schools* should do to improve. The results of teacher testing around the nation should make it abundantly clear what some *institutions of higher education* should do to improve.

Teacher preparation is a responsibility of the entire college or university, not just of the teacher education unit. The performance of aspiring teachers on the growing number of state-required teacher tests reflects on the policies and curriculum of institutions of higher education as a whole. If their performance is less than it should be, the institutions just act to improve that performance.

Some historically black colleges are taking the lead in this aspect of the reform of higher education. These colleges traditionally have prepared a large portion of America's black teachers. They are feeling the impact of the new standards reflected in the teacher testing movement, and so are their students. In collaboration with these historically black colleges, ETS held an invitational conference in December 1984 at which representatives from nine historically black colleges described how their institutions were tackling this new challenge. The approaches differ from college to college, but some common elements are evident:

- *Presidential leadership.* In each case, the college or

university president is visibly involved and strongly committed to sustained improvement.

- *Institutionwide responsibility.* The improvement effort draws on and requires the involvement of all academic departments. In one college, for example, a college wide faculty committee is taking the lead, with faculty discussions and seminars being conducted on an interdisciplinary basis. In one university, the steering committee includes the deans of education, sciences, and arts and humanities, as well as the vice chancellor for academic affairs.
- *Specified policies for student advancement or graduation.* Policies for admission to teacher preparation programs, for advancement from sophomore-level to junior-level courses, or for graduation have been reviewed, strengthened, and made more specific.
- *Student proficiency assessment.* Faculty-developed or standardized tests are being introduced for advancement of all students from sophomore-level to junior-level courses, or admission to the teacher preparation program, or for graduation. All students, not just those in teacher preparation, are now expected to demonstrate certain basic proficiencies.
- *Learning/developmental centers.* Centers are being provided for remedial study and instruction. Some institutions require attendance; in others, attendance is voluntary. One such center has an extensive instructional staff and a wide array of self-instructional materials. It is centrally located and has extended hours to encourage student use.
- *Curriculum review and modification.* Improvement efforts are focusing on curriculum and content, not just on tests. Faculty committees review the content of required tests and study their relation to the institution's strengths. But the main focus is on how to develop student proficiency and on how each department can contribute to reaching this goal. For example, in one institution, each department will sponsor a required writing seminar for its majors.
- *Cooperative outreach and talent identification.* One college, in cooperation with a city school district, has initiated an outreach program to identify talented students who might be interested in becoming teachers. The school district and the college will provide experiences introducing such students to the teaching profession.

These actions, and others like them, are promising developments in higher education and in teacher education.

A Challenge for Testers

At the same time, ETS is practicing what I am "preaching" here. We, too, must act and lead. We have and we

will. In cooperation with the presidents of historically black colleges, we have jointly initiated what is called the HBC/ETS Collaboration. A series of workshops drawing on areas of ETS expertise have been conducted to address needs that the historically black colleges identified for themselves. ETS is learning a great deal from this cooperative venture that will help improve ETS services to the entire education community. Workshops have included financial aid, academic use of computers, and program evaluation. We are now planning activities related to improving student performance on teacher tests—particularly the NTE. In a separate undertaking, ETS is cooperating with the Southern Regional Education Board to provide faculty workshops on the NTE and on faculty-developed tests.

ETS provides NTE item-summary workshops for interested colleges and universities. When an appropriate time and adequate support can be arranged, ETS staff members meet with interdisciplinary faculty committees to analyze item-by-item performance on the NTE tests by students from that institution. This helps faculty members analyze how well students in their institution perform on particular questions and allows them to compare the performance of their students with that of others across the U.S. Twenty-eight institutions of higher education have held NTE item-summary workshops over the past two years.

ETS has also acted to provide information to policy makers and teacher educators. I have already described our position on the proper use of tests in Texas and Arkansas. We have been more successful in constructively influencing public policy with regard to teacher tests in Tennessee and Florida. The two ETS research reports on the impact of state testing policies on teacher selection are yet another part of our effort to raise important policy issues in the teacher testing movement.

Another contribution just completed is the first comprehensive job analysis of the teaching role in American elementary and secondary schools.[7] Teacher tests in the U.S. have traditionally been validated on the basis of what is taught in teacher preparation programs *before* prospective teachers enter the teaching profession. In other occupational fields, validation of licensing examinations generally depends on their relevance to duties to be performed *after* a person is actually on the job. The role of a teacher, however, was considered so complex and diverse that standard job analysis has not been thought possible until recently.

ETS will soon be publishing the results of a 16-month job analysis project for teaching. An ETS research team, led by knowledgeable program scientists in the field of job analysis, has developed a job analysis model for the teaching profession. Some 3,000 classroom teachers representing elementary, middle, and high school levels and most subject-matter fields participated in the project. We will use this job analysis model to assist in developing and validating the NTE for state certification and other purposes. We believe that the model can make a contribution not only to test construction but also to teacher education.

The strength of education reform in the 1980s lies in the fact that its dynamism has come from across the land. It has been nationwide rather than national, and that is the way it should continue. While those in the "bully pulpits" of Washington, D.C., can help by constructive exhortation, the real leadership must come from the towns, cities, and states throughout the U.S. and from educational institutions. This is especially true for the improvement of the quality and spirit of the teaching force in American public education. Higher standards must be accompanied by better preparation if we are to produce the number and variety of teachers needed in the 1990s and beyond. Teacher education ought to be in the forefront of the next stage of education reform—that which will take place in the colleges and universities.

FOOTNOTES

1. J.T. Sandefur, *Competency Assessment of Teachers: 1984 Report* (Bowling Green: Western Kentucky University, 1984).

2. Alec M. Gallup, "The Gallup Poll of Teachers' Attitudes Toward the Public Schools," *Phi Delta Kappan,* October 1984, p. 107.

3. Margaret E. Goertz, Ruth B. Ekstrom, and Richard J. Coley, *The Impact of State Policy on Entrance into the Teaching Profession* (Princeton, N.J.: Final Report to the National Institute of Education, NIE Grant No. G83-0073. Educational Testing Service, 1984); and Margaret E. Goertz and Barbara Pitcher, *The Impact of NTE Use by States on Teacher Selection* (Princeton, N.J.: Educational Testing Service, 1985).

4. Ibid.

5. For a summary of these data, see Board of Trustees, *1984 Public Accountability Report* (Princeton, N.J.: Educational Testing Service, 1984).

6. The *ETS Standards for Quality and Fairness* meet or exceed the *Standards for Educational and Psychological Tests* (1974) of the American Educational Research Association, the American Psychological Association, and the National Council on Measurement in Education.

7. The term *job analysis* is used here in the context of the federal *Equal Employment Opportunity Commission Uniform Guidelines on Employee Selection Procedures.*

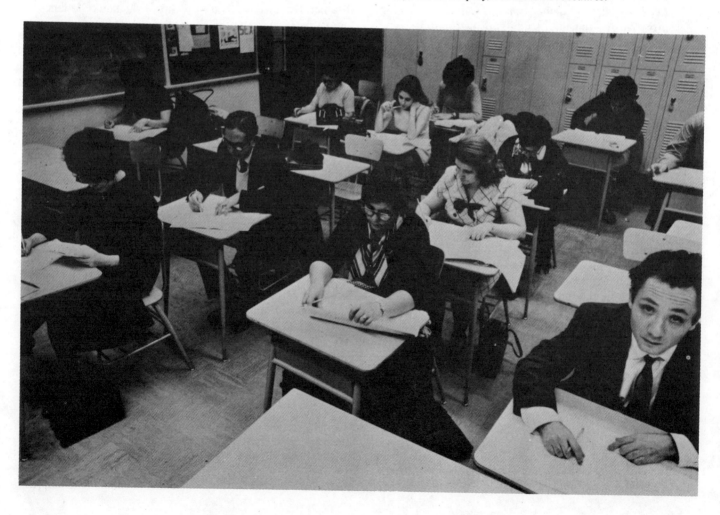

Chapter 24
What Do We Know About Teaching Effectiveness?
N.L. Gage*

Teaching is the central process in education. It comes after economic resources, physical facilities, and curriculum have been determined, and it is intended to lead toward learning. It is the social function through which societies foster achievement of their educational objectives, and it costs a great deal of money. And teaching can have great personal and emotional significance; a bad teacher can confuse us and make us miserable. Teaching is also intriguing as an object of scientific and artistic contemplation in its own right—worth trying to understand for the same reasons that we study the heavens or the impressionists.

But for several years in the late 1960s and early 1970s, the Coleman Report, the reanalyses edited by Frederick Mosteller and Daniel Patrick Moynihan, and the book on inequality by Christopher Jencks were interpreted as indicating that teaching was unimportant. Of course, those works never compared teaching with no teaching. Instead, they compared educational outcomes associated with different kinds of teachers and concluded that one teacher seemed to have about the same effect as another. The implication drawn from this finding was that it did not make much sense to try to improve teaching.

I do not intend to go into that story here, except to say that this body of work used unpromising independent variables, inappropriate dependent variables, and endlessly arguable correlational methods for determining causal relationships between the independent and dependent variables. Research and thinking since then have made most educational and social researchers reject the notion that it is pointless to try to improve teaching.

Reviewing What We Know

What kind of teaching are we talking about? I have in mind classroom teaching, especially as it goes on in elementary and secondary schools in the U.S. and, as it turns out, in many other countries where teaching has been observed. Classroom teaching does not mean lec-turing, exclusively, or discussing, exclusively, or tutoring, exclusively. Rather, it means the combination of all of these ways of teaching, as well as classroom recitation, or relatively rapid-fire teacher questioning and student responding, and so-called seatwork. Classroom teaching includes all of these and a variety of managerial activities that keep the whole process moving along in an orderly way.

So I am not dealing with anything very new or highly technological or revolutionary. I am considering what all of us experienced during most of the hours, days, and years we spent in classrooms between our sixth and 18th years.

The Art of Teaching

Many writers, including me, have said that teaching is an art. What does it mean to speak of an "art" of teaching?

Teaching is an instrumental or practical art, not a fine art. As an instrumental art, teaching departs from recipes, formulas, and algorithms. It requires improvisation, spontaneity, the handling of a vast array of considerations of form, style, pace, rhythm, and appropriateness in ways so complex that even computers must lose the way, just as they cannot achieve what a mother does with a 5-year-old.

The sense in which I use the term *art* includes any process or procedure whose tremendous complexity—resulting from the large number of relevant variables and the interactions among those variables—makes the process irreducible to systematic formulas. Thus an artistic process is not necessarily a *good* process: successful, cre-

*Dr. N.L. Gage is Margaret Jacks Professor of Education at Stanford University. This article is based on lectures delivered during 1983–84 at Oxford University, the University of Leicester, Harvard University, and the conference on "Teaching—Art or Science?" sponsored by the Swedish National Board of Universities and Colleges. Copyright © 1984, N.L. Gage. Reprinted with permission of the author and *Phi Delta Kappan*, October, 1984.

ative, productive of beauty, ingenious, versatile, or virtuoso. Bad art is nonetheless art; bad teaching is nontheless teaching.

Another view of what it means to consider teaching as an art was offered by Jay Wissot. He saw artistic activity as seeking "to remain faithful to the representation of particularized emotional experience," "idiographic in intent," intended "to make statements of utmost specificity about the subjective response to the physical world."[1] Accordingly, Wissot rejected the possibility of a science of teaching, and I agree. But he apparently failed to envisage the possibility of a *scientific basis* for the art of teaching. He saw an opposition between viewing teaching as a subject fit for scientific explanation and viewing it as a subject fit for artistic revelation, whereas I see teaching as amenable to *both* scientific and artistic scrutiny.

Wissot correctly viewed teaching as receiving and responding to "an enormous cascade of stimulation." From that fact he concluded that teachers have good reason for "limiting their reliance of rational anticipation" and relying instead on "their instinctive feel for emerging events."[2] Thus it would be futile to attempt to influence teachers to change their practices in the directions that empirical research suggests. Yet, as I will try to show below, such attempts have succeeded. Research has shown repeatedly that it is possible to change teaching practices—not for all teachers or for all practices, but for enough teachers and enough practices to make an educationally important difference.

The Scientific Basis

Let us turn now to the question, What is a scientific basis—especially a scientific basis for the art of teaching? My answer here is deliberately modest—perhaps overmodest. At the least, a scientific basis consists of scientifically developed knowledge about relationships between variables. In any issue of *Science,* the "Reports" almost always deal with relationships between variables. Even reports of case studies usually contain implicit references to relationships between variables.

Notice that I say nothing about theory, nomological networks, systems of postulates and axioms, or hypothetico-deductive relationships. In emphasizing relationships between variables, I am not denying the desirability of systematic theory; I am merely saying that, however desirable, systematic theory is not indispensable to any valid conception of science. The grand theories in the natural sciences and even theories of the middle range in the behavioral sciences may represent goals for us to aspire to, but they do not set minimum requirements as to what we must have before we can lay claim to scientific knowledge.

Table 1. Results of Hypothetical Experiment

Outcome	Receiving New Treatment %	Receiving Old Treatment %
Good	60	40
Bad	40	60
Total	100	100

Correlation = .2
Percentage of variance explained = 4%

I advance this modest conception of science in order to avoid claiming too much about where research on teaching stands today. As you will note later, we cannot make claims about relationships between variables without creating classifications, or taxonomies, of our variables. In research on teaching, the sets of relationships that we have available do, in fact, possess some semblance of order, organization, sequence, rationale, and meaning; they are not mere random collections of correlation coefficients or effect sizes.

Weak Relationships

In speaking of relationships between variables (relationships already identified and confirmed fairly well through research on teaching), I am not claiming that the relationships are strong ones. The coefficients of correlation fall between .2 and .5.

Are relationships of this magnitude useful? Until recently, many behavioral scientists were likely to look with scorn at values as low as .2. Readers of the Coleman Report and the reanalyses edited by Mosteller and Moynihan thought that relationships so weak betokened a kind of futility. Teacher characteristics that correlated at that level with student achievement were held to be useless. A correlation coefficient can be squared to obtain the percentage of variance in one variable explained by the other. Thus a correlation coefficient of .2 explains a mere 4% of the variance.

But, as Robert Rosenthal and Donald Rubin have shown, "(I)nterpretations like this may be very misleading. An appropriate measure of the size of an effect must be sensitive to the context of the data."[3] Rather than use the example of a correlation of .4, as Rosenthal and Rubin did, let me use an even weaker example, with a correlation of only .2.

A hypothetical experiment. Table 1 shows the results of a hypothetical experiment in which half of the subjects were randomly assigned to a new treatment while the other half were assigned to an old, or standard, treatment. The dependent variable is "good" or "bad." For

Table 2. Results of Beta-Blocker Trial

After 30 Months	Propranolol (N = 1,900) %	Placebo (N = 1,900) %
Dead	7.0	9.5
Alive	93.0	90.5
Total	100.0	100.0

Correlation = .045
Percentage of variance explained = .2%

Source: *Journal of the American Medical Association,* vol. 247, 1982, pp. 1707–13.

Table 3. Effects of Cholesterol Lowering

Result After Nine Years	Experimental Treatment (N = 1,906) %	Placebo (N = 1,900) %
Definite fatal or nonfatal heart attack	8.1	9.8
No definite fatal or nonfatal heart attack	91.9	90.2
Totals	100.0	100.0

Correlation = .03
Percentage of variance explained = .1%

Source: *Journal of the American Medical Association,* vol. 251, 1984, pp. 351–64.

example, one year after treatment, the subject may be alive or dead, or "still in school" as against "dropped out." Of the 50 persons who received the old treatment, 20 showed "good" results, but of the 50 persons who received the new treatment, 30 showed "good" results.

The coefficient of correlation for the relationship between treatment and outcome in this table is .2, and only 4% of the variance in the outcome is accounted for by the treatment. Yet the new treatment reduced the percentage of bad outcomes from 60% to 40%; that is, it caused a decrease of 20% in bad outcomes. Suppose we compare that decrease of 20% with the old treatment's bad-outcome rate of 60%. Then we realize that the new treatment has decreased the rate of bad outcomes by 33-1/3%. And all of this is true with a correlation coefficient of only .2.

Actual medical experiments. But these are only hypothetical data. What about the results of actual experiments with an important dependent variable, such as life or death? In 1982 news reached the public of the results of a large-scale experiment with a drug called propranolol, which was intended to increase the rate of survival of men who had already had one heart attack. The experiment was conducted with random assignment of about 3,800 such men to either the drug or a placebo. The investigators used double-blind procedures, and presumably the experiment, which cost about $20 million, was conducted impeccably in all other respects. The results of this experiment are shown in Table 2.

After 30 months, 9.5% of the men who had received the placebo had died, while only 7% of those who had received propranolol had died. The drug reduced the percentage of fatalities by only 2.5%. Such a result would almost certainly be regarded as trivial in research on teaching. But in the medical arena, the result was regarded as so important that the experiment was discontinued on ethical grounds; that is, the researchers felt that it was unethical to continue denying treatment to a control group. The results led to the recommendation that

propranolol be used—with a potential saving of about 21,000 lives per year in the U.S. alone.

In 1984 news of a similar experiment was released. This seven- to 10-year-long experiment cost $150 million and dealt with the lowering of cholesterol levels through diet and the use of a drug. The results are shown in Table 3.

Of the men who received the placebo, 9.8% had a definite (fatal or nonfatal) heart attack; of the men who received the experimental treatment, only 8.1% had a definite heart attack. The result was frontpage news in the *New York Times* and the *Boston Globe* and led to a cover story in *Time* (26 March 1984). An article in *Science* held that the results would "affect profoundly the practice of medicine in this country."[4] But the treatment produced only a 1.7% difference and accounted for only .1% of the variance in heart attacks.

Why this excursion into hypothetical and medical research? I am trying to defend the proposition that correlations or differences do not need to be large in order to be important. In education, we are not influencing life or death. But we are influencing dropout rates, literacy, placement in special classes, love of learning, self-esteem, and the holistic ability to integrate many facts and concepts in a complex way. The implications of research for practice depend not on the size of the effects but on the costs and benefits of any change in practice. And neither the costs nor the benefits of changes in teaching should be measured solely in monetary terms.[5]

Views of the Evidence

Thus what I see as a scientific basis for the art of teaching is the existence of one or more relationships between things that teachers do and things that students learn.

Now, given my definition of teaching, of an art of teaching, and of a scientific basis, can we say that we have a scientific basis for the art of teaching? Until about 1976, the consensus was that we could not. For several decades, one reviewer after another concluded that relationships between teaching practices and educational outcomes did not exist. This conclusion was due largely to the widespread fallacy of taking seriously the statistical significance of single studies that were statistically weak.

These studies dealt with intact teaching styles, such as open education and the mastery approach, or with discrete teaching practices, such as ways of asking questions or of reacting to students' responses. The literature on this kind of research is by now voluminous; it has been reviewed and synthesized repeatedly. Perhaps the most recent thorough review is that by Jere Brophy and Thomas Good for the *Third Handbook of Research on Teaching.*[6] Rather than attempt to summarize that review, let me merely quote the authors' statement that

> we now know much more about teacher effects on achievement than we did in 1963 or even 1973. . . . (T)he fund of available information on producing student achievement (especially the literature related to the general area of classroom management and to the subject areas of elementary reading and mathematics instruction) has progressed from a collection of disappointing and inconsistent findings to a small but well established knowledge base. . . .[7]

As everyone knows, however, correlation does not mean causation. So experiments have been done to determine whether actually changing teaching practices causes improved achievement, attitudes, and behavior on the part of students.

These experiments are fairly similar in some novel and important respects. First, the teaching practices that the experimenters tried to change in a specified direction had been derived primarily from previous correlational studies of the kind just described. That is, the behaviors were not derived from some ideology or from a theory based on laboratory experiments or from some kind of philosophical reasoning. They were derived from correlations between specific teaching practices and student achievement or attitude or both.

Second, these experiments were accompanied by classroom observations. These observations determined the degree to which the desired teaching practices were actually used by the teachers in the experimental group as compared with the control group. Third, the teachers involved in these experiments were volunteers who agreed to accept random assignment to either the trained group or the control group. The teachers or their schools were then randomly assigned to one group or the other. Such random assignment greatly enhances the validity of the experiments. Fourth, all teachers were regular teachers who were involved in the experiment for a whole school year or a whole semester—not merely for an hour, a day, or a week or two. Fifth, the students of the teachers took pretests of achievement and attitude at the beginning of the school year or term and then took comparable posttests at the end.

One final point before I discuss the results. Because of the way the teaching practices used in these experiments were derived, they did not represent any revolutionary, esoteric, or exotic ways of teaching. Instead, they were ways of teaching that other teachers in the same kinds of schools were already using—teachers in whose classrooms previous investigators had found better than average achievement, attitudes, or behavior.

Nine experiments of this kind have been reported.[8] In all except the one by Theodore Coladarci and me, the results were positive and substantial. For example, in the experiment by John Crawford and others,[9] 33 third-grade teachers in two school districts were randomly assigned, within each district, to a control group or a training group. The latter group received training over a period of a month; the former group did not. Both groups were observed before, during, and after the training. The results of the observations showed that the training was effective in bringing about significant change on the part of the trained teachers. The classes of the trained teachers had higher mean scores on achievement tests and attitude inventories. Indeed, the differences in achievement between the two sets of classes yielded an effect size of .69, which means that the mean class of the trained teachers scored at about the 75th percentile rank of the classes of the untrained teachers.

These experiments suggest that the progression from observational and descriptive studies through correlational studies to experiments has begun to pay off. We are beginning to have evidence that the correlations betoken causal relationships, so that changing teaching practices *causes* desirable changes in student achievement, attitude, and conduct. And the changes in achievement are substantial, not trivial. Moreover, the changes are brought about not by revolutions in teaching practice or school organization but by relatively straightforward attempts to educate more teachers to do what the more effective teachers have already been observed to be doing.

This kind of research is relatively independent of values. So far it has been conducted primarily to achieve the values implicit in achievement tests, attitude inventories, and classroom order. But there is nothing in the general approach to prevent the same gains from being made in achieving the values of those who believe in open education or in any other kind of education.

Applying What We Know

The problem of applying what we learn from research on teaching effectiveness is the problem of teacher education. In one sense, this problem is the same as that of teaching, but now we are dealing with the teaching that teachers *receive* rather than the teaching that teachers *do*. The similarity is apparent when we refer to the kinds of variables the process entails: I dealt above with teaching practices as *independent* variables and student achievement, attitudes, and behavior as dependent variables. Now I will deal with teaching practices, broadly defined, as *dependent* variables and with teacher education practices as the independent variables.

I take up three questions in turn. First, is teacher education important? In the 1980s, the U.S. is going through one of its perennial surges of concern with education, with many study commissions engaged in efforts to diagnose and prescribe for the nation's educational ills. Where does teacher education fit in? Is it peripheral or central?

Second, is there evidence that teacher education is possible? Or are teachers born rather than made? Many of us know good teachers who never went through a teacher education program. Does this mean that we should leave teachers alone, let them learn on the job, and hope for the best? Or is teaching something that *can* be taught and learned with a reasonable (and not too costly) investment of effort and skill? These questions apply not only to new teachers but to those already on the job.

Third, what kind of research on teacher training is likely to pay off best in view of the peculiar nature of the teacher's job? If teaching is an instrumental art, it cannot be taught in the same ways that we train assembly-line workers, aircraft mechanics, or medical technicians. Teachers need more autonomy and more freedom to use their judgment than many other kinds of workers. But teaching is an art with obligations to the society, with moral imperatives relating to the welfare of students and the body politic. So teachers cannot have the complete autonomy of creative artists who can choose to be surrealists, atonalists, Dadaists, or anything else. Thus we need approaches to teacher education that walk the path between unacceptable regimentation and unacceptable anarchy.

The Importance of Pedagogy

Is teacher education important? A great many factors work together in our educational system: finance, buildings, curriculum, and administration. It is hard to know where to begin in trying to improve that system. Harold Howe II considered several alternative emphases: more

equitable funding, desegregation for achieving greater fairness, and such vast changes as a voucher system. But he decided that these were "unlikely to produce the improved learning we want within a reasonable period of time."[10] And then he concluded that "the improvement of pedagogy is the most likely source of a real solution to the shortcomings of America's schools."[11]

A similar conclusion appeared in a searching and critical analysis of four recent reform proposals for American education. The reviewers, Lawrence Stedman and Marshall Smith, analyzed the report of the National Commission on Excellence in Education, appointed by Secretary Terrel Bell; the report of the Task Force on Education for Economic Growth, established by the Education Commission of the States; the College Entrance Examination Board's report, *Academic Preparation for College;* and the report of the Twentieth Century Fund's Task Force on Federal Elementary and Secondary Education Policy. Stedman and Smith found a serious omission in all four reports: they had "ignored the problem of pedagogy: namely, the question, 'How is it taught?' "[12]

Howe's statement and the review by Stedman and Smith emphasize the importance of pedagogy. Contrast these with the lack of concern about pedagogy in the four commission reports. This discrepancy suggests that we need to call more attention to the improvement of teaching practices through what we have learned from research. For whatever reasons, as the four commission reports demonstrate, much thinking about education has found it possible to focus on almost every conceivable part of the enterprise except its central process: the teaching function.

Improving Teacher Education

Is teacher education possible? Can we influence the ways teachers teach? Can we change their thoughts and actions? And, if so, can we consider the changes to be improvements?

These questions are worth asking because, as everyone knows, teacher education has for a long time been held in low regard. In 1963 Americans were surprised that James Bryant Conant, the former president of Harvard University, came back from a diplomatic assignment in West Germany to devote himself not merely to education, which would have been remarkable enough, but to teacher education, a pariah among pariahs. But Conant's effort, *The Education of American Teachers,* had an impact not at all like that of the Flexner Report on medical education. So, two decades later, the universities and many leaders of public education still have their doubts about the value of teacher education.

Even if we give pedagogy a modicum of respect, we find widespread doubt about the efficacy of teacher education, even (or perhaps especially) among teachers themselves—most of them graduates of teacher educating programs. We hear that teacher education courses are irrelevant, too theoretical. The courses are full of material about learners and learning, when prospective teachers want to know about teachers and teaching. The courses tell about the history, philosophy, sociology, and psychology of education, when prospective teachers want to know how they should teach. The courses give future teachers knowledge of the subject matter to be taught, when prospective teachers may already know far more about a subject than they will ever need in teaching third-graders or even 12th-graders. The evidence that knowledge of a subject is not enough to make a teacher is plain to anyone who has ever seen a Ph.D. in mathematics thoroughly confuse a freshman calculus class—or the holder of a bachelor's degree obfuscate the past tense in teaching third-grade reading.

Thus generations of teacher education students have been given inadequate grounding in how to teach. They have not been taught how to organize a course, how to plan a lesson, how to manage a class, how to give an explanation, how to arouse interest and motivation, how to ask various kinds of questions, how to react to students' responses, how to give helpful correction and feedback, how to avoid unfair biases in interacting with students—in short, how to teach.

Until recently, one reason for the neglect of these matters in teacher education programs has been the relative dearth of research-based knowledge about them. Only in the late 1960s and the 1970s did the findings of research studies begin to converge. Now these findings have accumulated into bodies of fairly well-confirmed knowledge—confirmed in the sense that teaching practices of certain kinds have been found to be associated with higher student achievement and more desirable student attitudes and conduct.

How Can We Improve?

It would be nice if the evidence on improving the performance of teachers through the use of research-based teaching practices could be drawn from work in regular *preservice* teacher education programs. But I, at least, cannot provide that kind of evidence. Instead I must refer to the experiments that I cited above, conducted with *inservice* teacher education programs. These experiments, now numbering at least nine, have dealt with teachers at several grade levels.

The main conclusion of this body of research is that, in eight out of the nine cases, inservice education *was* fairly effective—not with all teachers and not with all teaching practices but effective enough to change teachers and improve student achievement, or attitudes, or

behavior. Even in the unsuccessful experiment by Coladarci and me, it seemed that the recommended teaching practices, derived from previous correlational studies by others, were valid, because the scores of the teachers for conformity with these recommendations correlated with mean class achievement at about .4.

Before we conclude from these experiments that regular inservice education along the same lines will be equally effective, some caveats are in order. All nine of these teacher education efforts were conducted as research experiments, and it is not possible to say that similar education, conducted as part of routine staff development in the schools, would be similarly effective. In others words, the results of these experiments may be partly due to the well-known Hawthorne Effect; that is, a research undertaking fosters the kind of spirit and dedication that tends to make anything work better than it otherwise would.

We should consider this possibility in the light of three facts, however. First, two major reviews have concluded that the Hawthorne Effect is not at all widespread.[13] Second, one of the eight experiments gave members of the control group extra motivation to think more about their teaching.[14] In this experiment, the control group showed "marked improvement," but not as much improvement as the experimental group. Third, the findings of two experiments showed that the better a teaching practice was implemented, the more likely it was to correlate with achievement.[15] This suggests that the substance of the teaching practices, not the social environment in which they were used, was the cause of the improved achievement.

These three points notwithstanding, it may turn out that inservice teacher education as brief and relatively inexpensive as that used in these experiments will not work in routine staff development programs. If so, this kind of education will need to be strengthened in various ways. The problem of discovering and developing more effective ways of equipping teachers with pedagogical knowledge and skill is the same, in principle, as that of discovering more effective ways of teaching students.

Observe-Correlate-Experiment

In the history of science and technology, it is possible to discern a kind of progression from observation and description, through correlational work, to experimentation. This progression can be seen, for example, in the work on cholesterol.

I first heard about cholesterol as a possible factor in heart disease right after World War II. It was then a kind of conjecture or rumor that cholesterol had been observed, isolated, defined, and suspected or being a factor in heart disease. Then came correlational studies that showed that higher levels of cholesterol were associated with higher rates of heart attack. The medical community recommended that people watch their cholesterol intake. But this recommendation was only half-hearted, because no solid evidence existed that the correlation reflected a causal connection. Then came the massive $150 million, seven-to-10-year experiment that I cited above.

This same pattern—from observation to correlation to experiment—is beginning to develop in the case of some teaching practices and student achievement. Teaching practices have been observed, described, and measured. They have then been correlated with achievement. And most recently they have been "manipulated" in teacher education experiments and found to cause better student achievement, attitudes, and behavior.

For teacher education and staff development, the same general program seems to make sense. We have now had surveys of the practices used in teacher education and staff development programs. We have the theoretical analyses by such writers as Gary Fenstermacher and David Berliner, who have identified four facets of staff development activities that seem to them to be potentially important.[16] The four facets are:

- *Source of the initiative for staff development:* Is it initiated internally, by the teachers who will be involved, or externally, by some higher authority?
- *Target processes of the staff development:* Are they intended to effect compliance with laws and regulations? Are they intended to remedy deficiencies of the teachers involved? Are they intended to enrich teachers' knowledge and skills?
- *Size of the group involved:* Is is one teacher? A few teachers? Many teachers? Or is it all the teachers in a school, a school district, or a state?
- *Process of staff involvement:* Were the teachers involved of their own free choice, or were they required to take part?

We can readily conceive of a variety of staff development programs that would result from different combinations of these factors. At one extreme, we might have a program initiated by teachers themselves, aimed at enriching their knowledge, that would include only a few teachers who chose to take part. At another extreme, we might have a program initiated by a state superintendent, designed to effect compliance with a new law, and intended to involve all teachers in a state, by mandate from the state capital.

Such different staff development programs would obviously have different characteristics. Their processes would need to be described along different dimensions by different research techniques. Those processes would need to be correlated with different measures of success. And eventually, if the pattern of description, correlation, and experiment is followed, experiments that would test different staff development programs would need to be conducted.

We are now in the early stages of acquiring this kind of knowledge about how to educate teachers. Whether the work will ever be completed depends on whether policy makers decide that the investment is worthwhile. Some estimates indicate that staff development in recent years, including university courses for inservice teachers, has cost about $2 billion per year in this country. Divided by our approximately two million elementary and secondary teachers, this amounts to about $1,000 per teacher per year invested in the effort to improve teachers who are already employed. An investment of about 1% of the $2 billion in understanding and improving staff development would provide staff-development research with about $20 million a year. As the years go by, that research could make staff development the source of aid and comfort to teachers that it has never been but ought to be.

FOOTNOTES

1. Jay Wissot, "Teaching as an Art Form," *Educational Forum*, vol. 43, 1979, pp. 265–66.
2. Ibid., p. 268.
3. Robert Rosenthal and Donald B. Rubin, "A Note on Percent Variance Explained as a Measure of the Importance of Effects," *Journal of Applied Social Psychology*, vol. 9, 1979, p. 395.
4. Gina Bara Kolata, "Lowered Cholesterol Decreases Heart Disease," *Science*, vol. 223, 1984, p. 381.
5. N.L. Gage, "When Does Research on Teaching Yield implications for Practice?," *Elementary School Journal*, vol. 83, 1983, pp. 492–96.
6. Jere E. Brophy and Thomas L. Good, "Teacher Behavior and Student Achievement," in Merlin E. Wittrock, ed., *Third Handbook of Research on Teaching*, forthcoming.
7. Ibid., ms. p. 132.
8. Linda M. Anderson, Carolyn M. Evertson, and Jere E. Brophy, "An Experimental Study of Effective Teaching in First-Grade Reading Groups," *Elementary School Journal*, vol. 79, 1979, pp. 193–223; John Crawford, N.L. Gage, Lynn Corno, Nicholas Stayrook, and Alexis Mitman, *An Experiment on Teacher Effectiveness and Parent-Assisted Instruction in the Third Grade, Vols. 1–3* (Stanford, Calif.: Program on Teaching Effectiveness, Center for Educational Research, Stanford University, 1978); Theodore Coladarci and N.L. Gage, "Effects of a Minimal Intervention on Teacher Behavior and Student Achievement," *American Educational Research Journal*, in press; Thomas L. Good and Douglas A. Grouws, "The Missouri Mathematics Effectiveness Project: An Experimental Study in Fourth-Grade Classrooms," *Journal of Educational Psychology*, vol. 71, 1979, pp. 355–62; idem, "Experimental Research in Secondary Mathematics Classrooms: Working with Teachers," unpublished manuscript, 1981; Jane Stallings, Margaret Needels, and Nicholas Stayrook, *How to Change the Process of Teaching Basic Reading Skills in Secondary Schools: Phase II and Phase III* (Menlo Park, Calif.: SRI

International, 1978); Edmund T. Emmer et al., *The Classroom Management Improvement Study: An Experiment in Elementary School Classrooms* (Austin: Research and Development Center for Teacher Education, University of Texas, 1981); idem, *Improving Classroom Management and Organization in Junior High Schools: An Experimental Investigation* (Austin: Research and Development Center for Teacher Education, University of Texas, 1982); and Walter R. Borg and F.R. Ascione, "Classroom Management in Elementary Mainstreaming Classrooms," *Journal of Educational Psychology,* vol. 74, 1982, pp. 85–95.

9.   Crawford et al.

10.   Harold Howe II, "Improving Teaching: Solutions Close to the Classroom," *College Board Review,* no. 125, 1982, p. 13.

11.   Ibid., p. 14.

12.   Lawrence C. Stedman and Marshall S. Smith, "Recent Reform Proposals for American Education," *Contemporary Education Review,* vol. 2, 1983, p. 95.

13.   Desmond L. Cook, *The Impact of the Hawthorne Effect in Experimental Designs in Educational Research: Final Report* (Columbus: Ohio State University, 1967); and Shari Seidman Diamond, "Hawthorne Effects: Another Look," unpublished manuscript, 1974.

14.   Good and Grouws, "The Missouri Mathematics Effectiveness Project. . . ."

15.   Anderson et al.; and Crawford et al.

16.   Gary D. Fenstermacher and David C. Berliner, *A Conceptual Framework for the Analysis of Staff Development* (Santa Monica, Calif.: Rand Corporation, 1983).

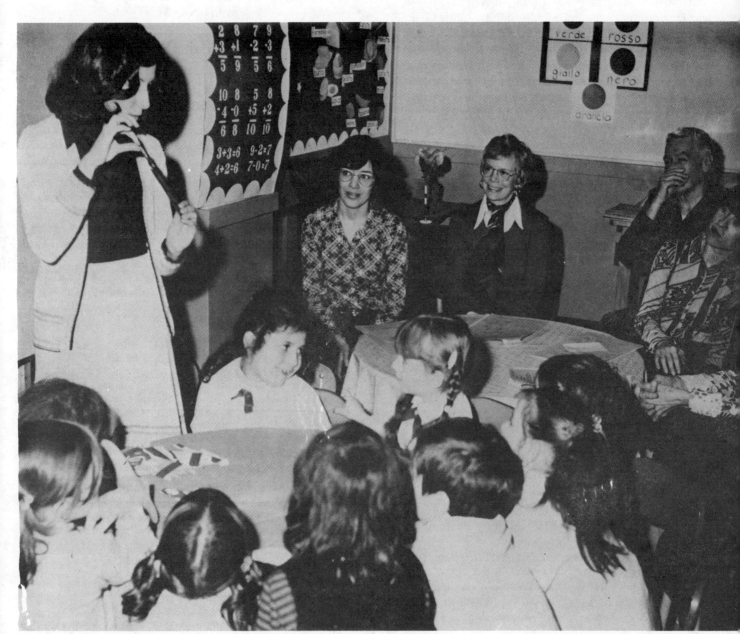

Superintendent Alfred Melov, NYC School Board 15

Chapter 25
Preparing the Preservice Teacher for Gifted and Talented Children

Teresa A. Trimarco, Rosemary M. Maher, and Donna M. Narducci*

Introduction

"The past twenty years have been a period of unparalleled affluence for public education and educational research in the United States" (Jensen, 1985). We finally dealt with racial desegregation. Large scale experimentation with compensatory education has been in vogue. Our nation has focused its educational resources on extending benefits of education to every segment of the population—especially to those groups that historically have derived the least benefit from the traditional system of schooling. Despite this energetic large-scale innovative thrust in the history of United States education, there have been signs of malaise (Jensen, 1985). Why? Whatever happened to curriculum innovations and special identification programs for the gifted and talented child? We have prepared preservice teachers who meet special state requirements. We have instituted preservice programs that, for the most part, are competency-based. These programs require preservice teachers to spend many hours in the field—on the front line—preparing students to teach in regular classes. These programs include courses in special education in order that the classroom teacher is knowledgeable and prepared to teach mainstreamed children. To date, no state or board of education has mandated any kind of preparation for the preservice teacher in the area of gifted and talented education. Why have we not adequately focused our educational resources on extending benefits to our gifted and talented children? Researchers clearly state the need for gifted education is great and we are not meeting present or projected needs (Johnson & Vickers, 1984).

In this paper, we will examine the issues in gifted and talented education with special focus on the preparation of preservice teachers. The "gifted and talented" of whom we speak will be those children who are identified by professionally qualified persons; who, by virtue of outstanding abilities, are capable of high performance; and who require differentiated educational programs in order to realize their contribution to self and society (Maryland, 1972).

Choosing Teachers for Gifted Education

Who then should be encouraged to pursue courses dealing with the gifted and talented? How are we to identify these preservice teachers who would have "necessary qualifications" for interacting with gifted and talented children? What are these extra qualifications?

Certainly these preservice teachers need to possess the characteristics of any good teacher. In addition, these teachers should be highly creative, that is, they should have the ability to stimulate and to motivate their charges in higher intellectual pursuits. The characteristic most often designated as desirable for a successful teacher of the gifted is facilitator of learning. However, a teacher need not be highly intelligent to work effectively with the gifted learner. But, that teacher should value intelligence, understand its implications and know how to nurture it (Clark, 1983). These preservice teachers also have to possess excellent managerial skills, and, at the same time, permit creativity to grow and to flourish in their classrooms.

"Students enrolled in gifted child education coursework need assurance that their training will be as qualitatively differentiated as the methodologies they are taught

*Dr. Teresa A. Trimarco is an Associate Professor and Chairperson of the Division of Education, Notre Dame College, St. John's University, New York. Dr. Rosemary M. Maher is a Teaching Fellow, Division of Education, Notre Dame College, St. John's University, New York. Donna M. Narducci is an Assistant Dean, College of Business Administration and Adjunct Instructor, Division of Education, Notre Dame College, St. John's University, New York.

145

to use with gifted children'' (Hershey, 1979, p. 13). On-site clinical experience is a most important component in the preparation of teachers for the gifted and talented. The actuality of working with gifted children is often very different from the reality. Successful teachers who had clearly managed mainstreamed classes effectively found themselves unable to allow children to be the dominant force, that is to permit children to take the lead, in the learning process. This is basic to gifted and talented education. The additional work involved in differentiating the curriculum for gifted students can be overwhelming. Inexperienced teachers frequently find themselves unable to handle this additional demand. For this reason, researchers have decided that the experienced teacher and the preservice teacher possessing some first-hand clinical experience are best suited for gifted and talented programs. In addition, experienced teachers have developed the facility for utilizing the talents of parents. Therefore, it is important in the education of preservice teachers that they also become aware of the wealth of experiences that can be provided by parents and community and that this knowledge comes by working in the schools.

Field Work Utilizing Community and Parents

Programs for the gifted are available in most cities but not at every school. Good public schools, whether elementary or secondary, have links with private institutions to explore and to utilize resources within the city. For example, a special project may be assigned to each grade. People—parents especially—from within the community should become involved. A law firm might have high school students spend the day with lawyers—touring offices, discussing cases and visiting with judges in courthouses. The parent-lawyer might eventually get interested students involved in a Mentor Program which could last for a semester or longer. Credit could be given to the high school students. At the elementary level, a third grade class might observe and help someone from a museum for a period of 4–5 weeks as part of a unit of study concerning museums and their offerings. Again, it would be beneficial to have a familiar parent who is involved with a museum at the helm of such a program (Fishman, 1986).

Colleges and universities might offer credit to preservice teachers who use expertise in conjunction with their course work. For example, credit might be given to a social science major for assisting the parent-lawyer and graduate credit to the inservice teacher for setting up a Mentor Program. Additionally, the elementary preservice teacher, who has knowledge about and interest in a specific museum, might use this site for field work. This could be a component of a required course dealing specif-

ically with gifted and talented children. The preservice teacher would assume partial responsibility for coordinating such a program.

Often preservice teachers go through an entire program without ever having any first hand experience with Parent Associations and their programs. Every good school has an active Parent Association or Parent-Teacher Association. Parents of today are interested in helping to create quality in their schools. They realize they cannot just sit back and think that tax dollars are enough. They raise funds via auctions, benefits and bazaars in order to purchase extras such as musical instruments, library materials, additional computers and audio-visual equipment. Some parents serve in the school library; others share their expertise developing enrichment programs for the gifted. Others are class mothers. In schools where many parents are participating on site, a special room is set aside for them.

Examples of enrichment programs which have been successfully developed by parents, teachers and the community working together include:

- *Culinary Arts Program*—children under the direction of parents participated in such activities as bread making from preparatory stages of recipe reading to the final stages of bread and jam;
- *Art Appreciation Program*—children guided by neighborhood Chinese water colorist used technique learned from demonstration lesson to create their own masterpieces.

Follow-up lessons included experimentation with other recipes, sampling of other foods and visiting galleries to view works of famous colorists.

When parents, staff and administrators are united, much can be undertaken. How many preservice teacher programs make it imperative that the students learn how to work with and how to utilize the expertise of parents and community? Are these intern teachers invited to Parent-Teacher Association meetings? Does the teacher training institution make this experience a requirement? Does the school administrator promote programs to facilitate a rapport between preservice teachers and parents?

According to research (Chapey & Trimarco, 1984), professional parents of gifted and talented children are not always involved in the education or their children. In a newspaper article (Chapey & Trimaco, 1982), it was reported that professional parents gave reasons for this lack of involvement. Their feelings: not enough time, baking brownies was of no interest. . . . If schools would just take the time to meet with parents informally to find out about their interests and talent, parents could become a part of special programs designed for the gifted and talented. If the school reaches out, the community puts forth all it has to offer. Preservice teachers might work with parents and community developing and carrying out enrichment programs *as part of* the field work required course dealing with the gifted and talented student.

Special Programs Are Needed for the Preservice Teacher

Researchers in the area of the gifted (Feldhusen, 1977; Renzulli, 1980) agree that not enough efforts have been made to develop programs to train classroom teachers for gifted and talented education. Educators do believe that through inservice training teachers can develop competencies on a temporary basis to meet the educational needs of the gifted. To date the greatest impact in the area of inservice training was made by the National/State Leadership Training Institute for the Gifted and Talented, which set up national conferences on gifted education (Curry & Sato, 1977). What national or state programs, institutes or conferences service the preservice teacher? It seems that specific field work courses with gifted children, offered as optional courses in some colleges and universities, are the only training they receive. The trend has been to offer graduate rather than undergraduate degree programs with some knowledge of gifted for all certified teachers (Seeley, 1979). Why aren't the experts concerned with the preservice teacher's training?

Preservice teachers need programs that provide simulated and real experiences so that gifted and talented behavior and characteristics would be better understood. Teachers need to know how to identify a gifted child. For example, the predominant view that intelligence testing will identify gifted and talented children is incomplete. Gifted and talented children must not only possess potential for academic success but must indicate some ability to achieve at their potential. Teachers must learn to look for leadership skills, performing arts ability, athletic excellence and demonstrated expertise in some specific subject area. In addition, the preservice teacher needs guidance in identifying behavior problems that are associated with gifted and talented children. These children frequently are disruptive or withdrawn because the curriculum does not challenge them. It is important to identify the behaviors associated with gifted children. Workshops designed to educate inservice teachers about the gifted and talented would be beneficial for preservice teachers as well.

The preservice teacher can certainly learn from mandated visits (built into a specific college course) to view special programs provided by various boards of education. This should be an integral part of teacher training programs. Often private schools provide worthwhile enrichment programs for the gifted. They should not be overlooked. For example, there is such a program in New York for gifted minority students. Another program in the New York metropolitan area provides opportunities on a college campus for identified gifted and talented students to enhance their particular talents and abilities on weekends. Observation and participation in these kinds of program will help to refine the preservice teacher's abilities concerning the identification process of the gifted and will provide a close-up look at the gifted in a less formal setting.

Legislation, Litigation and Research

In order to meet present and projected needs to care for the gifted, New York State's Commissioner Ambach in 1984 was responsible for the legislature's approval of monies that made gifted education in New York State a priority. (This is in keeping with P.S. 95–561, 1978, established by the Office of Gifted and Talented within the United States Office of Education. Inherent in the law was the principle of a team approach calling for active participation of parents with teachers and administrators, and where feasible, students, in planning, implementing and evaluating programs). Attention was focused upon staff development to allow personnel to develop skills to enable them to address needs of the gifted. It was suggested that a stronger thrust be placed on courses for the preservice teacher. These courses should be "on-site" courses as opposed to campus based courses.

Recent research indicates that parents, and in particular parents of the gifted and talented, have sought a new and expanded role as partners in school programs and activities in which their children are enrolled. For example, litigation in Pennsylvania mandated that parents of the gifted and talented share responsibility and decision-making with educators. Robinson, Roedell and Jackson (1979), based upon their experience in the operation of a university-affiliated program for young gifted children, observed that successful programs were directed towards parents as much as toward children themselves. Smutny (1980) notes that parents are expected to participate in designing and planning programs for the gifted.

A pilot study conducted by Chapey and Trimarco (1984), confirms the reports of administrators and parent leaders that contrary to the expanded role assigned to parents of the gifted and talented in recent legislation, litigation and the literature, these parents are not very involved in school activities. One alternative for resolving this concern might be closer partnerships between universities and local education for both preservice and inservice teachers since the major responsibility for public education rests with local and state governments.

Research development and leadership training have been provided by federal sources in fields other than education (e.g. health, agriculture). Other areas of education, such as the education of handicapped children, have received research monies resulting in higher and more consistent levels of quality. A dichotomy exists at the federal level of government in programs for exceptional children (Gallagher, 1986). By definition, exceptional children include gifted children in half the states and these states provide resources for their education. However, this is not true at the federal level. In 1985, over one billion dollars was spent for the education of the handicapped. Yet, P.S. 91-230, which established an Office of Gifted and Talented in the United States, provided a very small sum of money for this office. Their budget was not at all consistent with the budget of the Office of the Handicapped.

Conclusions/Recommendations

A lack of research on best ways and means of preparing the teacher of the gifted suggests a need for the universities, along with boards of education, to conduct studies in this most crucial field. Hesitation might reflect problems involved in adopting new curriculum requirements for existing programs or perhaps the desire to isolate gifted education as a separate program or graduate level concentration (Seeley, 1985). It does appear that curriculum innovations for gifted education are not being shared with the preservice teacher. State Education Departments have, to date, not mandated special preparations (via certification) for the teacher of gifted. Utilization of parents and community resources for gifted children by the preservice teacher is still in beginning stages. We should be encouraging the highly creative preservice teachers to pursue innovative courses for the gifted with built in field work involving parents and community. Local boards of education and individual states should be sponsoring conferences and institutes specifically designed for preservice training of those interested in gifted education. Gifted children have a right to be educated by teachers who are specifically qualified to teach them. There are few subjects in the field of educating today so important as the instruction of the gifted (Tannenbaum, 1983). What our nation provides for its best and brightest serves as an indicator of abilities toward the teaching and learning of all children. The rights of gifted children have, for the most part, been neglected. These children need spokespeople and lobbyists, but more than that, they need a network of support and this support includes help in preparing preservice teachers interested in gifted and talented education. Support, via certification for teachers of gifted and talented, would enhance the morale of present teachers and would en-

courage others at the preservice stage to pursue programs designed especially for gifted education.

BIBLIOGRAPHY

Bishop, W.E. (1966). Characteristics of teachers judged successful by intellectually gifted high achieving high school students. Doctoral Dissertation, Kent State University.

Chapey, G., & Trimarco, T. (1984). Participation of parents in programs or the gifted in New York City. *Journal for the Education of the Gifted, 7,* 178-191.

Chapey, G., & Trimarco, T. (1982, October 24). Professional parents find less time for school activities. *Staten Island Advance.*

Clark, B. (1983). *Growing up gifted.* Columbus: Charles E. Merrill.

Curry, J., & Sato, I. (1977). Training on the right track. *Gifted Child Quarterly, 21,* 195-200.

Feldhusen, J. (1977). Meeting the needs of gifted children and teachers in a university course. *Gifted Child Quarterly, 21,* 201-209.

Fishman, K. (1986). The middle-class parents' guide to the public schools. *New York, 19,* 20-31.

Gallagher, J. (1986). A proposed federal role: Education of gifted children. *Gifted Child Quarterly, 30,* 43-46.

Hershey, M. (1979). Toward a theory of teacher education for the gifted and talented. *Roeper Review, 1,* 12-14.

Jensen, A. (1985). Compensatory education and the theory of intelligence. *Phi Delta Kappan, 66,* 554-558.

Johnson, A., & Vickers, L. (Winter 1984). Teaching gifted children: A summer institute for regular classroom teachers. *Education, 105,* 193-200.

Marland, S. (1972). Education for the gifted and talented. Report to the Congress of the United States by the U.S. Commissioner of Education. Washington, D.C.: U.S. Government Printing Office, 2.

Renzulli, J. (1980). Will the gifted movement be alive and well in 1990? *Gifted Child Quarterly, 24,* (2), 3-9.

Robinson, H., Roedell, W., & Jackson, J. (1979). Early identification and intervention. In A. Passow (Ed.), *The Gifted and Talented.* National Society for the Study for Education Yearbook, 138-154.

Seeley, K. (1979). Competencies for teachers of gifted and talented children. *Journal for the Education of the Gifted, 3,* 7-13.

Seeley, K. (1985). Facilitators for gifted learners. In J. Feldhusen (Ed.), *Toward Excellence in Gifted Education.* Denver: Love Publishing Company.

Smutny, J. (Ed.). (1980). *Education of the gifted.* Evanston: Phi Delta Kappa, National College of Education Chapter.

Story, C. (Fall 1985). Facilitator of learning: A micro-ethnographic study of the teacher of the gifted. *Gifted Child Quarterly, 29,* 155–163.

Tannenbaum, A.J. (1983). *Gifted children: Psychological and educational perspectives.* New York: Macmillan.

Association of Science Technology Centers

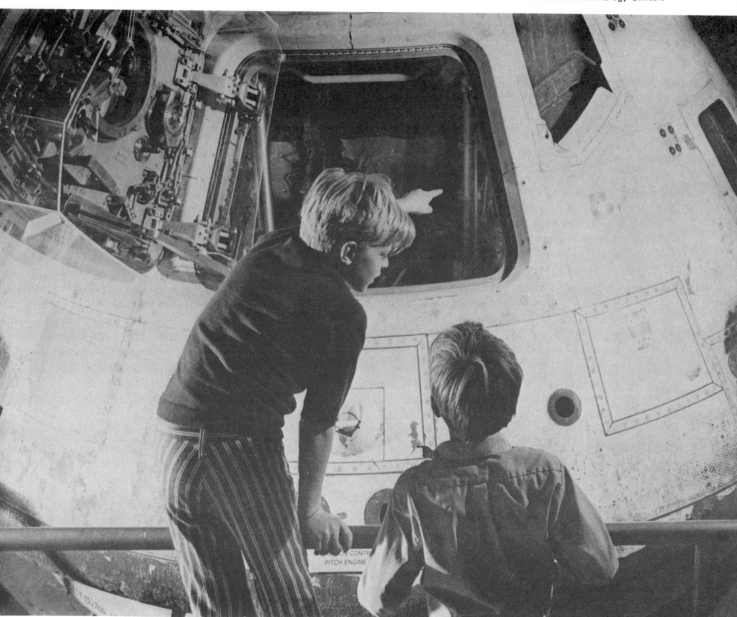

Chapter 26
Preservice Teacher Training–Promoting Effective Teachers
Irene S. Pyszkowski*

Educational reform, the agenda of the eighties, now appears to be gaining momentum. Preservice education must recognize the frenetic mood of our times and be prepared to respond with meaningful practices and policies. Currently, screening methods filter out marginal education students, but these same screening methods hire students with no educational background. State legislative acts and much publicized federal commission studies are just two of the many actions aimed at improving education in our schools. Students contemplating a career in education and educators responsible for preparing future teachers need to be aware of the trends in today's learning climate.

Testing Present and Future Teachers

State officials, sensitive to the criticisms about teacher effectiveness and teacher preparation programs, have turned to testing as a tool for instituting reforms. In March, 1986 more than 200,000 veteran teachers and administrators in the state of Texas were obliged to take a language examination to test reading and writing skills. This test was the result of legislation enacted in 1984 by the Texas legislature. It was mandated that teachers and administrators in Texas submit to this exam to determine whether they were competent enough to continue teaching in that state. Barring a teacher shortage, once a teacher fails a second time he will not be permitted to teach. He may, however, continue to take the test repeatedly and resume teaching once he succeeds in passing.

In 1985, 35,000 of Arkansas's 45,000 certified teachers were obliged to submit to math, reading and writing tests. Georgia, the only state testing its veteran teachers, requires that teachers be tested only in the subject they teach. However, Georgia will soon require all those teaching since 1977 to submit to a teachers' exam. Beginning teachers in forty-two states in our nation are expected to undergo some type of testing (N.Y. Times 3/16/86).

The most widely used testing instrument for the certification of incoming teachers is the National Teaching Examination (NTE), a Core Battery test designed by the Educational Testing Service. The NTE Core Battery is intended as an objective standardized measure to provide information related to the knowledge and skills developed in academic programs for the preparation of teachers (ETS, 1983).

The National Teacher Examination is administered at present to new teachers in twenty-eight states reports Gregory Anrig, President of ETS (Bowen, 1986). In New York State, Commissioner Gorden M. Ambach has mandated that, as of 1984,—all applicants for a provisional teaching certificate in New York State submit to the Core Battery of the NTE. Commissioner Ambach asserts that the Tests assess the general and professional knowledge provided in the teacher education programs in New York and expected of minimally qualified beginning teachers in New York (Memo 12/6/83).

Basics and Alternatives in Teacher Education

Teacher education provided by more than 1200 colleges and universities prepares approximately 140,000 new teachers each year according to Egbert (1984). Traditionally teacher education consists of several components: a general liberal-arts education, a major and minor in a specific area, and preservice training. Students preparing to enter the field of elementary education generally major in education and minor in another specific subject area. Those students who plan a teaching career in higher education major in their field of expertise and minor in education or select education courses as electives. Preservice training is comprised of courses dealing with foundations, philosophy, and psychology of education;

*Dr. Irene S. Pyszkowski is an Associate Professor, Division of Education, Notre Dame College, St. John's University, New York.

150

courses dealing with content and methodology of curriculum, and courses involving field and clinical experience in a professional setting.

Teachers learn to teach as an outgrowth of preservice training. Since elementary school teachers usually teach in self-contained classrooms, they are considered generalists or general practitioners in the art of pedagogy. They must instruct in the "three R's" plus spelling, science, social studies, and sometimes art, music, and physical education. Future elementary school teachers prepare for instructing in this broad expanse of subject matter by enrolling in courses dealing with the content and methods of elementary school subjects. These courses deal with the curriculum content and teaching strategies effective within the classroom. Students in these content and methods courses are required to prepare lesson plans, curriculum projects, instructional outlines, research projects, etc. to enhance their knowledge and understanding of the pedagogical process and subject matter.

Those educators responsible for the teaching curriculum may be part of a department, division, college, school or merely a few faculty members assigned to teach education courses and supervise student teachers. Supervising and observing the field experience of preservice teachers has long been considered a vital and integral part of teacher training. However, some voices have been speaking out for alternatives to traditional preservice field experience. According to Fagan and Merchant (1984), not all educators agree that early field experiences are professionally justified. Some question the insistence on early commitment to teaching by pointing out that immaturity, limited experience, or anomie may force out some of the best teacher candidates.

Others are proposing elimination of all education departments on the undergraduate level, eliminating the possibility of early field experience. College graduates who seek to enter the teaching profession would apply for admission to an internship program in a graduate school and would receive all preservice training as an intern without the benefit of preparatory teaching courses. Brodbelt (1985) reports that the governor of a northeastern state is attempting to bypass the state educational certification process by allowing B.A./B.S. graduates, with math or science major field of concentration, to be hired immediately as classroom teachers.

Rationale for Preservice Teacher Education

Gamble (1985) states that a training program spread out over a four year period gives students an opportunity to discover, early in their college careers, whether teaching is something they really want to do. In describing a program in an urban college, Gamble says students enter a preservice training program as early as their freshman year. They must spend two mornings per week in an inner-city school.

Fagan & Merchant (1984) point out that early field experiences help to identify borderline prospective teachers. Those students who appear to be undecided about teaching careers might seek counselling and choose to pursue other career goals. Extended field experiences allow the student to grow into teaching gradually and assume more responsibility as the assigned activities increase. Those students not suited for teaching will be helped to recognize their ineptitude and counselled accordingly.

Field experiences offer the students an opportunity to see theory taught in the college classrooms practiced in the class or learning programs. Lectures and assigned readings expose the students to a curriculum rich in educational pedagogy, but classroom exposure affords the student the opportunity to weigh the merits of educational theory with educational practice. The field experience provides a clinical laboratory in which theory and practice are compared.

Student teaching was generally the sole field experience provided in early teacher training programs. This course, required in the second half of the senior year, placed the prospective teacher in a school setting in which the primary professional contact was the classroom teacher (Egbert, 1985). This limited exposure to professional activities did not permit the student to experience a wide enough range of teaching programs or permit contact with a variety of teaching models. In recent years, teacher training programs have been expanded to include extended preservice field experience as pre-requisites to certification. In the data presented by Heald (1983) students must typically complete thirty hours of clinical experience before being admitted to teacher education, and they must complete from 50 to 100 additional hours before being permitted to enroll in student teaching. These figures are contained in a report on the field work requirements of students in a variety of colleges and universities offering teacher education programs.

The rationale for field experiences are manifold. These include:

1. Field work reinforces the preservice teacher's desire to teach.
2. Field work helps preservice teachers determine the level they wish to teach.
3. Preservice teachers experience many classroom atmospheres during field placement.
4. Preservice teachers observe many teaching styles and strategies during field work.
5. Field work enables preservice teachers to observe,

execute, and evaluate a variety of different learning experiences.
6. Field work enables preservice teachers to gain an understanding of:
   —how children learn, individually, in small groups, in large groups.
   —how children behave.
   —the interests and attitudes of children.
   —the capabilities of children.
   —how children respond to various instructional strategies and materials.

Practices in Preservice Teacher Education

Preservice field experiences cover a multitude of activities ranging from merely prosaic to highly academic. Some tasks assigned to beginning preservice students are so routine in nature as to appear dull and repetitious. However preservice teachers should be made to realize that, in teaching, the performance or those humdrum chores is vital and necessary and constitutes the operational phase of the classroom management. More exciting and challenging opportunities occur as the developing preservice teacher is involved in concrete teaching situations. Here the responsibility of the teacher-education institution is to foster field experiences that provide a link between educational foundation courses and on-site classroom activities.

The preservice phase of teaching is, by its very nature, limited in scope. Research on the preservice phase has focused on the limited amount of professional content and experience actually received by prospective teachers (Doyle, 1985). However, a number of teacher education institutions are beginning to realize the importance of more meaningful activities in the preservice years and are moving in that direction. One such program states that typically a preservice program is initiated in the sophomore year, combines course work and field experience (including early participation rather than observation), draws heavily on the service of experienced teachers, and is flexible and adapted to the needs and interests of individual students (Egbert, 1985).

In another effort to provide additional professional activities to prospective teachers, the staff of the Division of Education in an eastern university devised a program of preservice education that would be initiated in the sophomore year. This program was developed to provide an advantageous experience in the field that related to campus courses. With each education course, provisions were made for field experiences to observe a number of varied model programs of a relevant nature. In the junior year, field experience and a methods course were offered

as a pre-requisite for student teaching. This course combined campus based lectures with school based field work.

Lessons planned and taught in these early preservice experiences generally follow prescribed guidelines set by the methods teacher. By limiting the teacher experiences to a specific professional activity, the preservice teacher has an opportunity to realize early the carryover from theory to the practice. If topics addressed in the field are closely coordinated with topics in the campus classroom, preservice teachers can perceive a meaningful relationship between instructional strategy and assigned activities.

Preservice Experiences

While some strides are being made to increase professional participation in the preservice years, a random sample of activities generally assigned to students is tabulated in Table 1. The activities have been divided into three loosely defined categories of professionalism.

Are these activities professionally useful? Fagan and Merchant (1984) report that most activities assigned and performed by prospective teachers within their first field experience are necessary but mundane routines. These

Table 1. Field Experience Activities

Low Professional Involvement	Medium Professional Involvement	High Professional Involvement
correct paper	develop answer keys	construct instructional puzzle
make duplicates	make bulletin board	supervise independent seat work
take attendance	one-to-one tutorial	make transparencies
record student grades	read a story	log students' behavior patterns
collect & distribute	talk with school psychologist—assist in field trips	attend parent-teacher conference
collect & distribute notices		attend curriculum meeting

practices generally fall within the category of low professional involvement but must be performed for the smooth operation of the classroom.

Activities in the second category of medium professional involvement correspond to the working responsibilities of preservice training and might occur after a student has completed the initial field experience. These educational practices allow the student the opportunity to link field experience with foundation courses.

The third category enumerates those activities that are considered as having a high professional involvement. They are more likely to occur later in the preservice program just prior to actual student teaching and when the student has developed some confidence and know-how in the classroom.

Table 1 represents a cross section of tasks assigned and performed by preservice students. While this list is by no means complete, since the range of activities in preservice training is practically infinite, it does include some very traditional practices employed in schools of education, by colleges and universities. In view of the rapid rise of technology, no list would be complete without some mention of the increased use and application of technological aids in preservice training. Students planing to teach in the near future should be trained in the computer's basic operation and how it will help children learn. More thought should be given to expanding the role of the new technology in preservice assignments. States Hunter (1983) we must become computer literate to cope with the forthcoming revolution in education.

Teaching and learning are two functions that do not cease to operate when the classroom door is shut at the end of the school day. Rather they are functions which become integral parts of the human condition and need to be nurtured and replenished. Students pursuing teaching careers are not limited in their field experiences solely by courses described in college catalogues. There are many opportunities existing in the larger community for volunteers to work in situations which are closely allied to the public schools. Indeed some of these institutions (i.e. museums) train volunteers as docents who are then engaged to instruct classes both within and without the institution. Students should avail themselves of opportunities and enhance their experiential contacts in teaching related activities.

The Student Teaching Component

Student teaching, which usually occurs in the senior year of an undergraduate program, is the culmination of all the methods, content, and foundation courses. Students view this component as a joy: a coming together of all their acquired knowledge and skills. Hermanowicz (1966) reports teachers felt that the most valuable experience they had before beginning to teach was their student teaching. It was then they learned the most about being a teacher. In spite of the enthusiasm and eagerness to embark on this new experience, students do feel anxious about implementing practices and procedures consonant with those taught in methods courses.

It is the cooperating teacher who plays a significant role in effecting the transition from clinical field experiences to actual classroom teaching. Researchers of practice teaching (Zeichner 1980, Johnson 1979, Seperson & Joyce 1973, Yee 1969) agree that the primary influence on student teachers' instructional style is the cooperating teacher. It is not surprising, therefore, that prospective teachers view their cooperating teachers both as role models and mentors who will facilitate the road to professional success.

Cooperating teachers who participate in the student teaching component usually have agreed to do so. They are willing game players who wish to share their expertise and professional "know-how" with prospective teachers. In the selection process of student teachers, every effort is made to match the personality and interests of the cooperating teachers to that of the incoming student teacher. When an ideal match-up is not feasible, alternative procedures must be employed to prevent the student teaching experience from becoming difficult and frustrating.

Role of the Cooperating Teacher

Cooperating teachers serve as mentors, nurturing and training aspiring teachers and proposing approaches for optimal growth. When student teachers demonstrate deficiencies in specific areas, the cooperating teacher is there to offer remediation procedures. Since the primary responsibility of the cooperating teacher is continued progress of the pupils in the classroom, teaching errors or weaknesses by the preservice teacher must be corrected as quickly as possible. This intervention by the classroom teacher serves a dual purpose. It prevents damaging teaching strategies from continuing unchecked and provides instant re-play for the preservice teacher, something a preservice supervisor cannot possibly accomplish on a daily basis.

If rapport exists between the student teachers and the cooperating teacher, constructive criticism can be offered in a friendly spirit of give and take based on professional mutual interest. If the relationship between the two is less friendly, the same spirit of professional concern should prevail when criticism is offered.

Classroom teachers, like preservice teachers and the population at large, come equipped with differing personalities and competencies. Preservice teachers must be prepared to adapt to these differences as part of their student teaching experience. Ideally, the cooperating teacher as depicted in the literature is warm. friendly, open, supportive, and of a high professional caliber. But, in reality, these qualities are not always present in all cooperating teachers. The student teacher needs to be flexible enough to realize that one can profit from negative as well as positive situations. Learning to reject inappropriate teaching styles and techniques is equally as important as learning to emulate valid and appropriate procedures in the classroom.

Role of the Supervisors of Student Teaching

In the hierarchy of preservice education, the supervisor of student teaching acts as a facilitator and link between the campus and the classroom. On average, a student teacher is observed approximately four times during the student teaching practicum. It is on these visits that contacts with cooperating teachers and student teachers are established and pedagogical performance is assessed. The supervisor's specialized knowledge of teacher education can assist the student teacher in resolving problems and conflicts faced in the classroom environment while aiding the classroom teacher in making effective use of the student teacher.

During these observations, the style, methods and overall performance of the preservice teacher are evaluated and critiqued by the supervisor. Further analysis and assessment of the preservice teacher are discussed with the cooperating teacher and, ultimately, with the preservice teacher. This evaluation process affords the preservice teacher the opportunity to examine critically the strengths and weaknesses in his teaching technique as reflected in classroom observation lessons.

It has been argued by some that a supervisor of preservice teachers who has had some prior experience in the classroom is in a better position to analyze critically the professional temperament of a prospective teacher. Conant (1976) recommends that "the professor from the college or university who is to supervise and assess the practice teaching should have had much practical experience. His status should be analogous to that of a clinical professor in certain medical schools." Whatever the background of the supervisor, many existing practitioners of supervision feel that they serve their institutions as teachers, primarily; their students need much more clinical feedback by professional teacher educators than they are receiving (Koehler, 1985).

Student Self Evaluation

Preservice teachers should be required to keep a log which includes lesson plans, description of their experiences and evaluation of their teaching experiences. They should be encouraged to include insight about their growth, their students, their subject matter, and their use of materials, as well as including an evaluation of themselves as teachers. This provides additional communication between preservice teachers and college supervisors.

The log constitutes a valuable learning experience and helps students assess their effectiveness in interacting with their students and, thus, helps them gain understandings of how children learn. Frequently, preservice teachers lack introspection and self evaluation skills. To help students with self evaluation it is necessary to provide questions that will serve as guides, such as:

- Did the lesson go well?
- Why or why not?
- What would you change if you taught this lesson again?
- How did you feel about what you did?
- Were you well prepared and organized?
- Was the lesson appropriate for the students?
- Were the materials appropriate for the lesson?
- Was the lesson well motivated?
- How did the students respond to the lesson?
- Was the lesson understood?
- Were your explanations and directions clear?
- Was the lesson well integrated?
- Did the lesson provide for individualization and enrichment?
- Was the lesson well paced?
- Were the questions carefully thought out?
- Was information elicited from the children through good, clear questions?
- What disciplinary techniques did you use? Did they work? Were they appropriate? Could they have been avoided? How?
- Did the students take an active part in the lesson?
- Were major points of lesson reviewed?

Conclusion

Critics abound in the field of education both within and without the profession. Currently the caliber of students preparing for teaching careers is under attack. Increased efforts are needed to attract quality students. Conant (1963) urged that students with high academic quality be recruited by education faculties. Until recently, education majors were in poor supply because of low wages and bleak employment possibilities. Students of high academic standing shunned teaching in favor of more lucrative and rewarding professions.

Now that we are faced with an impending teacher shortage, action is necessary to once again attract candidates who will do justice to the teaching profession. Several programs have been initiated to complement a recruitment drive. One program involves the granting of scholarships and loans to make college tuition more accessible. Some states and institutions are offering tuition loans which will be forgiven after graduation if the students remain in teaching for a specified number of years. In other instances, attractive scholarships and tuition waivers plus stipends are being made available to qualified students.

While these efforts are being made to resolve the student population problem, teacher educators must continue in their efforts to insist on a quality product from their students. Preservice training which commences in the early years of preparation ensures a steadily maturing and learning process. Encountering more and more field experiences, the prospective teacher becomes more knowledgeable about the teaching community and whether teaching is really the appropriate choice.

REFERENCES

Ambach, Gordon, M. Memorandum to Chief Executive Officer of Institutions of Higher Education. December 6, 1983.

Brodbelt, S. "Considerations for Redesigning Teacher Education" *The Clearing House*. 1984, 58(3): 122-126.

Bowen, Ezra. Reported by Leavitt, Russel B. Atlanta. "Bad Medicine? Testing Teachers in Texas." *Time*. March 24, 1986, 127(12): 74

Conant, J.B. *The Education of American Teachers*. New York: MacMillan, 1963.

Doyle, Walter. "Learning to Teach: An Emerging Direction in Research on Preservice Teacher Education." *Journal of Teacher Education*. 1985, 36(1): 31-2.

Educational Testing Service, 1983-84 *Bulletin of Information*. Princeton, N.J. p. 5

Egbert, Robert L. *National Commission for Excellence in Teacher Education*. (A briefing document) Washington, D.C. American Association of Colleges for Teacher Education, 1984.

Egbert, R.L. "The Practice of Preservice Teacher Education." *Journal of Teacher Education*. 1985, 36(1): 16-22.

Fagan, E.R. & Merchant, L.J. "A Priority Assessment of Pre-Service Teachers' Field Experience Activities." *The Clearing House*. 1984, 57(8): 374.

Gamble, M.V. "Training Preservice Teachers for Inner-City Schools." *Phi Delta Kappan*. 1985, 67(4): 316-317.

Heald, J.E. *Report to the Profession*. Washington, D.C. American Association of Colleges for Teacher Education, 1983.

Hermanowicz, H.J. "The Pluralistic World of Beginning Teachers." *The Real World of Beginning Teachers*. Report of the Nineteenth National Teacher Education Professional Standards Conference. Washington, D.C. NEA, 1986.

Hunter, E. "What's the Low-Down on High Tech?" Some Questions for Teacher Educators." *Journal of Teacher Education*. 1983, 36(5): 26-28.

Johnson, J. "Changes in Student Teacher Dogmatism." *Journal of Educational Research*. 1969, 62: 224-226.

Koehler, V. "Research on Preservice Teacher Education." *Journal of Teacher Education*. 1985, 36(1): 23-30.

Seperson, M.A. and Joyce, B.R. "Teaching Styles and Student Teachers as related to those of their Cooperating Teachers." *Educational Leadership Research Supplement*. 1973, 31: 146-151.

The New York Times. "Texas Teachers Took It. Now You Can Test Classroom Skills." March 16, 1986, Sect. 4, p. 9.

Yee, A.H. "Do Cooperating Teachers Influence the Attitudes of Student Teachers?" *Journal of Educational Psychology*. 1969, 15(4): 327-332.

Zeichner, K.M. "Myths and Realities; Field Based experiences in Preservice Teacher Education." Journal of Teacher Education, 1980, 31(6): 45-46.

Chapter 27
Coping with Incompetent Teachers
Edwin M. Bridges*

Incompetent teachers represent a relatively small proportion of the teaching force, but the number of students who are being taught by such teachers is substantial. Even if only 5 percent of the teachers in public elementary and secondary schools are incompetent, the number of students being taught by these teachers exceeds the combined public-school enrollments of the 14 smallest states.

Students are not the only ones who are being short-changed by incompetent teachers. These poor performers tarnish the reputations of the vast majority of teachers who are competent and conscientious professionals.

Quite understandably, the problem of teacher incompetence has captured the attention of education reformers. They have advanced numerous solutions: cleansing the profession by dismissing all incompetent teachers; improving the attractiveness of teaching by raising salaries; restricting entry into the profession by means of competency tests; upgrading the quality of pre-service education by adopting competency-based preparation programs; and providing incentives for quality teaching by instituting merit pay.

Although there is no shortage of ideas about what should be done to redress the problem of teacher incompetence, virtually nothing is known about how local school officials are actually dealing with the problem. I have attempted to fill this void by conducting extensive original research that draws on a rich array of sources: interviews with administrators, documents from personnel files, a survey of local school districts, and a case study of a district that deals forthrightly with its poor performers. My aim has been to answer the following questions: What is the nature of teacher incompetence? How do administrators ascertain teacher incompetence? What are the perceived roots of incompetence? How do administrators respond to teacher incompetence? What determines how administrators respond? What is the bottom line in responding to the problem?

What Is the Nature of Teacher Incompetence?

Incompetence is a term without precise technical meaning; moreover, there are no clear-cut standards for determining whether a teacher is incompetent. This ambiguity is especially troublesome for school administrators. Approximately 75 percent of the teaching force has tenure. Tenured teachers may not be dismissed for poor performance unless the administration can prove to a hearing officer, a commission on professional competence, or a judge that the teacher is incompetent.

The lack of clear-cut standards, along with the extensive legal protections afforded tenured teachers, means that proving incompetence is a highly problematical, time-consuming, and costly undertaking for school administrators. As a result, I found, many administrators are inclined to tolerate the poor performer unless he or she is such a blatant failure in the classroom that no one doubts the appropriateness of the label "incompetent." Marginal teachers and teachers who are incompetent but are the target of few parental complaints are apt to be endured, if not ignored.

When teachers fail, they commonly exhibit a weakness in maintaining discipline. This particular form of failure is the leading cause for termination in all studies of teacher failure which have been conducted over the past 70 years. Besides manifesting a weakness in maintaining classroom discipline, incompetent teachers usually fail in one or more of the following ways as well: failure to treat students properly, failure to impart subject matter effectively, failure to accept teaching advice from supervisors, and failure to produce desired results in the classroom.

How Do Administrators Ascertain Teacher Incompetence?

Recognizing that most of a teacher's activities take place

*Dr. Edwin M. Bridges is Professor of Education, Stanford University, California.

behind closed doors, administrators use a variety of means to identify incompetent teachers. The most common methods, I discovered, are supervisor ratings and observations, complaints from parents or students, complaints from other teachers, and student test results.

Parental complaints play an extremely important role. Such complaints signal that something may be radically wrong in a teacher's classroom and may stimulate a closer look at what is happening. Parental complaints also exert pressure on the administrator to deal with the poor performer. As one administrator put it: "Parent complaints are the most powerful force that we have to deal with. Without parent complaints, we leave the teacher alone."

Complaints from teachers, though less frequent than those from parents, also alert supervisors to the poor performers on the staff. These complaints arise in part because of the interdependent character of teaching activities. The incompetent teacher creates several potential problems for colleagues. Most of the poor performers are unable to maintain discipline; if students become too unruly, the noise may disrupt the instruction taking place in other classrooms. The students who have been taught by these teachers may also create difficulties for subsequent teachers if the students have not mastered the concepts, skills, and material to which they have been exposed. Finally, incompetent teachers may become a source of frustration for their colleagues if they work together as members of a teaching team. Any one of these problems may prompt other teachers to complain.

What Are the Perceived Roots of Incompetence?

Most proposals for school reform assume that teacher incompetence is due to a lack of skill or motivation. But the roots of incompetence are much more complex, my research suggests, than reformers have assumed. Rarely is a teacher's poor performance due to a single cause, such as insufficient skill, ability, or effort. More commonly, unsatisfactory performance stems from other sources as well, such as emotional distress, poor health, marital problems, and financial difficulties.

The inadequacies of past supervisors also are partially responsible for the present difficulties being experienced by incompetent teachers. According to some of the administrators whom I interviewed, these supervisors lacked the ability to deal with incompetent teachers and were reluctant to confront them about their poor performance in the classroom. One administrator bluntly stated, "He had incompetent supervisors who didn't help him to improve." Another administrator blamed the teacher's current problems on supervisory passivity; in the words of the administrator, "Her supervisors were

aware of the problems but did nothing. If they had confronted her and given her assistance, she might have been salvaged and transformed into an adequate teacher."

Under these conditions, improving the performance of an incompetent teacher is a formidable challenge. It is unlikely that something akin to a miracle drug will ever suffice as a cure for teacher incompetence. The extent of an incompetent teacher's difficulties in the classroom and the causes that underlie these difficulties are simply too far-reaching.

How Do Administrators Respond to Teacher Incompetence?

Many school administrators, like their counterparts in business and in other professions such as law and medicine, are inclined to tolerate and protect the poor performer. In school districts, administrators manifest this tendency in several ways. They use classroom observation reports as occasions for stating glowing generalities (e.g., "I really enjoyed visiting your class") even though the teacher's performance is below par. They use double-talk to cover or to deaden the sting of their criticisms (e.g., "I know that a continued positive attitude toward change will only lead to her becoming a well-liked teacher"). They provide inflated performance ratings; ratings of satisfactory or better are commonplace despite the perceived inadequacies of the teacher. They rely on escape hatches (e.g., transfer) to skirt the problems posed by the incompetent teacher. Finally, they make minimal use of the most drastic sanction for poor performance—dimissal.

The prevelance of inflated ratings is particularly troublesome for administrators when they decide to get rid of the deadwood on the teaching staff. As one of our interviewees summed up the situation, "Most often the data do not support the dismissal of an ineffective teacher because the history of evaluation is too good." Prior use of glowing generalities, double-talk, and escape hatches adds to the difficulties of terminating incompetent teachers.

When an administrator does decide to confront a teacher about his or her poor performance, the administrator's efforts generally fall into two distinct stages. In the first stage, the administrator concentrates on trying to salvage the teacher. My analysis of these salvage attempts indicates that they are seldom successful, especially with a veteran teacher.

As one supervisor described such rescue efforts: "It is a frustrating process for the helper. We may save the teacher's job, but we're never sure whether it's best for the kids. The teacher rarely becomes anything better than low average." Another administrator bluntly stated: "The (incompetent) veteran teacher is near impossible to make a good teacher. I really question whether it's worth the grief and the aggravation." Improvement is limited, in part, because administrators lack the resources and training needed to diagnose and correct poor performance.

If the teacher fails to demonstrate sufficient improvement during the salvage stage, the administrator begins to concentrate on the next stage: getting rid of the teacher. The method of termination is largely determined by the teacher's employment status. Teachers without tenure are dismissed; those with tenure are generally induced to resign or to retire early.

In California, for example, temporary teachers may be dismissed at the expiration of their contracts without cause and without due process. Although temporary teachers constitute less than 7 percent of the state's teaching force, they accounted for approximately 70 percent of the dismissals for incompetence between September 1982 and May 1984. In contrast, tenured teachers are covered by a thick layer of legal protections and accounted for only 5 percent of California's dismissals during the period I studied—even thought they make up 80 percent of the teaching force.

Moreover, my research shows that when California's tenured teachers are terminated, they are 20 times more likely to be eased out than to be dismissed. Regardless of the termination method used, few tenured teachers are being weeded out of the profession for incompetence in our most populous state—less than 1 percent of the total tenured force in two years.

Inducing an incompetent teacher to resign or to retire early isn't easy. But it can be done, as I found in a case study of a school district that restored public confidence by inducing 20 percent of its teaching staff to leave during a period of declining enrollments and shrinking resources. These teachers, all tenured, were the weakest ones working in the district.

When incompetent teachers resign or retire early, they often are under intense pressure from administrators. The power of gentle persuasion (e.g., suggesting it may be a good time for the teacher to consider other options) does not seem to work. Incompetent teachers are unlikely to leave a district unless administrators communicate their dissatisfaction with the teacher's performance, buttress their criticism with specific instances of the teacher's shortcomings, give negative evaluations, and issue a legal notice of the district's intent to recommend dismissal if the teacher's performance does not improve. The road to an induced resignation is paved with emotional and procedural cobblestones and produces a bumpy, taxing ride for administrators and teachers alike.

A carrot, as well as a stick, figures in the induced resignations and early retirements of incompetent teachers. Districts commonly offer a wide array of induce-

ments to poor performers in exchange for their "voluntary" separations. The three most common kinds of inducements are medical coverage for a fixed period of time, employment as a part-time consultant, and cash settlements ranging from $5,000 to $15,000. What a teacher actually receives depends in part on the financial status of the district and his or her age, health, and perceived effort.

What Determines How Administrators Respond?

Several factors incline administrators to tolerate and protect the poor performer. The first of these factors is the desire of administrators to avoid unpleasantness. They prefer to be spared the emotional ordeal entailed in criticizing and finding fault with the behavior of others. Accordingly, administrators are inclined to suffer other people's shortcomings in silence and to "manage by guilt" (Levinson, 1964). The significant elements of management by guilt are disappointment in the employee; anger at his short comings; failure to confront him realistically about his job behavior; procrastination in reaching a decision about the poor performer; compliments to cover-up or ease the guilt of managerial anger; and finally, discharge (Levinson, 1964). According to this view, school administrators are inclined to withhold negative information from ineffective teachers until the moment when termination becomes the overriding issue. As I indicated earlier, that moment rarely comes.

The organizational context in which administrators work, along with the legal protections of teachers and the lack of agreement about what constitutes effective teaching, reinforces the tendency to suppress negative judgments. There are often contradictions between the legitimate and the expert power of the administrator; he often is expected to evaluate the performance of professionals whose competencies differ from his own (Trask, 1964). These contradictions breed self-doubt and strengthen the tendency to withhold criticism. Administrators also play multiple roles which limit the amount of time that they can spend on any one activity. Because they are unable to spend much time in a teacher's classroom, they hesitate to be critical of a teacher's performance. Moreover, criticism generates additional time demands and the need to work closely with teachers to improve their performance. Finally, lenient evaluations have functional value; they represent a potentially potent strategy for increasing the willingness of subordinates to comply with managerial initiatives. Under these conditions, the safest course of action is to follow one's instincts and avoid the conflict and discomfort that accompany confrontation.

Although the tendency of administrators to tolerate and protect the poor performer is a strong one, its strength may be diminished by several factors. Administrators are likely to confront incompetent teachers and pressure them to leave if the district attaches high importance to teacher evaluation. A district's commitment to a strong program in teacher evaluation is evidenced in three ways. First, the district provides its principals with remedial assistance that can be used in efforts to improve the performance of an unsatisfactory teacher. Second, the district provides principals with meaningful feedback and incentives in relation to how well they carry out their assessments of classroom teachers. Finally, the district takes steps to ensure that principals have the skills and knowledge required to evaluate teachers and to take formal action against those who fail to improve their performance in the classroom. Unfortunately, most school districts lack these three characteristics.

Administrators also are more likely to confront an incompetent teacher if their district is facing declining enrollments and is relatively small in size or is experiencing a financial squeeze. Declining enrollments confront administrators with the need to lay off teachers. State laws and collective bargaining agreements often mandate layoffs on the basis of seniority. The seniority principle creates problems for administrators because incompetent teachers are much more likely to appear among the most senior segment of the teaching force than among the least senior. The likelihood of this occurrence is not due to the age or the experience of the teacher. Rather, it is accounted for by the selection ratios (i.e., the proportion of applicants who were hired) in effect at the time the most experienced and least experienced teachers were employed. Individuals who are hired in a period of labor shortage are more likely to be unsatisfactory employees than individuals who are employed during a labor surplus (Taylor and Russell, 1939). Since the most senior teachers were hired during a period of labor shortage and the least senior teachers were hired during an era of teacher surplus, the odds are that the incidence of incompetence is inversely related to seniority. The odds are further strengthened by selective attrition; there's some evidence that academically able teachers are more likely to leave teaching than the less able (Schlechty and Vance, 1981).

Therefore, decreasing staff size on the basis of seniority is likely to necessitate releasing competent teachers and retaining the incompetent teachers. If administrators choose to reduce the size of there staffs through layoffs, they may be bombarded with complaints from parents who question the wisdom of this practice. When these complaints arise, school officials may be forced to adopt a more aggressive approach to teacher evaluation. Even if parents do not mount a campaign against layoffs on the basis of seniority, administrators may anticipate that staff reductions will eventually lead to complaints from parents whose children are being taught by incompetent

teachers. Wishing to avoid these complaints, administrators may tighten the evaluation procedures and put the pressure on these teachers to improve or to leave the district.

Declining enrollments do not necessarily result in the death of the inclination to tolerate the poor performers, however. If the district has adequate financial resources, administrators are likely to evade, rather that confront, the problems created by declining enrollments. As long as money is plentiful, administrators can afford to retain all teachers and to use a variety of escape hatches to avoid parental complaints. Incompetent teachers can be assigned to elective courses with small enrollments, to tutor students in their homes, and to work on special projects in the central office. If a district is strapped for funds, administrators lose these options and must confront the incompetent teacher.

The size of the district also affects how administrators respond to incompetent teachers during a period of declining enrollments. Large districts are able to cushion the impact of shrinking enrollments through attrition. The teaching staff can be decreased through naturally occurring events—deaths, retirements, and resignations. Large districts also are able to use between-school transfer and the roving substitute to avoid parental complaints. Small districts lack these escape hatches; as a result administrators in these settings are more likely to confront the poor performers and to weed our the deadwood on the teaching staff when enrollments begin to fall!

What Is the Bottom Line in Responding to the Problem?

The single most important personnel decision a school district makes is the decision to grant a teacher tenure. The tenure decision is the last opportunity a district has to enforce high performance standards. Once teachers acquire tenure they have to be unmistakable failures before the district can get rid of them. Every time a district makes a mistake in granting tenure, it creates scores of problems.

Teacher-evaluation systems should be redesigned to reflect the importance of the tenure decision. Resources—time, energy, people, money—are limited, and districts should allocate these resources where they are likely to receive the greatest return. With nearly one million new teachers expected to enter the profession over the next five years, districts should concentrate their scarce resources on the selection, evaluation, and development of probationary teachers. Moreover, if the anticipated teacher shortage actually develops, districts should resist the understandable temptation to grant tenure to marginal teachers on the grounds that "the next ones could be even worse."

Better yet, districts should make it as difficult for teachers to obtain tenure as to lose tenure once it has been granted. By adopting more stringent standards for awarding tenure, districts would be able to retain institutional flexibility in dealing with future fluctuations in enrollments and funding. More important, districts would be able to ensure that future generations of students will be taught by competent teachers.

In redesigning teacher evaluation systems to reflect the overriding importance of the tenure decision, school districts should be hard on the standards and soft on the people. Implementing high standards for awarding tenure will be especially difficult because the measurement of teacher effectiveness is an inexact science. No single source of evidence is an adequate and valid indicator of teacher effectiveness. Under such conditions, it makes sense for school districts to base tenure decisions on multiple sources of evidence, which when considered fairly and impartially, induce a reasonable belief that the teacher is fully competent.

The following types of evidence warrant consideration in the tenure review process: (1) observations by principals; (2) observation by peers who are expert in the subject matter and grade level being taught; (3) student ratings (grades 7–12); and (4) student test performance. When student test results are used, a school district needs to be sure that the tests measure knowledge and skills which match the teacher's instructional objectives. In addition, a district needs to rule out the possibility that a relatively poor or strong showing by students may be due to initial differences in the performance potential of the students.

To ensure that these various types of evidence are weighed carefully during the tenure review process, school districts should establish a Tenure Review Committee. This Committee would consist of three persons: an administrator, a tenured teacher who has knowledge or the probationary teacher's grade level, subject matter, and teaching context; and a teacher from within the system who is appointed by the teacher's union. The task of the Tenure Review Committee is two-fold: (1) to discuss the review of the teacher's performance to see if it warrants by a preponderance of the evidence the granting of tenure, and (2) to render judgments on this issue. Each member of the Committee is expected to declare an opinion (yes or no) and to state the reasons for his/her judgment. The Committee's report, along with the review prepared by the principal, would be forwarded to the Superintendent and the Board of Education for a final decision on tenure.

Being soft on the people means abandonment of the "sink or swim" philosophy that governs the practices of many school districts during a teacher's probationary period. Beginning teachers are usually left on their own to master the complexities of teaching. If these teachers are held accountable for meeting stringent standards when the tenure decision is made, they are entitled to receive intensive care and assistance during their probationary period. Although remediation does not seem to work well with veteran teachers, it may be beneficial for neophytes in the teaching profession.

There are two kinds of professional assistance which are reasonable for probationary teachers, and participation in these programs should be entirely voluntary. The first of these programs would be oriented to *groups* of teachers. This Professional Development Program (PDP) would focus on strategies and techniques for dealing with the common problems of beginning teachers: discipline, classroom management, lesson design, and lesson implementation. In addition, the PDP staff would demonstrate a variety of instructional strategies and introduce teachers to various ways of obtaining feedback from students about what is happening in the classroom.

The second program would be geared to *individual* teachers. This Instructional Assistance Program (IAP) would provide for tenured teachers to work with probationary teachers in their classrooms in whatever capacity the teacher and the staff member agreed was appropriate. Participation in the IAP, as well as the PDP, would be voluntary. Efforts to force-feed teachers have seldom been successful. Unless teachers want assistance and believe it is necessary, they are unlikely to profit from it. Districts have a responsibility to offer the assistance and to let teachers know what is available. Whether they elect to use it should be their decision and should not figure in their evaluations. Good performance, not a "good attitude," should be the overriding concern.

Since there appears to be no cure for teacher incompetence, districts must emphasize preventive measures: more careful selection, assistance during the probationary period, and substantially higher performance standards for granting tenure.

REFERENCES

Bridges, E.M. (1986). *The incompetent teacher.* Philadelphia, PA: The Falmer Press, Taylor and Francis, Inc.

Bridges, E.M., & G.B. (1984). *Managing the incompetent teacher.* Eugene, OR: ERIC Clearinghouse on Educational Management

Levinson, H. (1964), *Emotional health in the world of work.* New York: Harper and Row.

Schlecty, P., & Vance, V. (1981). Do academically able teachers leave education? The North Carolina case. *Phi Delta Kappan, 63,* 106–112.

Taylor, H., & Russell, J. (1939, October). The relationship of validity coefficients to the practical effectiveness of tests in selection: Discussion and tables. *Journals of Applied Psychology, 23,* 565–78.

Trask, A. (1964, December). Principals, teachers, and supervision: Dilemmas and solutions. *Administrator's Notebook, XIII, 1–4.*

American Federation of Teachers

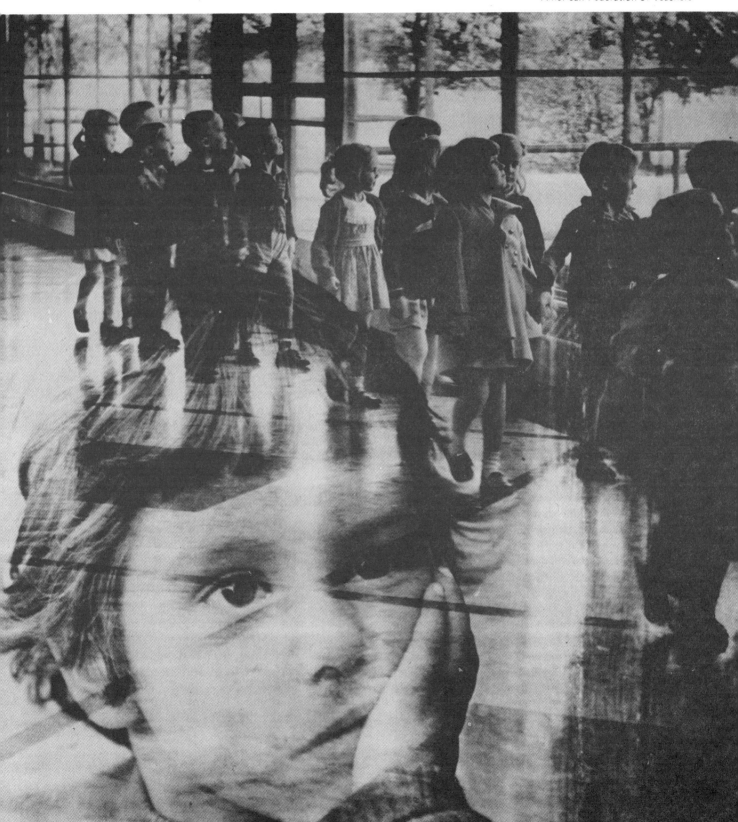

Chapter 28
Teacher Job Satisfaction
Paula E. Lester*

Because teaching is unique (Lortie, 1975), it is essential to explore the nature of the educational work setting and the characteristics or teachers themselves in order to understand teacher job satisfaction. Prior to the development of the TJSQ (Teacher Job Satisfaction Questionnaire), it was necessary to identify (a) the reasons people choose teaching as an occupation, (b) the characteristics of teaching, and (c) the reasons people leave teaching. This study consisted of the development of an instrument (TJSQ) designed to assess teacher job satisfaction in elementary, junior high (middle) schools, and senior high schools. The following procedures were conducted to develop the TJSQ:

1. *Conceptual.* A thorough review of concepts, theories, and approaches related to job satisfaction was conducted in order to develop a clear definition of job satisfaction.
2. *Job characteristics.* A list of different factors which might account for teacher job satisfaction was compiled after a systematic review of the literature. These factors were given operational definitions and an item pool was created.
3. *Psychometric characteristics.* Statistical procedures were followed to develop a representative sample of items. Tests of reliability and validity were performed.
4. *Pilot study.* A pilot study was conducted with subjects similar to the population in the final study to improve the instrument before the final study. Item analyses and tests for item discrimination were performed to eliminate undesirable items. An initial test of reliability was also conducted.
5. *Administration of the TJSQ.* An appropriate sample was randomly selected to complete the instrument. Factor analysis and reliability procedures were employed.

In order to generate a taxonomy for the development

of this instrument, the theories of Maslow and Herzberg were explored as sources of job satisfaction. These theories contain specific concepts that correspond to the factors logically found in the educational setting, and which were identified in the development of the TJSQ. Consequently, their theories provide a system of classification that supports the conceptual foundation of this study.

Review of the Literature

Of more than 35,000 occupations listed in the *Dictionary of Occupational Titles,* between 35% and 40% of all people in the professional services are grouped as teachers (Gould & Yoakam, 1947). There is no other occupation with a membership of over a million college graduates and tens of thousands with advanced degrees (Lortie, 1975). Because more college students prepare for teaching careers than for any other single area of work, it is important to study (a) why people choose teaching as a profession, (b) the characteristics or the teaching occupation, and (c) reasons for leaving teaching. Such background helps explain not only the choice of teaching as a career, but also what constitutes teacher job satisfaction.

Why People Choose Teaching as a Profession

Lortie (1975) examines the attractions of teaching and identified eight reasons (which he called *appeals*) for becoming a teacher. First is *interpersonal appeal*—people become teachers because they are interested in children and want to help develop a youngster's potential. In the second category is *service appeal*—people become teachers in order to perform a special mission in the community, teaching is an opportunity to serve society, and the teacher is a moral agent dedicated to serving the public. *Continuation appeal* is another category—people choose teaching because they enjoyed school as students. Mate-

*Dr. Paula E. Lester is an Assistant Professor of Educational Administration and Leadership at C.W. Post Campus of Long Island University, NY.

rial benefits, such as job security, prestige, and money form the fourth appeal. Five-day work weeks, short workdays, many holidays, and long summer vacations help make teaching an appealing occupation. Socioeconomic constraints make teachers' colleges economically accessible for many, thereby increasing the number of teachers. For others, teaching is a "safety net." People who cannot enter a more preferred line of work can become teachers without loss of status. Finally, teaching appeals to some as a second career after trying other work.

In a study conducted by the National Education Association in 1981, teachers were requested to choose three reasons (from a list of 19 items) for originally choosing teaching as a profession. At least 20% of the respondents reported the following eight reasons: (a) a desire to work with young people, (b) interest in a subject matter field, (c) the value or significance of education in society, (d) the influence of a teacher or advisor in elementary or secondary school, (e) the influence of family, (f) long summer vacation, (g) job security, and (h) never really considered anything else. Age, sex, and school level accounted for the major differences between groups in analyzing these reasons. Teachers under age 30 cited a desire to work with young people and the long summer vacation more frequently than did teachers over 30. Teachers under age 40 chose interest in a subject matter field more frequently than older teachers. The importance of job security was cited more frequently by teachers over 30. More males indicated a desire to work with young people and interest in a subject matter field than did females. However, more females than males indicated that they had never considered any other career and that they were influenced by their families. Elementary and junior high or middle school teachers selected a desire to work with young people more often than did senior high school teachers, whereas junior high or middle school teachers cited interest in a subject matter field more frequently than did elementary school teachers. Finally, more elementary school teachers than junior high, middle school, or high school teachers, indicated that they never really considered anything else (NEA, 1981).

A comparison of these two studies reveals that the primary reasons for selecting teaching as an occupation are love of teaching and of children, liking of subject field, desire to serve, financial benefits, and the influence of school and former teachers.

Characteristics of Teaching

In a study by England and Stein (1961), various occupational groups responded to items describing the following areas of the work environment: co-workers, company, communication, hours, pay, promotion,

recognition, security, supervision, type of work, and working conditions. The authors conclude that significant occupational differences make it necessary to identify important areas of interest for each occupational group. They recommend the development of scales that emphasize particular areas of importance for each occupation.

Teaching is unique (Lortie, 1975), and, as a career, offers "opportunities for service and for personal satisfaction which are equaled by very few professions" (Gould & Yoakam, 1947, p. 3). Lortie (1975) discusses three types of teaching rewards. The first type is *extrinsic reward,* which includes salary and prestige, and is seen as being independent of the teacher. The second type of reward is linked to the objective nature of the work as perceived by the teacher and is labeled *ancillary reward.* The final type of reward is *psychic or intrinsic reward,* which is subjective and varies from teacher to teacher. Lortie asserts that "the structure of teaching favors psychic rewards" (pp. 101–103).

According to Dorros (1968), the work climate of teaching entails a number of aspects. Professional status involves recognition and the opportunity to make decisions. Personnel policies signify the duties and responsibilities of the teacher, the teaching conditions, and the process for hiring teachers. Work load denotes the teacher's daily activities, such as class size, record keeping activities, and preparation of lesson plans. Instructional material and equipment include money for textbooks and supplies. Physical conditions are encompassed by the buildings themselves. Security of position refers to tenure and seniority. Academic freedom alludes to the right to teach the truth as perceived by the teachers. Personal freedom means engaging in activities outside school without fear of reprisal. Dorros identified problems in the work climate of the school involving a lack of teacher autonomy, inefficient administration, misassignment of teachers, excessive work load, extracurricular duties, and a lack of security in some school systems.

Other characteristics of teaching worthy of mention are income, status, and the work schedule. For Dorros (1968), the economic welfare of teachers consists of salaries, retirement benefits, fringe benefits, and other aspects related to working conditions. Lortie (1975) views teacher income in terms of a trade-off between the amount of money received and the amount of risk involved. Lower salaries are more expected in the public sector than in private industry.

Teaching has been considered a white-collar, middle-class occupation. Traditionally, teaching has offered its members an opportunity for upward mobility. Unfortunately, the teaching occupation has a low standing in the community (Waller, 1965), even though society values learning.

Finally, the work schedule of teachers has received much publicity. The average teacher works five short days per week with many holidays and long summer vacations. Women who become teachers view teaching as an in-and-out arrangement, dependent upon marital and maternal commitments (Lortie, 1975), with teaching as a secondary commitment, and family the primary commitment. Lortie found that women have time to perform household duties and have a work schedule that coincides with the schedules of young school-age children.

On the other hand, Lortie found that men view teaching as a means toward an end, seek administrative positions, or leave for better positions, more pay, and the higher standard of living that private industry can offer. In other words, for many people, teaching does not represent a full time commitment.

Following the recommendation made by England and Stein (1961), that particular areas of importance be emphasized for various occupations, the characteristics of the teaching occupation that seem to require further investigation are: (a) co-workers (colleagues, fellow teachers), (b) company (school), (c) pay, (d) promotion, (e) recognition, (f) security, (g) supervision, (h) type of work (instructional material, work load), and (i) working conditions (physical conditions).

Reasons for Leaving Teaching

Crane and Ervit (1955) identify 14 reasons for leaving teaching in New York State. Among the reasons given by female teachers, the researchers note (a) marriage, (b) married and moving to another state, (c) decision to have children, (d) pregnancy, and (e) home and children considered a full-time job. These reasons coincide with the view of teaching as an in-and-out arrangement dependent upon marital and maternal commitments.

Inadequate salary, not being granted tenure, conflict and/or dissatisfaction with administration, teaching situation, lack of discipline or respect by pupils, and teaching load are among additional reasons for leaving, as cited by Crane and Ervit (1955). Certification problems, geographic location or the community, and the feeling of being unsuited for teaching are other cited reasons.

Dillon (1978) has identified 10 factors that may influence the decision to leave teaching. They are: (a) long hours, (c) too much preparation for classroom teaching, (c) lack of student interest, (d) salaries, (e) personality conflict with school administration, (f) time, (g) lack of advancement opportunities, (h) inadequate knowledge of subject matter, (i) lack of variety on the job, and (j) poor fringe benefits.

Knight (1978), in a review of related literature, found seven major categories that influence teachers to leave the profession. The categories are: (a) student related

concerns, (b) time requirements of the job, (c) job characteristics, (d) personal concerns, (e) administrative and supervisory concerns, (f) preparation for teaching, and (g) factors outside the profession.

It should be noted that some of the cited reasons for leaving have also been found in studies of reasons for entering the profession of teaching. Women enter and leave because of marital and maternal commitments. Additionally, financial and material benefits are frequently cited as reasons for entering and leaving. Pay, job security, and prestige (status) are three rewards that teaching can provide. When they are present, they contribute to job satisfaction, whereas when they are absent, they contribute to job dissatisfaction, and eventually to the decision to leave teaching. Other aspects or the work environment that are potential sources of dissatisfaction are poor fringe benefits, lack of opportunity for advancement, administration, pupils, and the job of teaching.

Research Methodology

The population from which the sample was drawn includes teachers from New York City, Westchester, Nassau, and Suffolk Counties. Within each of these four geographic locations, a sample for two school districts was randomly selected by using a table of random numbers. Within each of the eight school districts thus identified, an elementary, junior high school, and a senior high school were randomly selected. Of the 1,600 instruments and personal data forms distributed to teachers in these schools, 631 returns were received from all eight districts, providing 620 usable returns.

Frequent distributions for items and for factor scores were obtained, and response patters examined to assess the variability of ratings.

The internal consistency of the TJSQ was examined by obtaining coefficient alpha for each scale and for the total score (.93).

Factor analysis was undertaken as an exploratory technique to help discover underlying factors and as a psychometric procedure for the development and refinement of the TJSQ. A terminal nine factor, orthogonal varimax solution was accepted using the criterion of Eigenvalues greater than or equal to unity. The nine factors are: Supervision, Colleagues, Working Conditions, Pay, Responsibility, Work Itself, Advancement, Security, and Recognition.

The data were classified by sampling procedure into system level variables of location (urban/suburban), school district size (small/large), county, school level, and district. Descriptive statistics were computed to summarize the similarities and differences of job satisfaction scores on the various scales (factors) in relation to the system level variables and the personal and demographic variables found in the personal data form (age, sex, marital status, total years of teaching experience, years in district, educational level, tenure, and union affiliation).

Similarities and differences among elementary, junior high schools, senior high schools, and the eight school districts on the nine factors were studied by obtaining the scale means and standard deviations and by examining the distribution of scores. One-way analyses of variance, with significance at the .05 level, were performed among the system level variables to test statistically whether the means of the groups were significantly different from each other.

Findings

One-way analyses of variance were performed with each of the system level variables and the nine factors of the TJSQ to identify differences among the various groups. Based upon location (urban or suburban), the five factors denoting pairs of groups significantly different at the .05 level were Supervision, Working Conditions, Pay, Work Itself, and Advancement. Suburban districts were more satisfied than were urban districts, except for the factor of Supervision.

Analysis by the variable of size (small or large district) showed that only the factor of Pay demonstrated significance between small and large districts with small districts being more satisfied than large districts. This finding is consistent with the findings of the National Education Association (1982) regarding the relationship between size of the school district and satisfaction. The National Education Association found that the larger the school system, the greater the dissatisfaction; that is, teachers in small districts are more satisfied than teachers in large districts. When analyzed by county (New York City, Westchester, Nassau, and Suffolk), Working Conditions, Pay, and Work Itself demonstrated significant differences. New York City was the least satisfied area on all three factors, whereas each of the three other counties were the most satisfied on at least one factor.

Analysis by school level (elementary, junior high school, and senior high school) demonstrated significant differences between groups on the factors of Supervision, Colleagues, Working Conditions, Pay, Responsibility, and Work Itself. Elementary school teachers were more satisfied than senior high school teachers on all these factors, except Supervision. This finding is also consistent with the findings of the National Education Association (1982), which found that elementary school teachers are the most satisfied, and senior high school teachers are the most dissatisfied.

Finally, analyses by the variable of the eight school districts showed evidence of significance at the .05 level

for differences between groups on the factors of Supervision, Working Conditions, Pay, and Work Itself.

Implications

College graduates are not choosing the teaching profession because of low salaries, increased violence in the schools, poor working conditions, and the large amount of paper work (clerical duties) involved. However, according to the present study, teachers are not as dissatisfied as expected. Teachers are dissatisfied with pay, advancement, and recognition, but satisfied with supervision, colleagues, responsibility, work itself, and security, except for a few elementary and junior high school teachers within specific districts. Working conditions is one area that shows dissatisfaction at the district level, as well as at the school level within specific districts. The fact that all but one of these results are within one standard deviation from the mean indicates that, regardless of location, size of district, county, school level, and district, teachers generally feel similarly about their jobs. Basically, those aspects of the job that are negatively perceived (pay, advancement, and recognition) are perceived as such by most teachers. However, their perceptions of those aspects of the job that are positive vary slightly.

School administrators can use this instrument to find out how their teachers feel about what they do. Administrators can gain valuable information about how their teachers evaluate their present teaching positions in order to determine teachers' expectations about the job and the work environment. Administration of the TJSQ to all teachers within a school district may promote the discovery of those aspects of the work setting that contribute to teacher job satisfaction. By careful examination of the results for each school within each level in a district, useful information may be obtained about the characteristics of the work situation and the characteristics of individuals. Such analysis may be utilized to redesign jobs to further strengthen the organizational fit between the job and the person. Educational policy decisions need to consider the importance of each aspect of the job to the individual rather than merely the level of overall job satisfaction. The results provided by the interaction between the nature of the work setting and individual teachers may facilitate effective job restructuring in order to maximize the achievement of organizational and individual goals and ultimately to improve teacher job satisfaction.

REFERENCES

Athanasiou, R., Robinson, J.P., & Head, K.B. (1969). *Measures of occupational attitudes and occupational characteristics.* Ann Arbor: University of Michigan, Institute for Social Research, (Draft)

Berdie, D.R., & Anderson, J.F. (1974). *Questionnaires: Design and use.* New Jersey: Scarecrow Press, Inc.

Borgatta, E.F. (1967). The work components study: A set of measures for work motivation. *Journal of Psychological Studies, 15,* 1–11.

Brayfield, A.H., & Rothe, H.F. (1951). An index of job satisfaction. *Journal of Applied Psychology, 35,* 307–311.

Crane, E., & Ervit, J. (1955). *Reasons why some teachers leave public school teaching in upstate New York.* New York: The State Education Department of New York, The University of the State of New York, Division of Research.

Dillon, R. (1978). Identification of factors influencing vocational agriculture teachers to leave teaching. *Journal of the American Association for Teacher Educators in Agriculture, 19*(3), 34–39.

Dunnette, M.D., Campbell, J.P., & Hakel, M.D. (1967). Factors contributing to job satisfaction and job dissatisfaction in six occupational groups. *Organizational Behavior and Human Performance, 2,* 143–174.

Dorros, S. (1968). *Teaching as a profession.* Columbus, OH: Charles E. Merrill Publishing Company.

Edwards, A.L. (1957). *Techniques of attitude scale construction.* New York: Appleton-Century-Crofts, Inc.

England, G.W., & Stein, C.I. (1961). The occupational reference group—A neglected concept in employee attitude scales. *Personnel Psychology, 14,* 299–304.

Gould, G., & Yoakam, G.A. (1947). *The teacher and his work.* New York: The Ronald Press Company.

Gruneberg, M.M. (1979). *Understanding job satisfaction.* New York: John Wiley & Sons.

Herzberg, F., Mausner, B., & Snyderman, B. (1959). *The motivation to work.* New York: John Wiley & Sons, Inc.

Hoppock, R. (1935). *Job satisfaction.* New York: Harper & Brothers.

Kerlinger, F.N. (1973). *Foundations of behavioral research.* New York: Holt, Rinehart, & Winston, Inc.

Knight, J.A. (1978). Why vocational agriculture teachers in Ohio leave teaching. *Journal of the American Association of Teacher Educators in Agriculture, 19*(3), 11–17.

Lester, P. (1984). Development of an instrument to measure teacher job satisfaction. *Dissertation Abstracts International, 44,* 3592. (University Microfilms No. 84–06,298)

Lortie, D.C. (1975). *School-teacher: A sociological study.* Chicago: The University of Chicago Press.

Maslow, A. (1954). *Motivation and personality.* New York: Harper & Row.

Miskel, C., & Heller, L. (1973). The educational work components study: An adapted set of measures for work motivation. *The Journal of Experimental Education, 42,* 45–50.

Nie, N.A., Hull, H.C., Jenkins, J.G., Steinbrenner, K., & Bent, D. H. (1975). *Statistical package for the social sciences* (2nd ed.). New York: McGraw-Hill.

Nunnally, J.C. (1967). *Psychometric theory.* New York: McGraw-Hill, Inc.

Scott, W.E. (1967). The development of semantic differential scales as measures of morale. *Personnel Psychology, 20,* 179–198.

Sergiovanni, T.J. (1967). Factors which affect satisfaction and dissatisfaction of teachers. *Journal of Educational Administration, 5,* 66–82.

Smith, P.C., Kendall, L.M., & Hulin, C.L. (1969). *The measurement of satisfaction in work and retirement.* Chicago: Rand McNally.

Status of the American public school teacher, 1980–1981. (1982). Washington, DC: National Education Association.

Waller, W. (1965). *The sociology of teaching.* New York: John Wiley & Sons.

Weiss, D.M., Dawis, R.V., England, G.W., & Lofquist, L.H. (1967). *Manual for the Minnesota Satisfaction Questionnaire* (Minnesota Studies in Vocational Rehabilitation: XXII). Minneapolis: University of Minnesota, Industrial Relations Center.

Chapter 29
Teachers as Philosophers
Edward A. Wynne*

Teachers and administrators are confronted with many philosophic issues in their work. Finding the proper answers to such questions is a challenging—and sometimes unending—task. But often the challenge is exacerbated by the denial that such philosophic issues exist. And so a first step in handling the challenge is to recognize its reality. Then, we can consider some of its implications.

My personal discovery of the centrality of philosophy in teaching occurred during the research my students and I have been doing in Chicago area schools. For example, one student, as part of his research paper, asked different teachers in the same school how they would handle a typical instance of student cheating. One respondent said, "My policy is to announce in my first class that any student I catch cheating on an exam will be flunked for the *course*. Then, I carry out my warning." Another respondent said, "I announce that any student caught cheating on an exam will be flunked for the *exam*." The last respondent said, "My students know that I will flunk—on that exam—any student I catch cheating. However, I will listen to any 'explanation' offered by guilty students." Information like this proved food for thought. To be precise, the three answers represent divergent philosophies. Let me explicate.

We can start our analysis with the middle answer—flunking for the exam. We should assume that oftentimes, students are not caught when they cheat. Suppose we speculate that ten percent of cheaters are caught. Then, "flunking on the exam" means that 90 percent of the time, "cheating pays." Indeed, assume a student does flunk an exam because he was caught cheating. Even so, the student might conclude that he might've flunked without cheating, so little has been lost. Thus, "flunking on the exam" assumes that almost all cheaters are caught, or that threats of comparatively mild punishment will deter most students from the potential profits of cheating. Are such assumptions realistic? The teacher who flunks for the course has a more negative view of human nature. He assumes that students will tend to

cheat unless they are confronted with severe sanctions. Are these assumptions realistic? The last respondent, who flunks for the exam but will talk things over, assumes that students will tend to be honest, and that students who are caught cheating after a warning will offer honest and good "explanations."

After my attention had been caught by such inconsistent patterns, my students and I began to ask and listen more carefully. Over the years, I have identified dozens of day-to-day issues where different educators have differing positions essentially based on philosophic premises.

Examples of Differences

What are some examples of areas of differing teacher opinions? Here are some questions my students asked teachers:

- How often should a principal visit a teacher's classroom? What different patterns of visits—if any—should apply to tenured and untenured teachers?
- How much recognition—apart from extra pay—should principals give to teachers they believe are performing well?
- What criteria should be applied in evaluating teachers? What weight should each evaluation give to teachers' away-from-class responsibilities (e.g., participating in faculty meetings, collegial relationships)? How carefully should written lesson plans be examined?
- How rigorous should be the performance pressures we put on students? Should one, in effect, grade on the curve? Should good pupil performance be conspicuously praised? How much homework should be expected of students? How much pressure should be

*Dr. Edward A. Wynne is a Professor, College of Education, University of Illinois at Chicago.

put on them to complete homework? Should exceptions be made, in grading, for pupils who appear to come from disordered homes?

- If pupils are performing substantially behind the level of others in their grade, should they generally be retained for another year?
- How much choice should pupils in departmentalized schools have in determining their courses?
- How active should teachers be in enforcing discipline—especially in the school, but away from the classroom?
- Should discipline codes restrict or prohibit student (male/female) handholding, cigarette smoking throughout the whole school, or rude language among students?
- Assuming it were legal and administered in a reasonably careful fashion, should corporal punishment be applied to pupils who violate discipline norms?

The questions were presented in a special perspective: What *should* the practice be? "Shouldness" is a philosophic matter. Many respondents simply recited back the policies of their school (which supposedly controlled all its teachers). But we then asked them, "Do you think this practice is ideal?" Eventually, they articulated their own opinions—which was sometimes the same as the school policy, and sometimes differed with it. The contents of responses were also affected by the grade levels taught by teachers, their years of experience, and the kinds of communities in which their schools were located. Still, after all these qualifications, my graduate students—who were often teachers themselves—could recognize patterns of difference which were independent of such "externals." The nub of the matter is that different teachers, under the same circumstances, have different philosophies about how to handle basic components of their work.

The effects of these differences in opinion are more than philosophic. My own research, and that of many others, has emphasized the importance of staff coherence in operating effective schools. Thus, a typical study of more- and less-effective high schools included:

> The faculty and administrators at effective high schools share a common sense of purpose that guided the development of curriculum, influenced classroom and administrative procedures, and related instructional methods to measurable outcomes. In contrast, principals and faculty in low-performing schools had difficulty articulating their school's mission, and when they did express a goal, faculty and administrators at the same school frequently disagreed with each other.

Staff coherence is important because pupils—and teachers too—work better when they receive consistent fair, supportive, and demanding treatment from all the people in a school. Then, appropriate attitudes are developed, and transformed into habits. This promotes improved learning. Contrarywise, when different teachers apply conflicting philosophies, pupils are tempted to engage in frequent "testing," especially since such tests often succeed. Take the example of my cheating story. When different teachers apply different policies against cheating, pupils will wonder whether cheating may pay in some particular class, and try their luck. Then the frequency of cheating rises, and the job of even the strong anti-cheating teachers is complicated.

A personal example of the ramifications of teacher inconsistency recently occurred to me. A graduate student who had produced miserable work complained to me about the grading procedure I used. I pointed out that my procedure was fully outlined at the beginning of the term. He could have chosen, early on, to drop my class. He agreed that he had been put on notice. But than he said, "All professors talk about their firm grading procedures. However, they then change them when students face difficulties or raise questions. The trouble with you is that you mean what you say! That's not fair." To his credit, the student smiled when he said this. I can imagine students making arguments which exaggerate the styles of other professors—to their personal advantage. Still, the student involved had gotten a college degree, and showed me very little propensity to study. Probably the student was right when he said many professors do not mean what they say.

Consider the effects if all teachers consistently apply the same policy. For example, suppose a school maintains a strong anti-cheating rule. Then, many pupils, after a year in school, will decide that cheating doesn't pay, and simply concentrate on getting good grades via doing good schoolwork. Indeed, some of the better schools I have studied have taken steps to attain this uniform effect; they have promulgated thorough, clear, written anti-cheating rules with strong penalties, which are to be enforced by all teachers. But even such clear rules do not settle the matter. Some teachers who oppose such policies may simply fail to enforce the rule. Thus, as one part of the process of attaining philosophic coherence, good schools work to try and enlist the hearts and minds of their faculties.

As we continued our research and sporadic questioning, my students also discovered that many layperson's also hold divergent opinions about what should be done in education. Often, such opinions are poorly formed. This is not too surprising. The topic is complicated. Furthermore, my lay interviewees usually had only limited information about school policies—as they admitted—or had not deliberately considered the matter. Given this ambivalence among the public, it is understandable why new teachers, or education students, might hold incoherent, or conflicting opinions about education issues. Indeed, perhaps the naivete of newcomers in education is typical of most professions. For example, I have personally passed through several different careers, and can recognize my own progression from naivete to philosophic sophistication about these fields as my experience grew. The striking thing about education is not that recruits to teaching hold discordant views. Rather, it is that the discordant views of new teachers often persist far into their careers. A number of reasons are responsible for this persistence of philosophic disharmony.

Why Incoherence Persists

The first thing to consider is how teachers are trained to be teachers. An important aim of any pre-employment training process is to give all potential workers a common philosophy to apply on their first job. Consider, for example, the formal training—or socialization—offered to initiates in the professions of law and medicine. Such socialization is supposed to produce a shock effect—and dramatically demonstrate to apprentices that being a lawyer or doctor means thinking in a very special way. The movie *Paper Chase,* or the numerous movies and television shows about medical internships, suggest some of the pressures which afflict such beginners. The aim of such a socialization process is to cause students to either quit, fail, or learn the profession's way of thinking—a new philosophy. And so recently graduated doctors and lawyers usually share important common values with other members of their profession. Contrarywise, very few graduates of teacher education programs feel they have been put through a powerful pressure-cooker. Apart from some trouble with student teaching, the whole thing is pretty relaxing. But such relaxation means that many education students graduate with the same haphazard philosophies about their future careers that they came in with. Thus, they're poorly prepared to philosophically comprehend their work—or share common perspectives with their senior colleagues.

But in many work situations, much of the transmission of a common philosophy occurs on the job site. New employees often come in with divergent philosophies about their work. Then the pressures of their job, and the intervention of their peers and supervisors, moves them towards philosophic coherence. Unfortunately, schools are different from many other job sites.

Public schools are not engaged in a business. They are not governed by profit-and-loss principles. Thus, the pressures on workers for philosophic coherence are low. Conversely, in many business situations, immediate decisions are ultimately determined by their economic implications. If a fast food chain introduces a new item, and it does not sell, it is abandoned. And if a business persist-

ently ignores the messages of the marketplace, it will expire. These principles do not always tell business people what to do in many immediate situations, but they establish generally accepted guidelines. In contrast, almost no public school has gone out of business for losing money. Indeed, schools are not supposed to make money—they are supposed to "do good." The problem is that there are usually generally agreed accounting conventions which enable a business to know if it's making money; what constitutes "doing good" is more problematic. That's where philosophy comes in.

In some educational situations, it seems easy to separate the good outcomes from the bad; presumably, literacy is better than illiteracy, and pupil order is better than gross indiscipline. But a high proportion of education decisions have elaborate ramifications. All the teachers in my earlier anecdote were presumably against cheating. However, their different answers about punishment were undoubtedly the result of giving different weights to other aspects of the problem—the effects of different policies on students' attitudes, the hassles teachers were prepared to bear, the priority each of them gave to communicating a commitment to honesty to pupils, and different theories about how pupils learn.

Workers and supervisors in profit oriented businesses are under pressure to develop coherent group philosophies. As a result, new workers are pressured into harmony, or invited to leave. Conversely, in education there is less incentive—or pressure—for the organization to pursue the development of philosophic harmony among workers (new or old).

Inadequate Answers from Research

Some observers may assume that many pedagogical questions have been settled by research. Thus, even though we cannot tell if an educational practice is economically profitable, we may hope that research will provide an objective evaluation; if teachers' opinions conflict, the teachers only need more scientific information. This assumption is a half-truth. More accurate information about the effects of education programs is desirable, and teachers are sometimes uninformed. Still, speaking as a researcher, much research itself rests on problematic philosophic premises. For example, in the Chicago city public elementary schools, heavy emphasis is given to a system called Continuous Progress Mastery Learning. The approach was developed with the help of important researchers. Supposedly, it is an ideal means of teaching. Actually, it poses important—and semi-ignored—philosophic issues. The approach assumes that almost all pupils can attain certain optimum levels of learning. It directs teachers to focus their efforts on getting all pupils to such levels. But in the process, as other researchers have emphasized, the more able students are often left to stand by, or engage in repetitious desk work, while their lagging classmates catch up. Now, mastery learning may be very good (or not so good), but that evaluation will not be settled by research. It is largely a matter of philosophic values. It is probably impossible to simultaneously teach all pupils in a class or school at each one's ideal pace. Some compromises are needed, and surely justified. But exactly how much teacher time and attention should one group of pupils be asked to surrender so another group can be benefited? That is not a research question, but a philosophic issue. And, similarly, innumerable other education issues are, in the end, essentially matters of *opinion*.

This is part of the reason why education is recurrently swept by fads—*opinions,* by definition, are mutable or transitory. Or, to mask our need to rely on opinion, modest pieces of evidence are inflated beyond their legitimate significance. Of course, there are more and less thoughtful opinions—and so there is nothing wrong with preferring one opinion over another. However, it is still good to label opinion as opinions, and not "truths."

One additional reason for frequent philosophic differences affecting jobs of all sorts is that our philosophies help determine how hard we have to work. Suppose a teacher philosophically believes that pupils should be given rigorous, well monitored homework. Then, that teacher's workload will increase. Conversely, teachers whose philosophies favor less homework, less stringent grading, less stress on out-of-classroom discipline, and so on, are incidentally favoring policies which will lower their short-run work demands. And we should recognize that "work" not only involves putting in more hours. It also includes policies which compel teachers to face increased pressure, as they confront erring students, parents, and colleagues. Undoubtedly, such tensions—due to philosophic conflict—are part of the causes for teacher burnout. In all job situations, there are natural tendencies for some employees to prefer philosophies which shelter them from work; the unique thing about education is that these self-interested on-the-job philosophers are more sheltered from pressures to conform while working in schools than in many other jobs. Many factors produce this sheltering effect. Most teachers are subject to less intense supervision on their jobs than many other workers: principals have more subordinates to supervise than supervisors in most other work sites, and the typical enclosed classroom leaves teachers relatively out of contact with their colleagues' activities. In addition, the prevalence of tenure provides many teachers with more means of resisting supervisory pressure than workers in many other activities. As a result, teachers have less need to harmonize their philosophies and practices with those of co-workers than many other em-

ployees. Sometimes the term "professionalism" is presented to justify such noncomformity. However, this is an ironic use of the term. The relatively low level of philosophic conformity often displayed by teachers is really one reason why they are not, technically speaking, "professionals." True "professions" have fairly clear norms which govern the conduct of all their members.

Contradictions

One effect of these factors is what can be termed fuzzy thought. Of course, that characteristic is diffused throughout the human race. Still, I have suggested reasons why it is more prevalent among educators than some other groups. Let me instance my point. A respondent was asked, "How should a principal go about visiting a classroom?" He replied, "Well, I do not believe he should use a checklist. However, he should see whether the pupils were attentive, whether the teacher was presenting the material in a clear and interesting fashion, and so on." But, of course, *a principal should never use a checklist*. Obviously, the respondent's reply is inconsistent. If the principal is going to systematically look over the class, it is immaterial whether he actually physically holds a checklist in his hand. Indeed, if the observation is going to be systematic, it probably is better that there be a checklist, so it can be used as an advance guide by the teacher.

It was common for my interviewers to present five and ten page typed reports where an interviewee would present replies on page eight which contradicted the positions on page two. Sometimes, my interviewers would point out such contradictions to their interviewees, and invite them to give further explanations. About half the time, the interviewees would recognize their inconsistencies, and either change their positions, or admit that they had never given the topic significant reflection before.

Such fuzzy thought is common because: people come into education with obscure ideas of what they are to do, and why, and then receive inadequate help—for the reasons just discussed—to elevate their perspective. It's not that teachers never change their views; it is that the changes are too often sporadic, unreflective, and unsystematic. And so school faculties often do not fit together.

Many of the teacher interviewees had rarely before been asked to think and talk about the basic principles governing their work. And, when such discussions had presumably occurred, they had not been governed by an intellectual framework—such as we tried in my class. Thus, the teachers we interviewed were really handicapped by powerful external forces. It is also my belief that many organized groups concerned with education have a stake in maintaining teaching as an unintellectual activity. As a result, teachers are too often unprepared to talk or think deeply about much of their work. But what benefits could such groups derive from this effect? And why would some teachers buy such a line?

The groups would benefit because they could tell many teachers what they would like to hear and thus win their friendship, i.e., they could peddle specious philosophies which justify low teacher job commitment. The messages might also add to the prestige of certain messengers, e.g., education research will supply many answers. Why would teachers buy such lines? Well, most of us are sympathetic to philosophies that seem easy to learn, and propose that we should work less, and be paid more. Furthermore, I have already pointed out the weak communication and supervision factors which handicap teachers in evolving consistent philosophies.

There is a final cause for the current situation which largely lies outside of the education system. In a brilliant piece in *The American Scholar,* Diane Ravitch pointed out that many of our most recent education policy conflicts were over questions of equality versus a stress on excellence. Everyone is for excellence, and most people are for equality. However, people are beginning to realize that such goals are not always compatible in an imperfect world, with limited resources. One American technique for handling such controversies is to deny that such ends are incompatible in any way. Then, everyone is happy—for a while. But, we are now discovering that we are pursuing non-parallel lines, and that there may be a collision. Oftentimes in such situations, the teacher becomes the scapegoat.

Some Prescriptions

In a complex situation, I can only offer qualified prescriptions. Still, they may be of some use to readers:

- "Good" education philosophy is important to managing classes, and running effective schools. It is therefore worth the trouble to pursue, and attain.
- Schools of education, and other groups interested in teacher preparation, should develop more rigorous programs of teacher preparation. Each such program should be based on a relatively integrated philosophy of education. And that philosophy should finally be related to very practical, concrete school questions, such as were discussed earlier in this article. The program should be managed so that if students can't learn and apply its philosophy, or strongly don't agree with it, they won't stay and graduate—just as is the case in medicine and law.
- Teachers should become more self-conscious in identifying the philosophic elements of their work. Oftentimes, some of those elements are governed or affected by external forces, eg., school policies, union

contracts, local or state laws. Still, a teacher should try and decide, "Is this policy or practice sound? Why, or why not?"
- Teachers and educators—including school administrators—should more openly discuss the philosophic elements of their work, and try and articulate the rationales for their conclusions.
- In heightening one's philosophic understanding, consistency is one useful criterion. Clarity is another. The two criteria mean that the different parts of one's philosophy fit together, and that someone can easily understand their operating implications. It was evident that, even when some of my graduate students (who were teachers) disagreed with the philosophy of particular interviewees, the students were semi-persuaded by clear, consistent statements.
- "Good" education philosophy can partly be evaluated through studying its application in particular schools. Even though many of my students disagreed about each-other's individual philosophies (on particular issues), it seemed that they generally could identify a well-run and effective school. My opinion is that the philosophies applied in those schools are all relatively congruent. And so, teachers can learn philosophy not only by reasoning, but by observing the philosophies applied in healthy organizations. (This is partly how I have developed my own education philosophy.) Unfortunately, too many teachers have never worked in really well-run schools.

Personal Values

Let me conclude with a few words on my own educational philosophy—although I am far more interested in transmitting processes to people than communicating my particular values:

We human beings are a mixed bag, and necessarily need the support and direction of others to live happily, and do right. Many teachers apply such principles in the management of their own classrooms: they *govern* their students. Still, I am sometimes surprised to see how the same adults often display considerable hostility towards similar control being exercised over them by principals or colleagues. Of course, these "other adults" are sometimes in the wrong. But teachers, too, are sometimes wrong in handling pupils, and yet the policy of adult control of the young is still maintained.

As for our pupils—and I am a teacher too—we owe them a demanding, supportive education. As human beings, they all have certain inalienable rights. However, the capabilities of students—depending on their age—are varied; and some students will never do as well academically as others. There is nothing wrong in making demands which separate pupils according to academic ability, as long as we recall that school does not measure all talents, and that human dignity exists independent of academic attainment.

Human societies have had a lengthy, and largely successful, history of transmitting their culture to their descendants. Education is largely a subset of this process of transmission. In situations where there is conflict, I am disposed to look to the broad-sweep tradition and see what it implies for our philosophic options. I am pessimistic about philosophies which heedlessly disregard such traditions. I tend to call them "utopian." It is a term of strong derision.

In questionable or disputed philosophic issues, the best rule for a teacher is to opt for the philosophy which subjects him to stress and hard work. Sometimes such pressures are unjustified, or grossly inefficient. But, there is a widespread human disposition to avoid strenuous demands. Thus, the principle of first putting burdens on ourselves is a plausible counterweight.

Finally, the rights of individual pupils, parents, and teachers are largely defined by the rights which we grant to others. In other words, oftentimes when we provide a right to "A" we may diminish the rights of "B." To pick up a term of the 1960s, there are not many victimless crimes—nor are there cheap rights. Thus, I often am constrained to inhibit the potential rights of certain individuals to maintain or enlarge the rights of some group or collective. This general principle affects many of the school policies I support.

Chapter 30
Implementing a Quality Circle in an Educational Setting
Brian R. Metke*

Today a cry for a sense of direction in education is coming from many groups and individuals in society who see education mainly in terms of the vast spiraling costs pouring into educational services. As budgets for these services go higher, both the public and its representative legislative bodies are insisting upon more credible reporting of the results.

The cry for a sense of direction in education is also a result of change in society and the need for an accompanying change in educational structure. During such periods of rapid social change, the institutions of society tend to lose their bearings, and therefore, education, too, needs to regain a sense of direction.

One problem or issue in education seems to be the dilemma of the school as an agency of social change. For instance, should schools provide leadership in the promotion of change or, rather, reflect the transmission of cultural heritage along with its attitudes for change. Another dilemma for education is the conflict between quality education and mass education with all its concomitant problems.

As evidenced in many recent investigations on education, there has emerged a need for a solid conception of innovation based on realistic diagnosis of educational needs and systematic planning, development, and evaluation. The National Commission of Excellence in Education, *The Nation At Risk,* has prompted educators to revise curriculum, reconsider graduation requirements and ask for additional funding within school districts.

But attainment of excellence may not be well addressed by such action alone, for some educators believe that the key to higher quality lies in the people in the organization. The most significant thing about Quality Circles is that they are *people building*. The kind of skills and knowledge and experience gained by people in a Quality Circle process becomes their skills and knowledge and experience as well as those of the school district.[1]

"If educators are to have some leverage in increasing productivity and quality in America's schools in the next few years, we must focus our energies on the most potent and expensive resources under our control—the people who work in our schools."[2]

American education has adopted industrial trends in several ways over the years: labor unions, organizational development practices, collective bargaining and the emphasis on accountability. Recently, American management has considered a Japanese Quality Circle technique to save costs and increase productivity. Quality Circles are small teams of employees who meet regularly to discuss "the little things" that go wrong in an organization and suggest means of improving productivity and quality control. The human organization is an important concern. It seems possible that educators could also look at this development in industrial management as a potential tool for education institutions.

A Quality Circle within an educational setting is far more than product quality control in the industrial sense; it enables schools to implement change at a faster pace than tradition dictates provided goals are set and objectives are clearly defined. The term "Quality Circle," then, has two meanings; it refers to both a structure and process and to a group of activities they undertake. A Quality Circle is to be understood as a pattern of situations which are interconnected by communicative and collaborative activity within an organization.

The concept of Quality Circles recognizes the intelligence and creative capacity of people within the school organization. This approach taps the creative intelligence of employees and provides them the means to use their minds, not just their hands. Quality Circles differ from the participative management ideas tried in the 1960s. Circles work with management in solving problems, however the acceptance or rejection of solutions rest solely with management.

*Dr. Brian R. Metke is Assistant Principal and Quality Circle Facilitator, Burns Union High School, Burns, Oregon.

An informal method of providing staff and student input into decision-making to supplement the formal organizational school structure is seen to be a necessity. Quality Circles provide an opportunity for everyone to participate in decision-making. This does not imply involvement for its own sake, but specifically for the purpose of providing optimum educational experience and opportunity for all participants. When disparity is found between what a school is doing for its students and what various groups—the lay public, students, and administration—feel the school should be doing, concerned groups feel a need to develop and administer programs. The whole purpose, then, of a Quality Circle is to provide functional direction to decision-makers.

What attracts people to Quality Circles? What helps them to sell the concept to others in their organizations? What is it that holds management's continuing support as it operates? What is it that keeps the Circle members enthusiastic? Why should educators implement a Circle program?

The answer is *results*—positive results that pay off in terms of improved quality and better attitudes. Quality Circles are not a panacea, but a combination of known management concepts that work. The reason for Quality Circle acceptance is: they offer practical solutions because they are philosophically based with a pragmatic foundation.

John Dewey

To completely analyze and document the quality benefit of implementing a Quality Circle program in an educational setting, the program need be examined as a social change agent. A comparison of John Dewey's educational pragmatic philosophy to the Quality Circle activity can provide educational and democratic perspective for the advancement of educational management structure and development within American schools.

For Dewey, the proper concerns of philosophy are social conflicts, especially those found in a scientific industrial democracy. Educators are reminded of Dewey's participatory concepts (Activity, Problem, Data Gathering, Hypothesis, Testing) which represent for him a complete act of thought. His "Instrumental" theory of learning is embodied within the Quality Circle decision-making process (Problem Identification, Problem Selection, Data Collection, Problem Solution and Evaluation). His main conviction was that education should not be simply instruction in various subjects but rather a coherent unified effort to foster the development of citizens capable of promoting the further growth of society by employing intelligence fruitfully in a social context.

Dewey maintained that from the scientific side, it is demonstrated that effective and integral thinking is possible only where the experimental method in some form is used. For Dewey the complete act of thought is the same for a child in school, a worker in industry and a scientist working on a problem in a laboratory. All go through the same process which may be described in five steps: (1) Activity, (2) Problem, (3) Data Gathering, (4) Formation of a Hypothesis, and (5) Testing.

Quality Circles are involved directly in evaluating John Dewey's theory of social change by reflective and instrumental thinking due to the Quality Circle "five step" implementation process.

The Quality Circle Process

The beauty of the Quality Circle process is that it requires each educator to be his own strategist. One can be perfectly pragmatic and eclectic in choosing tactics that best fit one's style and experience in the situation in which one finds oneself. The "strategy" selected is not paramount, it is not the sole method, rather, the Circle *path* is critical. The following essential components of the Quality Circle process must be fulfilled in the order listed here to ensure successful implementation of a Circle program:

1. Problem Identification,
2. Problem Selection,
3. Data Collection and Analysis,
4. Problem Solution, and,
5. Management Review and Evaluation.*

The following flowchart (Figure 1) was obtained from The Productivity Center, Lane Community College, Eugene, Oregon (the process is summarized in this concept).

An administrator's first impulse is to map-out a timeline of target dates summarizing the whole program in one visual display. Do *not* do this! Quality Circles must "run their own course." A Quality Circle is not a "quick fix"—two week operation, but rather, is an open-ended process to maximize input, data-gathering and analysis which ensures the best solution for each problem considered. Ownership of each Circle rests with the Circle members, not management. Quality not quantity, should be

*Prior to implementing a Circle program, managers should obtain (and familiarize themselves with) a manual describing in detail the Quality Circle process and measurement techniques. Two excellent training manuals are:

Dewar, Donald L. *The Quality Circle Handbook*. Red Bluff, California: Quality Circle Institute, 1980.

Ingle, Sud. *Quality Circles Master Guide*. Englewood Cliffs; Prentice-Hall, Inc., 1982.

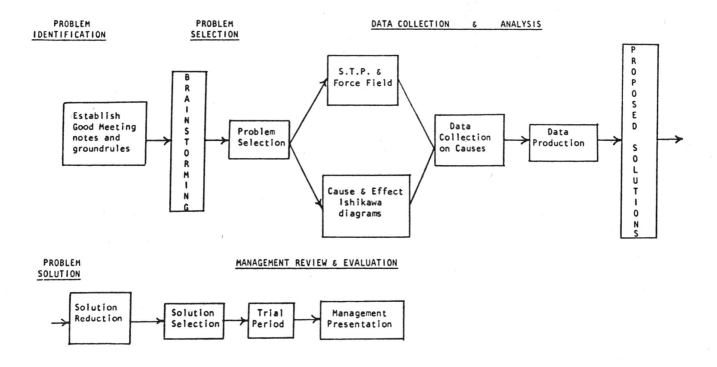

PROBLEM
IDENTIFICATION

PROBLEM
SELECTION

DATA COLLECTION   &   ANALYSIS

Figure 1. Quality Circle flowchart in an educational setting.[4]

of first consideration. Expansion will come of its own accord as word of mouth spreads success stories. Two Circles that function properly within a school setting and accomplish positive results are better than many unfulfilled Circles designed to get everybody involved, languishing for lack of skilled leadership, participant motivation and managerial support.

The basic premise of the Quality Circle process is that when employees and students are given the opportunity to meet regularly on a *volunteer* basis to discuss problems, they will indeed devise solutions. A Circle meets and begins by identifying school related concerns and/or problems. The team prioritizes and selects one or more problems to investigate. This is followed by data-gathering, problem analysis, and solution identification techniques; brainstorming, Pareto chart, cause and effect diagrams, and force-field analysis (see Figures 2, 3, 4, and 5 for typical examples). Finally, a recommendation is presented to management. Because the problem is one chosen by the group, there is a greater chance that participants will be motivated to arrive at a practical solution.

Since school organizations already possess a highly educated population, there is no magic involved in this effort to improve school districts through the Quality Circle process: just a great deal of hard work in establishing objectives within a school program and designing a detailed plan for achieving results through proven Circle technique. Once solutions to problems are implemented, those not directly involved in the Circle activities begin to make inquiries and some ''outsiders'' will volunteer to participate in next year's program. Once implemented correctly, a well organized and facilitated Circle program will model the following governing and driving principle: ''Success breeds additional success.'' In other words, nothing succeeds like success!

Many people feel that they really don't have the time for Quality Circle work. They are already busy with their work and sense an edict from above burdening them with another responsibility. Management must adhere to *voluntary* participation. Each individual sets his or her own priorities. Only when the potential of Quality Circles is realized by individuals do they realign their list of priorities each day to include Quality Circle participation.

Those unfamiliar with Quality Circle techniques might cynically feel that nothing new has been created here: ''These are nothing but glorified department-head meetings.'' In one respect they are correct; only when participants representing *all* areas of the school organization (Quality Circle idiom labels this vertical organizational arrangement as a VERTEAM) come together for the mutual benefit of the institution will the ultimate social change within schools be realized.

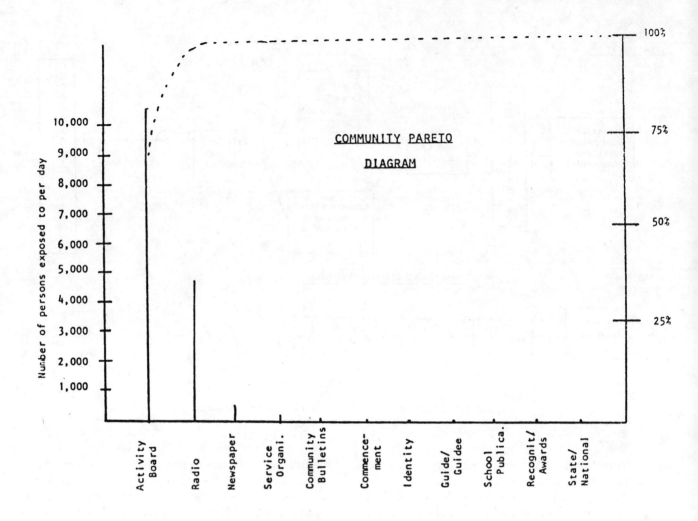

Figure 2. Data collection through use of a Pareto chart.

Vilfredo Pareto was an Italian engineer-sociologist who, in the nineteenth century, studied the numbers of people in various income classes and diagrammed his findings in the manner described above. Present-day applications of the technique compare frequencies of different forms of violent crimes, demonstrate the relative amounts of time office workers spend on various tasks, organize defective-part data according to type of defect, or indicate which of several similar machines produce the largest numbers of defective parts. In every case, the most important classes are identified so that corrective action can be directed where it will do the most good.[5]

The above Community Pareto Diagram graphically illustrates that communication through a school activity board will reach the largest community population. It makes sense to pursue an activity board solution (reaching the largest population) rather than other communication device alternatives.

Reactions from Circle Participants

To meet a specific level of satisfaction, a fundamental discipline is essential to an effective quality program. To implement lasting results within any organization, Qual-

ity Circles must be accepted as a *social change agent* rather than as a short-term novelty arrangement. The ultimate challenge for educators within any school arrangement, is the change and improvement they foster for the good of society. Schools are valued when they can

```
 11, 400   Activity Board:  7,600 @ day vehicle count from the State High-
                            way Department, La Grande, Oregon; 1½ person
                            occupancy per vehicle.

  4,600    Radio: Radio employee, Sam Toy, estimates 1,500 more daily listeners
                  than who read the Burns Times Herald.

    473    Newspaper: 3,300 weekly circulation

    100    Service Organizations: Kiwanis, Lions, BPW, Elds, Rotary, PEO,
                                   ZetaEpsilon, Booster Club, Music Society,
                                   Chamber, etc....approximately 700 total
                                   membership.

      9    Community Bulletins: 14 church bulletins, 2 grocery; 3,500 citizens

    2.3    Commencement: 900 in attendance

    2.0    Guide/Guidee:  Staff (50), Freshman/Sophomore Students (185),
                          Parents (350).

    1.2    School Publications:  Annual (350), Bagpipe (0), Tam-O-Shantar (100)

    .75    Awards: Student (Athletic/Bard/Month) - Approximately 252 students

    .7     Graduates: Reunions (200), School Visitations (43)

    .3     State/National/International: Oregonian (2 @ week), Edu-Gram (1 @
                                         month), State Dept. (1 @ month)
```

Figure 3. Pareto factual explanation by category.

bring about a better life. A Quality Circle program offers a viable alternative for school managers to not only resolve local school issues, but ultimately, society as well.

Quality Circles hold limitless potential within a school setting because they foster a conservative, evolutionary, approach (as opposed to revolutionary) to social change which school decision-makers prefer. Furthermore, educators can ensure the proper growth of this nation's democratic heritage by promoting the democratic ideal through the implementation of Quality Circles within an educational setting.

Quality Circles are a step in this direction; listen to these reaction statements offered by student members within Circle G and Pete's QC (two Quality Circles operating at Burns Union High School, Burns, Oregon, 1985):[6] "Everyone was fairly equal, the Circle process ensured so . . ."; "The circle process teaches respect for the other person"; "I liked how all opinion were given uninterrupted . . . each person understood that they had the floor for their given moment"; I liked the idea that everyone had an equal say . . . one vote/one person"; "Teachers usually dictate . . . whereas the Quality Circle

has all components on an equal basis . . . everyone was equal." An adult Quality Circle member felt the student participation was the most successful outcome of the Circle process. "Students got the most benefit. They received training and respect, and were treated like adults. They provided excellent input. I liked, especially, how they promoted enthusiasm and creativity within the group . . . they forced my mind to wonder—to look around oneself at our environment." "They (students) were good for the adults."

Quality Circles not only pursue the "democratic ideal": They also effect a change in school organizational structure, management behavioral attitude, leadership style, and an expanded role for staff and students. Successful reforms—those that endure—make structural and organizational additions or changes within a school system.[7]

No doubt the discussion of organizational management theory will retain the popularity it has held with both the public and professionals since John Dewey. But the real test of the effort will be in moving it over from an end in itself into significant revision of schools practice to

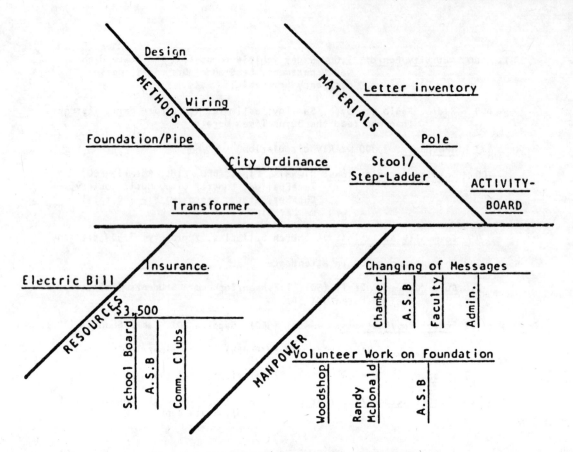

Figure 4. Using a Fishbone (Ishikawa) diagram.

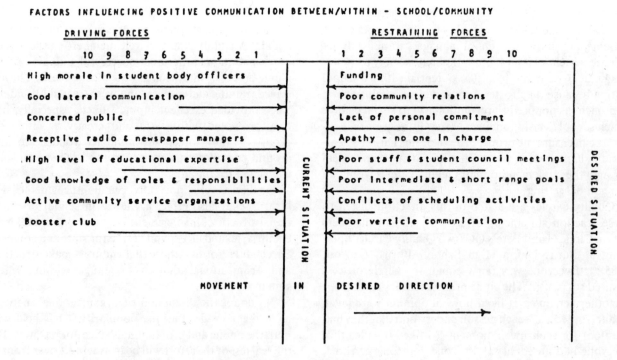

Figure 5. Determining driving and restraining forces with a Force Field Analysis.

serve the goal intent. The test of any theory is not in final agreement of their relative worth by their respective writers but rather in the attempt to apply them to the school setting.

Summary

The public demand for accountability in education has provided good reason to innovate, to look for plausible solutions to please both educator and layman alike. No proposal for change is of much use unless there is some practical means for getting from where schools are to where it might be well to be; the object is to consider how our education system can be upgraded.

School systems mirror industrial advancements in many ways. It is reasonable to expect school districts to examine a newly developed industrial Quality Circle technique within an educational setting. Quality Circles are an attempt to provide solutions for education's call to accountability by using input from staff and students involved in the educational process to improve the quality of the school. Quality Circles are a step aimed in the direction of establishing and fulfilling objectives while creating a democratic atmosphere within the organization.

Implementing a Quality Circle within a school setting will ensure an ongoing review of the purpose, procedure and evaluation (inherent in Dewey's five part "complete thought") of various school programs because of the successful five-step Circle process mentioned earlier.

John Dewey reminds educators that intelligence is to be alertly critical of outmoded methods in society, in government, in feeling, and in thought. He promotes "Faith in the capacities of human nature, faith in human intelligence and the power of pooled and co-operative experience."[8] Educators are further charged with a commitment to uphold and promote our democratic heritage within schools. The challenge to school leaders is to improve their organization by democratically mobilizing the human resource within their school setting through the use of Quality Circles.

A "people-building" climate fostering trust is due to the unique design of the Circle process to ensure voluntary participation; allow freedom of participants to select and pursue Circle objectives and goals; ensure review of the purpose, procedure and evaluation of various school programs; provide an alternative decision-making process within the school setting; and provide an evolutionary pace for school change within an organization while nourishing and promoting the democratic ideal.

First that the person have a genuine situation of experience—that there be a continuous activity in which he is interested for its own sake; secondly, that a genuine problem develop within this situation as a stimulus to thought; third, that he possess the information and make the observations needed to deal with it; fourth, that suggested solutions occur to him which he shall be responsible for in an orderly way; fifth, that he have opportunity and occasion to test his ideas by application to make their meaning clear and to discover for himself their validity.
—John Dewey,[9]

FOOTNOTES

1. David Hawley, "Quality Circles," *Oregon School Study Council Bulletin.* 28(September 1984): 1 and 20.
2. L. Chase, *Quality Circles in Education—Decisions for Excellence.* (Arlington Heights, Illinois: Illinois Revival Institutes, 1983).
3. Sud Ingle, *Quality Circles Master Guide.* (Englewood Cliffs, New Jersey: Prentice Hall, Inc., 1982), p. 50.
4. Julie Aspinwall-Lamberts, "Quality Circle Process Flowchart," *Productivity Center.* (Eugene, Oregon: Lane Community College, 1983).
5. Sud Ingle, *Quality Circle Master Guide.* (Englewood Cliffs, New Jersey: Prentice Hall, Inc., 1982), p. 108.
6. Brian R. Metke, *A Study Describing the Implementation of a Quality Circle in an Educational Setting at Burns Union High School According to the Pragmatic Philosophy of John Dewey.* (Ph.D. dissertation, Walden University, 1985), p. 159–160.
7. Ibid., p. 143–190.
8. John Dewey, *Problems of Men.* (New York, N.Y.: Philosophical Library, Inc., 1946), p. 59.
9. C. Max Wertheimer, *Productive Thinking.* (New York, N.Y.: Harper and Brothers, 1943), p. 190–191.

SELECTED BIBLIOGRAPHY

Chase, L. *Quality Circles in Education—Decisions for Excellence.* Arlington Heights: Illinois Revival Institute, 1983.
Cole, Robert. "Quality-Control Circles." *Across the Board.* 16(November 1979): 72
———. *Work, Mobility, and Participation: A Comparative Study of American Japanese Industry.* Berkeley: University of California Press, Ltd., 1979.
Dewar, Donald L. *The Quality Circle Guilde to Participative Management.* Englewood Cliffs: Prentice-Hall, Inc., 1980.
———. *The Quality Circle Handbook.* Red Bluff, California: Quality Circle Institute, 1980.
Dewey, John. *Democracy and Education.* New York: MacMillan and Co., 1916.
———. *Experience and Education.* New York: MacMillan and Co., 1938.
———. *Reconstruction in Philosophy.* New York: Henry Holt and Co., 1920.
———. *The Quest for Certainty.* London: Unwin Brothers, Ltd., 1929.
Ingle, Nima and Sud. *Quality Circles in Service Industries.* Englewood Cliffs: Prentice-Hall, Inc., 1984.

Ingle, Sud. *Quality Circles Master Guide: Increasing Productivity With People Power.* Englewood Cliffs: Prentice-Hall, Inc., 1982.

Ouchi, William, "Defining the Quality Control Circle." *Modern Office Procedures.* (April 1982): 14.

———. *Theory Z: How American Business Can Meet the Japanese Challenge.* New York: Avon Books, 1981.

Pachin, Robert I. *The Management and Maintenance of Quality Circles.* Homewood, Illinois: Dow Jones-Irwin, Inc., 1983.

Superintendent Alfred Melov, NYC School Board 15

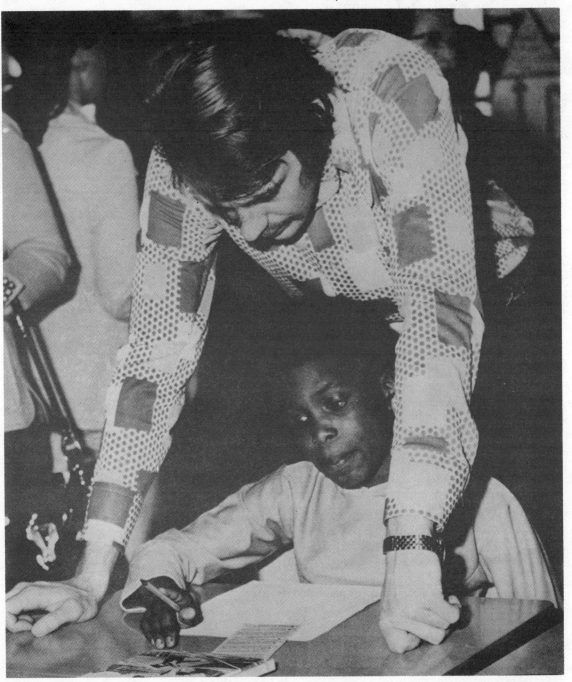

Section V
Curriculum Issues
Introduction by Paula E. Lester*

What is curriculum? Curriculum refers to subjects and subject matter. It is a set of subjects offered, required, and/or recommended. It is the dominant design whereby subjects are taught by teachers and learned by students. Curriculum refers to all elements in the experience of the learner. Curriculum refers to objectives; it is instruction—a means of attaining the ends or objectives. Curriculum is a plan that is tailor made for a school system. It is a plan for providing sets of learning opportunities to achieve broad goals and related specific objectives for an identifiable population. Curriculum is a system that is concerned with all relevant factors. The students to be educated represent the input. The educational planning, implementing, and evaluating represent the process. The graduates represent the output. Curriculum is the sum total of living experiences for which the school is responsible.

The curriculum planning process begins by examining external factors that influence the curriculum. Some of these external factors are: national curriculum projects, tradition, accreditation, preparatory syndrome, public opinion, special interest groups, testing programs, and philanthropic foundations.

Curriculum planning spans the national (guidelines); state (board of education, textbook adoption, accreditation, examination system, prescription of subjects to be taught); and local (priority goals) levels. Students, teachers, and the community participate in local curriculum planning. Students are actively involved in their own personal curriculum continuum. Teachers are the final decision makers about the opportunities to be provided. Teacher teams set goals for grades and subject sections. Curriculum councils serve as a clearing-house to plan general policies. Curriculum committees may be ad hoc to address specific tasks. Community participants may provide work experience programs and assist parents.

The major sources of data for curriculum planning include: students, society, the learning process, legal structures, resources and facilities. Data about students may be obtained from pupil population data, growth and development characteristics (physical, emotional, and social development, psychological needs, intellectual and creative development, and personal traits), home, family, and community conditions and career planning (vocational preparation). Social and cultural factors cannot be ignored. Schools serve social functions such as transmission of the culture, socialization of the young, preservation of the society as a nation (development of loyalty to the values and structures of the social group), preparation of the young for adulthood (teaching skills and competencies), and personal development of the young. Society makes demands on the school in terms of values, local mores, expectations, political power structures, trends of the times, occupations, and family status and conditions. The learning process encompasses the nature of learning, theories of learning, motivation, self-concept, readiness, and the transfer of learning. Legal structures control the schools, which were established under national, state, and local laws. The federal system, the U.S. constitution and constitutional rights, and the roles of the federal, state, state education department, and local boards of education, all affect how schools are established and operated. Finally, resources and facilities such as school staff, buildings, equipment, instructional materials, and professional literature must be considered in curriculum planning. Data must be obtained for a particular group of students and for individual students who are to be educated for membership in a particular social group at a particular time in history.

The components of the curriculum are: curriculum domains, curriculum designs, instructional modes, and evaluative procedures. Goals are the basic elements in education planning that are grouped into do-

*Dr. Paula E. Lester is an Assistant Professor at C.W. Post Campus of Long Island University, N.Y.

mains (large groups of learning opportunities, broad in scope, that are planned to achieve a single set of closely related major educational goals). Subgoals for each general goal are identified and then objectives that will contribute to the attainment of the subgoals are developed.

The next step is to select an appropriate curriculum design. Curriculum designs focus on specific competencies (performance based objectives), disciplines (subjects), social activities and problems (the life situation), process skills (learning process), and individual needs and interests. No one curriculum design can be adequate for the total curriculum plan.

The implementation of the curriculum plan involves a variety of instructional modes: lecture, discussion, questioning techniques, practice and drill, viewing, listening and answering, problem solving, laboratory or inquiry, role playing, simulation and games, and independent learning.

The final step is the evaluation for the curriculum, which involves the determination of what is to be evaluated, the kinds of data needed in making these decisions, the collection of these data, the definition of criteria for determining the quality of the materials being evaluated, the analysis of the data in terms of these criteria, and the provision of information for decision makers.

Now is the time to plan for schools in the future based upon the predicted changes in American life. We can expect that population will grow, more extensive opportunities for formal education will be sought, family life will change, population will become more urbanized, technology will continue to change modes of living, the work year will decrease, occupational patterns will change, government will become more omnipotent, and citizens will be better informed.

To meet the needs of this society, the schools in the future will be called upon to provide the fullest personal development, equality of opportunity, a personal counselor, a compassionate staff, a comprehensive curriculum, relevant subject matter, varied teaching modes, cumulative growth experiences, and a center for coordinating learning.

The articles in this chapter are truly representative of the range of curriculum issues facing our schools today. Five articles deal with subject areas (math and science education, learning to read, and computers); three deal with specific populations (all-day kindergarten, mainstreaming, and learning disabled). The other articles deal with the participants in the curriculum process (models of the learner, and school-home partnership), effective schools, curriculum change, and the "adultification" of children.

Chapter 31
Literacy: Trends and Explanations
Jeanne S. Chall*

For almost every statement on literacy, one can find another that directly opposes it, from the status of literacy—what it is today and whether it is getting better or worse, to how and why we got there. The universally accepted idea that it is good to be literate is even being questioned, and by some very sophisticated people. One argument is that TV, computers, and other interactive media may be viable substitutes for those who find it difficult to learn to read and write. Yet others claim that because of computer technology, a higher level of literacy is needed. This expression of doubt was not as prevalent during the 1970s when there seemed to be a greater optimism and a more intensive national effort to improve the literacy of children and adults.

It was a time of much activity: the National Right to Read Effort, Reading is Fundamental, The Office of Basic Skills, Sesame Street and The Electric Company, Head Start, Follow Through, Title I, and other national programs to improve literacy; increased federal funding of research on reading through individual grants, through research and development centers, and more recently through the Center for the Study of Reading at the University of Illinois; the beginning of nationwide testing by the National Assessment of Educational Progress (NAEP); the National Academy of Education's Reading Committee and its report, *Toward a Literate Society,* an analysis of the national reading problem with recommendations for its solution (Carroll & Chall, 1975). During the 1970s there was also a significant growth in professional associations concerned with literacy and its research, and in the number of articles and professional journals on reading and writing (Chall & Stahl, 1982).

Professionals concerned with research and practice in literacy included reading specialists, classroom teachers, administrators, reading and learning disabilities specialists, and educational publishers. Psychologists and linguists were engaged in much of the basic research. The medical field also was concerned with basic research and practice, particularly with the neurological basis of severe reading and learning disability. Adult educators in the United States and in developing countries worked on problems of adult basic literacy. Some lawyers were concerned with malpractice suits concerning attainment of inadequate literacy by high school graduates of normal intelligence. Other lawyers were concerned with the legal aspects of contracts that were unreadable to their audience. More recently, the legal professions have been involved in suits regarding the validity of state minimum competency tests for high school graduation, particularly whether they test what the students were taught (Madaus, 1982).

There was also much discussion during the past decade as to whether there was indeed a literacy problem. Some surveys found that a small percentage of adults was completely illiterate, and that this was rapidly declining. At the same time, substantial numbers of adults were estimated to be functionally illiterate (i.e., unable to read well enough for adequate functioning at work, for citizenship, and for personal needs). One estimate in the early 1970s was that almost half the adult population was functionally illiterate (Hunter & Harman, 1979).

A Harris survey commissioned by the Right to Read Office in the early 1970s reported substantial percentages of adults lacking "survival literacy;" that is, they had difficulty reading and filling out application forms for employment, a driver's license, medicaid, and the like. Other studies (Sticht, 1975) found that when the level of job-related reading materials in the army was compared to the level of reading ability of those who needed to use them (e.g., technical and job manuals), many adults in those jobs were unable to use them effectively.

Apparently, then, most surveys and interpretations of the past decade, although they disagreed about numbers,

*Dr. Jeanne S. Chall is Professor of Education, Director, Reading Laboratory, Harvard University, Graduate School of Education. Her specializations are Reading Development, Reading Disability, and Readability. Reprinted with permission of *The Educational Researcher,* November, 1983.

did agree that the status of adult literacy was far from adequate, particularly in terms of the growing technical nature of available jobs and the growing complexity of knowledge.

Although the problem of literacy among adults is extremely important, I would like to focus the remainder of this paper on literacy among students: those still in school or recently graduated. I do this for several reasons. First, there are more reliable data on the reading achievements of students. Most are tested regularly with standardized reading achievement tests from elementary through high school. Second, the testing program of the NAEP has made it possible to make comparisons nationally over time.

Literacy Trends Among Elementary, High School and College Students

What have been the broad literacy trends? I think we can approach some answers using the various reports from the NAEP, the standardized achievement scores reported in newspapers, particularly for the larger cities, and the verbal scores on the SAT.

When these scores are analyzed for the previous decade one finds different trends for different age groups, with the younger making greater gains over the 10-year period than the older.

These trends are found on the NAEP and similar trends have been reported in newspapers from standardized reading achievement test scores, particularly for large urban centers. The standardized test scores also seem to show gains during the decade in the early grades, particularly among children from low income and minority families. These gains seem to taper off in the middle and upper grades, and they seem to decline during the high school years.

The trends for writing at elementary and high school are not as clear cut as for reading. This comes from various factors, among them the relative novelty of "objective" assessment in writing. Although there is still much difference of opinion on the assessment of reading, there is even more disagreement as to how writing is best evaluated. Yet there appears to be greater agreement than there is for reading that writing is at a very low level of accomplishment at all levels of schooling.

Further evidence for the low state of literacy among high school students comes from the steady decline in SAT verbal scores (Wirtz, 1977).* Reading and vocabulary scores of freshmen were found to be significantly lower on a test originally administered 50 years ago in a midwestern university.

*The scores stopped declining in 1981 and increased slightly in 1982, although the higher scores are still relatively behind where they were before the present declines.

Because these comparisons were generally based on tests similar in content, form, and difficulty, the differences found may represent some realities, over time, in the state of literacy during the past decade. Before we examine some of the factors behind those trends, it is well to note that the trends are not accepted by all analysts. For example, Roger Farr, former president of the International Reading Association, has a more optimistic view. In his report to the Subcommittee on Education, Arts and Humanities on Basic skills (Basic Skills, 1979) he noted, "the trend has been for a consistent increase in reading achievement at all grade levels since the time that test data information in the United States was first recorded" (p. 424). However, he too reported that the most pronounced increases have been at the youngest ages.

Some Uses of Literacy Trends

I will use the literacy trends of the past decade, particularly those in reading, to help us understand what might be behind them. Hopefully, they will give us some explanations, or at least some suggestions, as to what seems to be working, what isn't working, and how it might be turned around. First, I will consider the effects of educational changes and emphases during the past decade. Second, I will consider the effects of individual development.

From the NAEP Tests

According to the 1980 test results from the NAEP, 9 year olds (Grade 4) were significantly ahead of 9 year olds tested in 1971 on all tests of reading: literal comprehension, inferential comprehension, and reference skills (NAEP, 1981). The 13 year olds (Grade 8) in 1980 did somewhat better than their age-mates in 1971, but they tested significantly better only on one reading test: literal comprehension. The 17 year olds (Grade 12) in 1980 tested lower on most of the reading tests. but *significantly lower* only on inferential comprehension (see Table 1).

Why the different trends for the different grade groups? One hypothesis is that we teach reading better in the early grades than in the upper elementary and high school grades. This has some merit and was found in several surveys of schools and teachers (Austin & Morrison, 1961; Morrison, & Austin, 1976). There is a general consensus, too, that knowledge about early reading is greater than knowledge about later reading (Resnick & Weaver, 1979). Indeed, this was one of the major reasons for the creation of the Center for the Study of Reading by the National Institute of Education in the middle 1970s. Its main function was to conduct research on reading comprehension at the middle and higher grades, consid-

Table 1. National Assessment of Educational Progress Gains in Reading Scores, 1971–1980

	Grade 4 (Age 9)	Grade 8 (Age 13)	Grade 12 (Age 17)
Total Reading	+ 3.9[a]	+ 0.8	− 0.9
Literal Comprehension	+ 3.9[a]	+ 1.6[a]	− 0.2
Inferential Comprehension	+ 3.5[a]	− 0.6	− 2.1[a]
Reference Skills	+ 4.8[a]	+ 0.9	+ 0.8

Grade 4 Scores	Grade 8 Scores	Grade 12 Scores
1971 cohort, in Grade 1, 1967	1971 cohort in Grade 1, 1963	1971 cohort in Grade 1, 1958
1980 cohort, in Grade 1, 1976	1980 cohort, in Grade 1, 1972	1980 cohort in Grade 1, 1968

Note. From NAEP, 1981
[a]Significant

ered to be more difficult to teach and learn than the word recognition and decoding usually taught in the early grades. But these hypotheses, although reasonable, do not seem to explain the trends sufficiently, particularly the increase in fourth-grade scores in 1980 as compared to those of 1971.

Let us look at still another hypothesis, one that may help explain both the recent increases in the earlier grades and the declines in higher.

I would like to propose that the gains and losses in reading achievement on the NAEP tests, and on others, reflect the changes in reading instruction that began in the late 1960s and that have been continuing in the 1970s and the early 1980s—changes largely brought about by the research and development efforts in literacy and directed more to younger children than to older ones. These included an earlier start, more and earlier phonics, harder basal readers grade for grade, more home instruction, more help to those who needed it, and the like. Thus the significant gains of fourth graders on all reading subtests in 1980 as compared to 1971 on the NAEP tests partly may be attributed to the stronger reading instruction in school and to the stronger home reading environment of the 1980 cohort as compared to the 1971. The fourth-grade cohort of 1971 was in first grade in 1967, before the stronger reading programs of the 1970s, and before Sesame Street and The Electric Company and the trend toward teaching of reading in kindergarten and in the home (Chall, 1983b). The fourth-grade cohort tested in 1980 were first graders in 1976, when they had the stronger school and home experiences in reading. Therefore, I believe that the significant gains over the 10-year

period can be explained partly by some of these instructional changes.

The Grade 8 gains from the 1971 to the 1980 testing period suggest some influences from the cumulative effects for the stronger early reading programs of the 1970s. The one significant reading gain from 1971 to 1980 was in literal comprehension. Since the 1980 cohort was in Grade 1 in 1972, when some would have participated in a stronger reading program and environment, the improved scores in literal comprehension may reflect this stronger beginning. The 1971 eighth-grade cohort, on the other hand, was in Grade 1 in 1963, before the changes in early reading instruction were widely practiced.

That no improvement took place for 12th graders from 1970 to 1980 may also be viewed in terms of their early instruction. Both cohorts were in Grade 1 before the 1970s when most readings changes took place. The 1971 cohort was in Grade 1 in 1958; the 1980 was in Grade 1 in 1968. Neither seemed to have a stronger beginning. Thus, it would appear that the changes in beginning reading attitudes and reading characteristics of the national literacy effort of the 1970s "passed" both 12th-grade cohorts. It would be questionable, therefore, to attribute the decrease in inferential comprehension of the 1980 12th graders to the stronger skills emphasis of their early reading instruction, since there is little evidence that they received it. If there were changes from 1958 to 1968, they were probably toward a lighter skills emphasis in 1968. And yet, increasingly researchers proclaim that the early skills emphasis of the 12th graders is responsible for their low scores on inferential comprehension.

That some early instructional programs may have substantial, constructive, long-term effects also was suggested in an exploratory study that we conducted several years ago on the relation between SAT verbal scores and textbook difficulty. At the request of the Advisory Panel on the Scholastic Aptitude Test Score Decline and sponsored by the College Board and Educational Testing Service, we analyzed textbooks used over a 30-year period by six cohorts of students taking the SAT (Chall, Conard, & Harris, 1977).

We found compelling evidence that the difficulty of the textbooks used by the six cohorts over a 30-year period was associated with their SAT scores—the harder the textbooks a cohort used from Grade 1 to 11, the higher their verbal SATs; the easier the textbooks, the lower their SAT scores. The level of challenge of the first-grade reading textbooks seemed to have a particularly strong association with the SAT scores:

those cohorts that were in first grade when the reading programs were more challenging did better on the SAT 10 years later. Those who were in first grade when the reading programs had become less challenging, had lower SAT scores 10 years later. (p. 61)

Why are the beginning reading textbooks so important? Why is beginning reading so important? Because it usually requires direct instruction, because most children cannot generate their own rules of print to speech, and letters to sounds. The children are thus more dependent on their teachers and on their textbooks than in later grades. Once the children have mastered the basic recognition and decoding skills and can read simple books on their own, much of their learning can be self-generated. In the sixth grade, good readers who have access to a library probably read more words, on a higher readability level, in a month than they read all year in a textbook. Even if their textbooks offer limited challenge, their own free reading can make up for some of the difference (Chall et al., 1977; also see Chall, 1983a).

That textbooks and reading methods affect reading achievement has long been accepted. What is not sufficiently recognized, I think, is the cumulative nature of this influence. Most would tend to agree that methods and materials for the higher grades influence abilities in the higher grades. Fewer would acknowledge that the instruction and materials of the early grades also influence higher level reading achievement. (We are continuing to study difficulty level of textbooks for the development of reading and other verbal abilities and for the acquisition of information.)

Developmental Changes in Individuals

The current literacy trends on the NAEP—greater gains in the earlier than in later grades—have been found in other studies. A deceleration of reading scores after the primary grades long has been noted, particularly for children of low-income families (Coleman, 1966; Deutsch, 1965).

In a recent study of the influences of families on literacy among low SES children in Grades 2, 4, and 6, we found the same phenomenon for reading, writing, and word meaning (Chall & Snow, 1982). At Grade 2, the scores were generally equal to the norms for a middle-class population. At Grade 4, the scores of the low-income children began to slip somewhat. At Grade 6, there was a considerable drop, as compared to the middle-class group, particularly in word meanings and in writing.

Why the relatively high scores among these children in the primary grades and the deceleration trends beginning after Grade 4? A likely hypothesis, I believe, is a view of the reading process as developmental, changing in characteristic ways from the beginnings (and prebeginnings) to highly advanced, skilled reading (Chall, 1979, 1983a).

If reading is divided into levels or stages (Chall, 1983), a major break seems to be at about Grade 4. Pre Grade 4

reading can be said to represent the oral tradition, in that text rarely goes beyond the language and knowledge that the reader already has through listening, direct experience, TV, and so forth. We can view reading beyond Grade 4 as comprising the literary tradition—when the reading matter goes beyond what is already known. Thus, Grade 4 can be seen as the beginning of a long progression in the reading of texts that are ever more complicated, literary, abstract, and technical, and that require more world knowledge and ever more sophisticated language and cognitive abilities to engage in the interpretations and critical reactions required. The materials that are typically read at Grade 4 and beyond change in content, in linguistic complexities, and in cognitive demands.

The decelerations in reading achievement often found after Grade 4 may be explained, at least in part, by the different demands made on the reader. While the earlier grades require proficiency in word recognition and analysis, and in fluency or automaticity in these, it requires relatively little stretching in tasks of linguistic and cognitive capacities. In the upper elementary grades, high school and college, the challenge becomes primarily linguistic and cognitive. Yet, it should be remembered that without the fluent recognition of words, the so called lower level skills, the higher cognitive skills do not function in reading comprehension.

Thus, we need to be concerned with at least two kinds of reading: reading for the early grades and reading for the higher grades. Children in the early grades presently seem to be succeeding. The higher are not.

Unfortunately, few changes have been implemented at the higher levels. Many propose that the higher level skills be taught earlier. Some go even further to claim that it is the lower level skills now taught in the primary grades that are responsible for poor achievement in the higher level skills.

It would seem to me that both these hypotheses need empirical testing before they become general practice. Indeed, the data that do seem to offer some direction for improvements at the higher levels suggest that we need to have strong skills at the beginning as well as higher order skills at upper elementary, high school, and college.

To Sum Up Some Recent Trends in Literacy

When various school populations are compared over a 10-year period—from about 1970 to 1980—the greater gains have been found for those below about grade 4. High school and college students have not fared as well. Indeed, most surveys have shown significant declines when compared to earlier populations of the same age.

Similar trends of deceleration with age or grade have been reported for children of low-income families—relatively good achievement in the early grades, with increasing losses from about grade 4 on.

Why? I have tried to show that explanations for both trends may lie in a consideration of history: the environmental history of how children were taught in school and at home, and how this environmental history fits with the course of development of reading in the individual.

When there are improvements or declines in literacy over time, it is well to look at what and how students were taught, not only at the time the decline is observed, but how they learned to read initially and over the long haul. It would seem important to keep records of the literacy environment, from the early grades through high school and college. Thus the periodic testing of samples of children as now done by the NAEP needs to be supplemented by periodic indices of reading and writing instruction—indices that have been found over the years to be reliably associated with literacy achievement. For reading, such factors as reading methods, book exposure in school and at home, the level of challenge of textbooks used in the different grades and content areas, the number and level of books read to and by the pupil, time on task, have proven useful. We do this for research (e.g., IEA Study), but not for describing on-going conditions. We would be doing no less than the economists who rely on all kinds of indices of production, investments and the like for their analyses.

Making inferences as to whether we are teaching correctly from achievement results alone, without relating them to what indeed was taught, is risky. Finding agreements on the minimal indices to record may not be easy either. Yet if we believe that literacy is learned, that children and adults can be educated, and that literacy is not mainly a natural phenomenon, then we should find some ways to reach a consensus or at least a compromise.

The development of literacy in individuals also needs to be examined carefully to help explain the highs and lows in the long progression from elementary school through college. It would seem therefore, that tests used to measure the national status of literacy might focus not only on the ultimate, expert tasks of mature reading, such as literal and inferential comprehension and reference skills, but on the more elemental knowledge and abilities of the novice—the beginning reading skills that are important in the development of higher skills—such as word recognition and decoding. The evidence indicates that they are necessary, although not sufficient, for more advanced reading. But the evidence is also strong that a lack of such skills is often behind the failure to progress by many children.

Development of reading through the various levels or stages, in relation to given learning conditions, may give us a better insight into solutions that might work over-time for the individual, for definable groups, and for

schools and school systems. It seems wasteful to cry for a different instructional program whenever scores drop, when we have so little evidence as to what brought it about and whether the different program will improve matters. It can make matters worse.

Thus the proposal of many that the emphasis on basic skills in the early grades during the 1970s produced the decline in 12th grade in the 1980 cohort as compared to the 1970 cohort is puzzling, for neither cohort had the heavier skills emphasis. Indeed, the NAEP data tend to show that those who did get the stronger skills emphasis did better. In Grade 4, in fact, they did significantly better, not only in literal comprehension, but in inferential comprehension and in reference skills.

I am mindful that my suggestions to look toward history (of instruction and of the individual's development) will meet with no easy consensus. They touch on long-held, strong, differing views on reading that have tended to overwhelm us—in theory, research, and in practice. And yet the gathering of systematic data on literacy practices (and expectations) and on the growth of literacy in individuals over time may help us speak to each other there a bit more productively as researchers, and as researchers with teachers, with parents, and others who depend on our expert knowledge.

How Much Literacy—Recent Trends

There is much difference of opinion as to what constitutes literacy. The confusion well may stem from the fact that the nature of literacy has changed and continues to change over time. Historically, the definition of literacy has changed from an ability to write one's name, to an ability to use reading for every day function in (4th-grade reading level, World War II, to an 8th grade), and to that needed for a high school equivalency diploma (Chall, 1983a).

The NAE Reading Committee report, *Toward a Literate Society,* suggested a 12th-grade reading level as essential literacy for today an ability to read the *New York Times* or a news magazine such as *Time* critically and analytically (Carroll & Chall, 1975). The state minimum competency tests for high school graduation, at Grade 11, seem to define minimum literacy lower, closer to grade 8 reading level.

An analysis of eight tests of minimum competency in reading for Grade 11 published in the late 1970s (Chall, Freeman, & Levy, 1982), half developed by state departments of education and half by publishing firms, revealed a wide range of reading ability needed to ''pass'' from a 5–6 grade level to an 11–12 grade level, with most of the texts requiring about a 7–8 grade level.

Analyses of the maturity of the reading selections (by Chall's reading stages) and the level of cognitive processing required to answer the questions (from Bloom's Taxonomy) confirmed that the level of literacy required by these minimum competency tests was characteristic more of the upper elementary grades than of high school.

While these lower competency levels may seem generous to those students who lag behind, we cannot overlook that the most important jobs today require higher abilities. (The largest percentages of unemployed youth seem to be among those with lowest levels of literacy.)

Reading Disability, Dyslexia, and Learning Disabilities

There is still another problem area that is of importance to a consideration of the status of literacy. Various government committees basing their estimates on a long history of research, have reported that about 10–15 percent of children and adults have severe difficulty in learning to read (Carroll & Chall, 1975). The Federal Handicapped Law, however, recognized only about 2 percent having learning disabilities needing special diagnosis and treatment.

This is unfortunate, for persons with severe reading difficulty represent a substantial proportion of the population, and because of greater understanding and adjustment made in curricula for those with learning disability, there are growing numbers of such students in high schools and colleges.

Can those with severe reading difficulty learn to read? There is considerable research indicating that they can. Although popular opinion, including that of many educators, is that if those with reading problems have not learned by high schools, they will never learn, the research indicates significant gains from remedial instruction. Comparisons with control groups indicate that there are immediate and long-term gains when remedial treatment is given (Smith, 1979).Remedial programs in community and 4-year colleges are also effective (Cross, 1981).

Status of Research

I would like to conclude with a few words on the status of research on literacy. There has been a tremendous growth in the amount of research over the past two decades. The research has also become more theoretical and "basic." In comparison, less seems to be directed toward solving the practical problems of literacy.

There is a growing tendency to cut up the field so that each part seems to invent anew what the other already knows. For reading, there seems to be several groups doing the major research and development:

- educational researchers and reading specialists do the major research on reading instruction;

- clinical psychologists and reading specialists are concerned with reading disability;
- special educators and various medical specialists, particularly neurologists, are concerned with reading/language/learning disabilities;
- adult educators are primarily concerned with adult literacy;
- cognitive psychologists and linguists are mainly concerned with basic research and theory.

A likely scenario follows on how students with learning problems might be viewed by each in turn: In Grade 1, students with reading difficulty might be classified as low in readiness (and as low achievers in the higher grades) by researchers on reading instruction. If the students have severe difficulty and are sent for a full evaluation, they will probably be classified as learning disabled by the reading/learning disability (medical) specialist. If they drop out of high school with reading ability below minimum competency, and enter an adult literacy program, they would probably be classified as being functionally illiterate. Most basic researchers would offer few explanations or classifications, only perhaps that instruction did not follow one or another of the theoretical models of the reading process.

The fastest growing research area is perhaps writing. As with the several groups in reading research, writing researchers seem to have produced many kinds of research, and a kind of separation from reading. As with reading subgroups, some of the researchers on writing seem to be discovering again what has been accepted knowledge in reading, still the most researched of the school subjects. On the whole, the status of research in writing seems better than it was a decade ago.

Overall, the research on literacy seems to be ready for a better balancing of the theoretical with the problem oriented, particularly for those children, young people, and adults who are having great difficulty with literacy; the poor, minorities, dyslexics, bilinguals, and the many high school and college students who are poorly prepared by their earlier experience. A greater recognition and use of the accumulated knowledge and wisdom of teachers would also help. So would a better appreciation of the cumulative effects of what is done in the school, the home and the community.

REFERENCES

Austin, M.C., & Morrison, C. *The torch lights: Tomorrow's teachers of reading.* Cambridge, Mass: Harvard University Press, 1961.
Basic Skills; 1979: Hearings before the Subcommittee on Education, Arts, and Humanities of the Committee

on Labor and Human Resources, United States Senate. Washington, D.C.: U.S. Government Printing Office, 1979.

Carroll, M.B., & Chall, J.S. *Toward a literate society.* New York: McGraw-Hill, 1975.

Chall, J.S. The great debate: Ten years later, with a modest proposal for reading stages. In L. Resnick and P.A. Weaver (Eds.), *Theory and practice of early reading.* Hillsdale, N.J.: Lawrence Erlbaum, 1979.

Chall, J.S. *Stages in reading development.* New York: McGraw-Hill, 1983.(a)

Chall, J.S. *Learning to read: The great debate* (2nd ed.). New York: McGraw-Hill, 1983.(b)

Chall, J.S., Conard, S.S., & Harris, S.H. *An analysis of textbooks in relation to declining S.A.T. scores.* New York: College Entrance Examination Board, 1977.

Chall, J.S., Freeman, A., & Levy, B. Minimum competency testing of reading: An analysis of eight tests designed for grade 11. In G. Madaus (Ed.), *The courts, validity, and minimum competency testing.* Boston: Kluwer-Nijhoff, 1982.

Chall, J.S., & Snow, C. *Families and literacy: The contribution of out-of-school experiences to children's acquisition of literacy.* A final report to the National Institute of Education, December 22, 1982.

Chall, J.S., & Stahl, S.A. Reading. In H.Mitzel (Ed.) *Encyclopedia of educational research* (5th ed.). New York: The Free Press, 1982.

Chomsky, C. Stages in language development and reading exposure. *Harvard Educational Review,* 1972, *42,* 1.

Coleman, J.S., Campbell, E.A., Hobson, C.J., McPartland, J., Mood, A.M., Weinfeld, F.D., & York,

R.L. *Equality of educational opportunity.* Washington, D.C.: U.S. Government Printing Office, 1966.

Cross, P. *Adults as learners.* San Francisco: Jossey-Bass, 1981.

Deutsch, M. The role of social class in language development and cognition. *American Journal of Orthopsychiatry,* 1965, *35,* 78–88.

Hunter, C.St.J., & Hartman, D. *Adult illiteracy in the United States.* New York: McGraw-Hill, 1979.

Madaus, G.F. Minimum competency testing for certification: The evolution and evaluation of test validity. In G. Madaus (Ed.), *The courts, validity, and minimum competency testing.* Boston: Kluwer-Nijhoff, 1982.

Morrison, C., & Austin, M.C. The torch lighters revisited—a preliminary report. *The Reading Teacher,* 1976, *29,* 647–652.

National Assessment of Educational Progress. *Reading, thinking, writing: A report on the 1979–80 assessment.* Denver, Colo.: Author, 1981.

Resnick, L.B., & Weaver, P.A. *Theory and practice of early reading* (3 vols.). Hillsdale, N.J.: Lawrence Erlbaum, 1979.

Smith, L. *An evaluation of studies of long term effects of remedial reading programs.* Unpublished master's thesis, Harvard Graduate School of Education, 1979.

Sticht, T.G. (Ed.) *Reading for working.* Alexandria, Va.: Human Resources Research Organization, 1975.

Wirtz, W. *On further examination: Report of the advisory panel on the Scholastic Aptitude Test score decline.* Princeton, N.J.: College Board Publications, 1977.

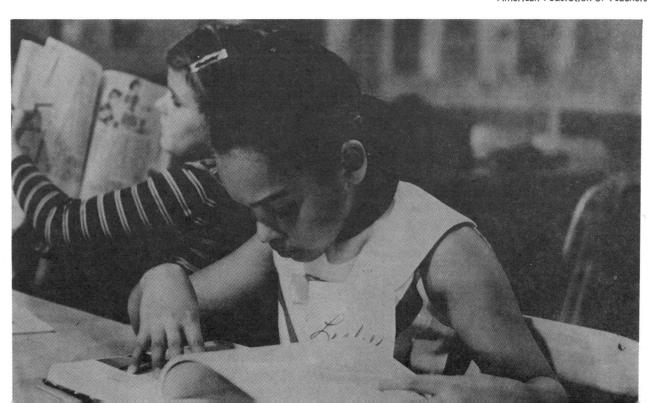

Chapter 32
Models of the Learner
Jerome Bruner*

Topics, including the topics of keynote addresses to learned societies, have a hermeneutic history. The hermeneutic history of a topic, we are cautioned, must be taken into account if we are fully to interpret its meaning. The topic of my paper, Models of the Learner, is no exception. It has such a history and has a proximal origin in a set of exchanges—first as a conversation and then as the topic of a more formal learned discussion.

Let me set forth the beginning narrative of that hermeneutic circle (or spiral) and continue it in the discussion that follows. The setting was an international conference in the not very Orwellian summer of 1984, a coherence ostensibly on the vexed subject of how to improve the quality of education. Sponsored jointly by the Van Leer Jerusalem Foundation and the Aspen Institute, it took place in a handsome mansion overlooking one of the scenic lakes on the outskirts of Berlin—a mansion that had been reconstructed on the ruins of the residence of the infamous Goebbels, Hitler's Minister of Culture, or was he the Minister of Propaganda? The participants were appropriately distinguished: some Deans of famous faculties of education, more than a sprinkling of great names in what everybody would agree is educational research, and a handful of psychologists and associated behavioral scientists whose work bore that tangential relation to the process of education that excites the optimism of educators with respect to the relevance of "pure" research. We were perhaps two dozen in number, and it was a convivial company.

After a day and a half of discussion on topics of great generality, all conducted at a level of striking knowledgeability, someone proposed that we could really not get to the heart of the matter unless we had more clearly in mind some working model of what a learner was, how he or she operated and, above all, what we thought to be an adequate learning environment for our putative learner. It was proposed to the plenary session that we give over the next morning to these issues.

I was among those asked to prepare some sort of state-ment on the matter. The discussion that ensued was lively. What it left behind in my mind and what several of us discussed later was the flat-footed impossibility of ever settling institutional questions of education without first making a decision—yes, a political decision—on the nature of learning and learners. Yet, for all that, the decision about learning and learners was perforce a decision about an ideal, about how we conceived what a learner *should* be in order to assure that a society of a particularly valued kind could be safeguarded. There is no completely naturalistic way of resolving the question about what model of the learner we want to enshrine at the center of our practice of education. For there are many ways to learn and many ways of encouraging different forms of learning with different ends in view. At the heart of the decision process there must be a value judgment about how the mind should be cultivated and to what end.

While I wish to consider alternate models of the learner, I have no illusion that I can do so just in the spirit of a naturalist or as a student of the learning process. In fact, models of the learner that are on offer in the psychological literature, in the cognitive sciences, or in AI are themselves constructions based on a selection not simply of data, but of the conditions under which learning is studied. As I tried to say a few years ago, it is possible to construct not only experimental studies but "real life" situations that make people (or pigeons, for that matter) look stupid or clever, generative or passive, combinatorial or rote (Bruner, 1982). Then the theoretical model that is constructed becomes, as it were, the text of the culture, and life is made to imitate text in the same subtle ways in which, in another closely related domain, life imitates art.

*Dr. Jerome Bruner is a George Herbert Mead University Professor at the New School for Social Research, New York, NY. His area of specialization is Educational and Cognitive Psychology. Reprinted with permission of The *Educational Researcher*, June/July, 1985.

Please do not interpret what I am saying in the relativistic sense that all theories or models of the learner are equally true or even equally right. Rather, what I wish to say is that any model of learning is right or wrong for a given set of stipulated conditions, including the nature of the tasks one has in mind, the form of the intention one creates in the learner, the generality or specificity for the learning to be accomplished, and the semiotics of the learning situation itself—what it means to the learner.

This is *not* to say that a new or different model of the leaner is needed for every task or situation in which learning takes place. To put it in the current jargon, it is absurd to insist that each and every theory of learning is utterly domain specific, that nothing general can be said about learners or learning or learning environments. You do not quite need a different model of a learner to talk about learning how to play chess, learning how to play the flute, learning mathematics, and learning to read the sprung rhymes in the verse of Gerard Manley Hopkins. Even if I do have to say it in folk psychology rather than in programming talk, all of them will involve attention and memory and courage and even, *pace* AI, some heuristics for maintaining frustration tolerance. The issue, as we shall see yet again, is that learning is indeed context sensitive, but that human beings, given their peculiarly human competence, are capable of adapting their approach to the demands of different contexts. But I am tipping my hand, for it is only later that I wanted to talk about a general model of a learner as one equipped to discriminate and deal differentially with a wide variety of possible worlds exhibiting different conditions, yet worlds in which one can cope.

Let me now take a fast gallop through the landscape we surveyed that day from the phoenix nest on the site of Goebbels' house in the exurbs of Berlin when we got down to our formal discussion of "models of the learner."

Models of the Learner

Tabula rasa. The first, and perhaps the most ancient is really based on the Aristotelian notion of *mimesis*. In its 18th century version, it rested on the premise that experience writes on the wax tablet of the mind. One learns from experience (rather than through divine revelation or through received texts). Or as Locke put it, nothing gets into the mind save through the senses—but as Leibniz countered, nothing except mind itself. This view takes as a central premise that such order as there is in mind is a reflection of the order that exists in the world, and that is why the concept of association is always so central to empiricist theories. Things that are together in space and time in the world succeed, under the sway of this principle, in being together in the mind. I need not go into the

troubles of empiricism. They have been raked over historically by everybody from Aristotle (whose *sensus communis* was something of a constructivist takeover bid) through the School-men, from Kant through Wittgenstein and Chomsky. I want, rather, to take it as a given, a cultural text in Geertz's sense, to be examined for its cultural significance in shaping our practices. I want to note only that, given belief in associationist empiricism, we adopted ideas about learning procedures to fit and constructed learning environments that in fact made people look like little empiricists—averting our eyes from all instances where it didn't, as for example in the acquiring of a language. and when we were forced to look at that, we concocted Augustinian theories about it and devised nonsense syllable research in support of them.

The formula for success in empiricism is to have experience.

Hypothesis generator. There is a class of learner models that represents a reaction against the rather passive view of empiricist, *tabula rasa* notions. They have in common a notion of intentionality at their center. The learner, rather than being the creature of experience, selects that which is to enter. The principle of selection varies from theory to theory: from the *sensus communis* of Aristotle and the *vis integretiva* of Aquinas that sorted the associated input of experience in the light of the principles of reason, to the principles of wish-fulfillment and ego defense of Freud that permitted us to experience (or interpret) only those parts of experience that were adequate compromises between the demands of conflicting needs. What exactly generates hypotheses or programs the filter, which selects and organizes what gets through the senses into the mind, varied widely and was always seriously underdefined. Even such towering learning theorists as Edward Tolman, Lev Vygotsky, and John Dewey, all of whom took the view that experience came shaped by hypotheses rather than by the world, were grandly vague in their specification of how hypotheses came into being—though Dewey and Vygotsky gave special pride of place to the role of language as a hypothesis-generator, a place that promised more than it delivered.

It was never altogether clear how to extrapolate an educational posture from hypothesis theories, save in one respect. Emphasis was on an active curiosity guided by self-directed projects—a feature of Progressivism in American and in the unrealized pedagogy of Vygotsky's followers in the Soviet Union, unrealized save in the discipline of "defectology."

The formula for success in learning, according to the hypothesis formulation, is to have a good theory.

Nativism. At least three forms of muted nativism have shaped our models of the learner. One derives from Immanuel Kant. A second comes from Gestalt theory. The third, derivative of Descartes, is still with us in

Chomsky's theory of mind. In a deep historical sense, they are all inheritors of the tradition of Platonism. All share one central concept: Mind is inherently or innately shaped by a set of underlying categories, hypotheses, forms of organizing experience. The task of the learner is to work his or her way through the cluttered surface structure of sense to an underlying or ideal or deep organization that provides a richer or righter or more predictive or more generalizable representation of reality. Where evolutionism entered this view (as with ethnologists and, in a shriller form, in sociobiology) it is assumed that the fit between the categories or hypotheses of mind and the world that they represent is a product of natural selection.

For all their disagreements on details, Nativist theories have one big thing in common: The opportunity to use and exercise the innate powers of mind is all. That is the formula for success as well.

Constructivism. Probably the most powerful expression of this view comes from Jean Piaget, although a more rigorous and considered expression of it can be found in the writings of the philosopher Nelson Goodman. The tenet of Piaget's constructivism is that the world is not found, but made, and made according to a set of structural rules that are imposed on the flow of experience. By structural rules it is intended to emphasize that knowledge is not local but derived from a structure of the whole—that local operations reflect universal operations of the system as a whole. Learning is bound within the limits of the rules of the system; it consists of realizations of the general rules in application to particulars. Development consists of a series of stage-like progressions, stage change consisting of a change in the rules of the system and later rule systems absorbing earlier ones as special cases. The learning dynamic of the system at any stage is provided by an unstable equilibrium or dialectic between assimilating experience to the rules and accommodating the rules to experience. When the equilibrium becomes unstable enough, the structure changes.

The constructivist model of the learner places strong emphasis on self-propelled operations on the world as the way to mastery—a pretty wide-band conception. Its formula for success is that nothing succeeds like a theoretical system, and one succeeds supremely only by going to a higher system that subsumes it.

Novice-to-Expert. This view of the learner has so recently emerged that is hard to characterize. It is very practical, in some respects highly anti-theoretical. It operates within domains, almost at times denying the utility of a general theory—or perhaps that is a sign of its immaturity. It begins with the premise that if you want to find out about learning, ask first about what is to be learned, find an expert who does it well, and then look at the novice and figure out how he or she can get there. To aid

in this task, simulate the novice's performance and the expert's in a computer program, and see what transformations and heuristics will get you from the one to the other. You may even be helped by studying and simulating some typical mid-stages. Such generality as may be present in learning different tasks will eventually show up in the simulations. The immediate challenge is to get the novice to be an expert as quickly and as painlessly as possible, and never mind high theory.

The formula for success is "be specific and be explicit." Or, a computer programmer is a better friend than a philosopher of mind. Or, it is more important to get through the keyhole than to see the sky. Or, and perhaps more seriously, subordinate the learner to the steps he must take to attain expertise.

In sketching these views about the model of the learner, I have omitted an important issue, one that had better be treated independently of each, for it is curiously extrinsic to all of them. It is the issue of the carrot and the stick—the role of motivation in learning. It has been a source of embarrassment in the history of the subject from the Stoics to Skinner. Let me state its dilemma in the starkest way. How can knowing something be affected by whether the knowledge gained leads to reward or to punishment? If the theory of reinforcement related to the acquisition of knowledge, God would not have had to expel poor Adam and Eve from the garden for eating of the tree of knowledge. He would have arranged, Huck Finn style, for them to have developed a very bad stomach ache from the consumption of green apples. Instead, He knew that knowledge, once attained, is irreversible and for better or for worse. And so, if I may be Miltonian, he had to condemn them to a new way of life where that knowledge could be put to use.

It is the use of knowledge rather than knowledge itself that is affected by the nature of its consequences. Use implies performance; performance entails action. The carrot and the stick are instruments for affecting action, not thought. Thus the degree to which models of the learner feature reinforcement is the degree to which they concentrate on the behavior of the learner rather than on his or her mind. It is not surprising, then, that even in the heyday of the Empiricists (who thought of themselves as philosophers of mind) virtually nothing was said about carrots and sticks. Indeed, as Crane Brinton reminded us a generation ago in his classic *Anatomy of Revolution,* the precepts of Empiricism (particularly in John Locke) were designed to justify man's freedom from the authority of King and Clergy. He was, in this new dispensation, his own knowledge getter. Thus Jonathan Edwards could preach to his flock in Northampton on the frontier of the Massachusetts Bay Colony in the late 17th century that they too, like Isaac Newton, could by their own efforts of mind unlock the secrets of God.

It is interesting, then, that most theories depicted the learner, either implicitly or explicitly, as self-motivated— at least while they concentrated on learning as a means of acquiring knowledge. Indeed, we can say that the carrot and the stick—reinforcement—have to do not with learning but with morality: how one acts on the basis of what one knows. Even then, the connection between reward and punishment on the one side and virtuous action on the other remains as obscure as ever. The debate over the effectiveness of, say, prisons rages as incoherently as ever. And the thought controls imposed by dictators are much more concerned with censorship and other means of stopping the flow of information than they are with tinkering with schedules of reinforcement.

A Model of Models

I have already tipped my hand, as I confessed in passing. There is no reason, save ideology and the exercise of political control, to opt for a single model of the learner. We *do* learn from experience, when that is all we have to go on. On occasion we act like induction machines, though it is rarely so dark out that we can't do better than that. Indeed, given half a chance, we generate hypotheses that take us way beyond the information given—often with good effect, and always with some risk, which requires courage and the buffering of a support system. There is every reason to believe that a nervous system evolved in nature and more latterly and swiftly in culture endows us with a set of useful presuppositions about both nature and culture. How else can we account for the swift mastery of language and other symbolic forms to which we take so easily and with insufficient knowledge for proper induction? How can we doubt that a culture that regulates its moods and acts according to such abstract inventions as interest rates, social slights, gross national products, and loyalty to Alma Mater is made up of people who not only construct the world in which they live but share it as an ontological given? It is even true that if you want to be a postman or a trust officer, you would do well to look closely at how they go about their business and then try to simulate them as a clever clone,

hopefully keeping your tongue in your cheek and your powder dry the while.

What it amounts to, as I have already hinted, is treating all models of the learner as stipulative, and then inquiring into the condition under which they might be effective or useful or comforting. If you genuinely believe that it improves a nation's confidence in its control over things to keep children in schools for a good part of the day, then do so. Or if you think formal schooling is structurally inevitable in a society with more disensus than consensus, again keep them in school. These are reasons of politics, and they plainly have a place in any debate, for education is political too. But if you see children learning mathematics by rote, you can also say (this time on more naturalistic yet practical grounds) that somebody got confused about models and slipped in an empiricist one in place of a constructionist one. In a word, the best approach to models of the learner is a reflective one that permits you to ''go meta,'' to inquire whether the script being imposed on the learner is there for the reason that was intended or for some other reason.

There is not *one* kind of learning. It was the vanity of a preceding generation to think that the battle over learning theories would eventuate in one winning over all the others. Any learner has a host of learning strategies at command. The salvation is in learning how to go about learning before getting irreversibly beyond the point of no return. We would do well to equip learners with a menu of their possibilities and, in the course of their education, to arm them with procedures and sensibilities that would make it possible for them to use the menu wisely.

Here the hermeneutic circle ends. You cannot improve the state of education without a model of the learner. Yet the model of the learner is not fixed but various. A choice of one reflects many political, practical, and cultural issues. Perhaps the best choice is not a choice of one, but an appreciation of the variety that is possible. The appreciation of that variety is what makes the practice of education something more than a scripted exercise in cultural rigidity.

Chapter 33
Effective Schools, Classrooms, and Instruction: Implications for Special Education

William E. Bickel and Donna Diprima Bickel*

This article reviews the literatures on the characteristics of effective schools, classrooms, and instructional processes. Central findings from these literatures are summarized, as are important cautions in interpreting this knowledge base. The implications for special education of the effectiveness literatures are discussed. It is the position of the authors that both special and regular educators can learn much from recent research in order to design more powerful and integrated instructional programs for students with special needs.

Since 1970, formal knowledge about the characteristics of effective schools, classrooms, and instruction has grown to a considerable degree. In this article, we summarize some of the most salient features of this emerging knowledge base and consider its implications for special education.

Procedures and practices found to be powerful in stimulating student achievement in basic skills (i.e., mathematics, reading/language arts) at the elementary level are the primary foci of our review. This admittedly narrow range is also a pragmatic one. The research literatures that are the subjects of this review have focused heavily on elementary school basic skills achievement as their major outcome measure. We confine our comments to the programs for academically handicapped students (e.g., learning disabled, emotionally disturbed, educable mentally retarded).

This review is organized into three major sections, beginning with a discussion of what is commonly known as "effective schools" research. In the second section, we turn to effective teaching practices and procedures for organizing and supporting classroom instruction. In the third section, we consider the implications of the effective schools, effective classroom/instruction literatures for special education.

In each section we have taken a "review-of-reviews" approach, in deference to space limitations, and in recognition of the many reviews published during the past 5 years. Our discussions will, perforce, be brief surveys of findings. For more detail, the reader is referred to the review cited, and to the original studies.

What Is Known About Effective Schools?

Some schools are unusually effective in teaching basic skills to underachieving poor and minority children. These effective schools share a number of characteristics that are correlated with their success and that lie well within the boundaries of what educators can reasonably manipulate. The correlates of the effective schools are being used in many educational settings as a framework, as "ends in view," for improving schools currently not deemed effective (e.g., Clark & McCarthy, 1983).

The reform movement based on the effective schools literature has two basic domains of activity: research studies that identify characteristics of effective schools and school improvement projects that use this research to promote change. The growth of these activities has been remarkable. For example, Mackenzie (1983b) reports that the 1983 meeting program for The American Educational Research Association included 25 separate entries in this area, as compared to only 4 in 1978. (Over 40 entries appeared in 1985). Similarly, Odden and Dougherty (1982) noted that most states in recent years

*Dr. William E. Bickel is Senior Scientist, Learning Research and Development Center, University of Pittsburgh, Pittsburgh, PA. Donna Diprima Bickel is School Consultant and Doctoral Student, Department of Special Education, University of Pittsburgh, Pittsburgh, PA. Reprinted with permission of the authors and *Exceptional Children*, Vol. 52, No. 6, pp. 489–500. Copyright © 1986 The Council for Exceptional Children. The authors wish to gratefully acknowledge Mary Margaret Kerr and Naomi Zigmond for their reviews of earlier drafts of this paper.

had initiated school improvement programs explicitly structured using the characteristics of effective schools identified through recent research.

The research that is at the core of the school improvement activity is surprisingly diverse, in both methodologies and results (Purkey & Smith, 1983; Reynolds & Sullivan, 1981). Approaches have included case studies (e.g., Brookover & Lezotte, 1979; Rutter, Maughan, Morimore, Ouston & Smith, 1979; Venezky & Winfield, 1979; Weber, 1971); program evaluation (e.g., Armor, Conry-Oseguera, Cox, King, McConnell, Pascal, Pauly, & Zellman, 1976); and outlier studies (e.g., Austin, 1979; Brookover & Schneider, 1975; Edmonds & Frederiksen, 1978).

What was generally shared across this diverse body of work was a focus on the search for school level variables that are associated with basic skills achievement and a conviction on the part of the researchers that schools do make a difference in a child's educational performance. This conviction has been a powerful motivating force behind the research. It was an attempt to refute the impression left by some earlier major research studies (e.g., Coleman, Campbell, Hobson, McPartland, Mood, Weinfield, & York, 1966) that schools are relatively powerless when compared to the effects of social background.

Characteristics Associated with Effective Schools

Most reviews include discussion of the following variables as key characteristics of effective schools: (a) educational leadership, (b) orderly school climate, (c) high achievement expectations, (d) systematic monitoring of student performance, and (e) an emphasis on basic skills (cf. Austin, 1979; Clark, Lotto, & McCarthy, 1980; Edmonds, 1979; Mackenzie, 1983a, 1983b; Purkey & Smith, 1983; Reynolds & Sullivan, 1981). These same variables have appeared in countless improvement efforts, partly as a result of their convergent strength in the literature and certainly as a reflection of their "intuitive appeal" (Mackenzie, 1983a).

In effective schools, the principal (or other appropriate administrative personnel) provides leadership by demonstrating commitment to goals, coupled with flexibility in pursuing them. There is also an emphasis on outcomes over procedures, the presence of high levels of informal interaction and the use of problem-solving and evaluation techniques to monitor performance objectives. There are clear and consistent school policies in effective schools; the policies emphasize shared responsibility for the overall school climate. There is also evidence that administrators and teachers communicate expectations for success in effective schools.

The notion of positive expectancy is perhaps the most fundamental message emanating from the effective schools literature. It is not only a specific finding in many of the studies, in a sense, it is the philosophical orientation driving the research. A conviction that "some schools work and more can" (Edmonds, 1979, p. 28) is at the core of this research. Similarly, continual monitoring of individual and class progress (Purkey & Smith 1983) and timely, accurate assessment for student progress (Mackenzie, 1983a), are reported as significant correlates of school success. A clear sense of the mission of schooling is exhibited in effective schools and it is consistently communicated to students and to the large school community; the goals of this mission are sharply focused on basic skill achievement.

Cautionary Notes

This very brief overview of some of the central themes that have emerged from the effective schools research cannot be shared without important cautions. Like any body of research that is as recent and as divergent as the effective schools literature, there are serious criticisms to be considered in the current state of knowledge. It is beyond the scope of this article to discuss these in detail; more complete discussions are available in the literature (e.g., Edmonds, 1982; Frechtling, 1983; Madaus, Airasian, & Kellaghan, 1980; Purkey & Smith, 1983; Rowan, Bossert, & Dwyer, 1983). However, we will briefly mention several of the most serious issues.

Several classifications of criticisms have been raised about the effective schools literature. One concern is the nature and strength of the findings themselves. Partly as a result of ambiguity in how a particular variable is defined, partly because many different research agendas and methodologies have been employed, the power of a specific variable is not clear across studies. How specific school level variables influence individual student achievement outcomes, and how one school level variable relates to others deemed to be important to school effectiveness is also unclear. Furthermore, there is uncertainty as to how school level variables interact with classroom level factors (e.g., those discussed in the next section) known to facilitate student achievement.

Another class of criticisms concerns the basic outcome criteria and measures typically used to judge effectiveness. We have noted that much or this literature focuses on achievement of basic skills as measured by standardized tests. This emphasis overlooks important aspects of the school curriculum and the educational agenda of society. The basic skills focus may force an unfortunate narrowing of the educational process. Further, it is worth asking whether the strategies that are helpful in meeting basic skills achievement goals are complementary or anti-thetical to success in other outcome areas (e.g., higher order cognitive skills, social skills).

A third major area of criticism concerns the utility of school effectiveness findings for the work of school improvement. The evidence is not yet in on this point. Hundreds of improvement projects around the country have modeled their efforts upon this literature. To the extent that these efforts are well documented, in the next few years we will learn much about whether this has been a good idea.

Commentary on Effective Schools

Notwithstanding all of the important cautionary notes previously cited, the literature on effective schools has made very important contributions to the way educators think about schooling and its outcomes. These contributions sort out along two fundamental dimensions: One concerns hope; the other involves how we focus our reform energies. The hopeful message of this literature is powerful and overdue. The way schools are organized can make a difference in the education of students, even if those students happen to be poor, minority, or exceptional children behind in their achievement. While many educators never lost this sense of hope (and responsibility), some did. The school is not the only important variable to be sure, but it is one important factor. As two perceptive critics of this literature noted:

> Having expressed our reservations about the available research . . . we nevertheless find a substantive use emerging from the literature. There is a good deal of common sense to the notion that a school is more likely to have relatively high reading and math scores if the staff agree to emphasize those subjects, are serious and purposeful about the task of teaching, expect students to learn, and create a safe and comfortable environment in which students accurately perceive the school's expectations for academic success. Such a mixture creates a climate that would encourage, if not guarantee, success in any endeavor. (Purkey & Smith, 1983, p. 440–441)

The second contribution of the effective schools literature, as we judge it, is its powerful reminder that instruction and learning take place in a larger social environment. As an important expression of that social environment, the culture of the school has a significant role to play for good or ill. Turning our attention more certainly to the school's role, and to how one can improve it is a major contribution indeed. We will return to this issue at a later point when implications for special education are discussed.

What Is Known About Effective Classrooms and Instruction?

Some procedures for organizing the classroom are unusually effective for basic skills achievement. Some teaching methods have similar results. In this section, we will highlight what has been leaned about such effective procedures and methods. In order to do this, we will draw upon a body of literature that is equally diverse as the effective schools research and that extends over a greater period of time.

Studies of teaching and of classroom processes have converged in important ways on concepts and practices that have an impact on the effects of instruction. This research has focused on the details of the classroom as the environment in which learning and instruction most directly take place, and on student/teacher interactions that define and influence learning tasks and outcomes.

This emphasis on a fine-grained analysis of what occurs inside classrooms represents an important shift away from the input/output evaluation studies of an earlier time that heavily emphasized major national educational programs as treatments (Cicirelli, Evans, & Shiller, 1970), and earlier research on teaching that emphasized the characteristics of teachers (Bloom, 1980). The research we review in this section is on how effective instruction is organized, on teacher strategies in effective classrooms, and on how teacher strategies can be supported. Again, we will use a review-of-reviews strategy in summarizing this literature. For more complete discussions, the reader is referred to Berliner, 1984; Brophy, 1983; Cooley and Leinhardt, 1980; Gage, 1983; Glaser, 1977; Hunter, 1984; Leinhardt, Bickel, and Pallay, 1982; and Rosenshine, 1983.

Characteristics Associated with Effective Instruction

Berliner (1984) organized his review of research on effective teaching into three broad categories involving preinstructional, during instruction, and post instructional factors. Rosenshine (1983) focused on specific teaching functions that take place during the instructional process that seem or be particularly effective. Leinhardt et al. (1982) primarily reviewed educational practices that seem to be effective for the organization of instruction.

Mackenzie (1983a) reviewed procedures for organizing instruction, some specific teaching functions, and some supportive activities that begin to integrate elements of the effective schools research with research on effective classroom instruction.

In structuring this discussion, we have sorted the complex set of findings related to organizing classroom instruction and teaching processes into three broad categories. These include variables related to teaching behaviors, the organization of instruction, and instructional support. These categories are offered as tools for surveying a complex terrain, not as rigid categories. They overlap in important ways. Indeed, in the case of instructional support, we argue that these findings are the beginnings of the bridge necessary to link the effective schools research with the effective classroom/instructional processes work.

In each area we highlight examples of major findings. The list is not exhaustive, but rather suggestive of the kinds of variables that are being found to be associated with basic skills achievement.

Teaching behaviors. In his review, Rosenshine (1983) focused on six instructional functions found to be essential for effective teaching behaviors. These functions concern:

1. Reviewing, checking previous day's work (and reteaching if necessary).
2. Presenting new content/skills.
3. Initial student practice (and checking for understanding).
4. Feedback and corrections (and reteaching if necessary).
5. Student independent practice.
6. Weekly and monthly reviews.

In her discussion of teaching behaviors, Hunter (1984) wrote of "designing needed practice . . . using reinforcers that enhance a student's self-concept, relating new academic learning to a student's own life" (p. 172–173). Hunter also stressed the importance of providing guided practice, modeling the new process or product a student is expected to learn, and checking for understanding as critical teacher behaviors.

What emerges across various commentaries is the image of effective teachers taking an active, direct role in the instruction of their students. These educators give many detailed and redundant instruction and explanations when introducing a new concept (Rosenshine, 1983). They give ample opportunity for guided practice with frequent reviews of student progress (Berliner, 1984). They check for understanding, using such techniques as questioning, consistent review of homework, and review of previous day's lessons before moving on to new areas. Such teachers move among students when they are involved in practice seatwork. Feedback is provided frequently and with meaningful detail. Effective teachers use feedback strategies for positive reinforcement of student success. Feedback also provides the basis for reteaching where necessary. Effective teachers take an active role in creating a positive, expectant, and orderly classroom environment in which learning takes place. To accomplish these climate objectives, effective

teachers actively structure the learning process and the management of time, building in such things as signals for academic work and maintaining student attention by group alerting and accountability techniques and through variation in educational tasks (Berliner, 1984).

Organization of instruction. The activist view of the teacher, directly engaged with students in the learning process, is further structured and sustained by a series of decisions about the way the instructional environment is organized. These decisions are often teacher made, although at times they may also lie in the larger domain of school leadership and are legitimate areas for action by the "principal as instructional leader" as envisioned in the effective school research. In either case, the implications of the classroom process literature are clear. Decisions about the use of time, the pace of instruction, the way the curriculum is structured and delivered, the way students progress through the curriculum, and the way students are grouped for instruction can directly affect basic skills outcomes. Understanding of the use of instructional time and its relationships to instruction and learning outcomes has grown considerably during the past decade. In examining these relationships, Berliner (1984) distinguished among allocated time, engaged time, and academic learning time. Allocated time involves basic decisions about subject matter focus and, within subject matters, areas of high and low priority for instruction. How much time in the elementary school year, in the school day, should be devoted toward reading instruction versus instruction in mathematics or science? And, within reading, how much time should be allocated for work on comprehension versus decoding skills? There is considerable empirical evidence that at these macrolevels, the allocation of time varies greatly across classrooms, schools, and curriculums and that this variation is related to student outcomes.

Taking one step further toward the instructional process, Berliner's (1984) concept of engaged time focuses on what students are doing within the time allocated. Time on task is related in important ways to student achievement. To state the apparently obvious, students learn more when they are attending to the learning tasks that are the focus of instruction. We say that this is stating the "apparently obvious" because there is strong empirical evidence of considerable variation in student engaged time across classrooms and that this precious resource is often an unmanaged one.

The concept of academic learning time (ALT) adds several facets to the time-on-task emphasis in the literature. At its core, ALT refers to student time on task when that task is directly "related to the outcome measure being used (often an achievement test), (and) during which a student experiences a high success rate" (Berliner, 1984, p. 60). Embedded in the concept of ALT is the larger notion of "content overlap among teaching, learning, and criterion" (Leinhardt et al., 1982).

> When teachers spend their time and energy teaching students the content that the students need to learn, students learn the material. When students spend their time actively engaged in activities that relate strongly to the materials they will be tested on, they learn more of the material. (p. 409).

Similarly, the student success emphasis of ALT is related to the broader concept of mastery. Rosenshine (1983) emphasizes the importance of students reaching success rates of 90% to 100% in their practice activities before moving on. Berliner (1984) argues that, especially for "younger students and for the academically least able, almost errorless performance during learning tasks results in higher test performance" (p. 59). These authors are focused on student learning tasks, especially when such tasks are ones where the student is working independently. More broadly, a master learning emphasis is built into the structure of the curriculum, generally, so that on the completion of discrete blocks of instruction here is formal assessment of student progress (Leinhardt et al., 1982). The mastery concept at this level is linked to the monitoring and feedback teacher behaviors discussed in the previous section.

What does not turn up as an important variable in the use of time are manipulations of the length of the school day or year (Mackenzie, 1983a). The critical point here is that such lengthening is clearly related to what use is made of the time. And, given the tremendous variation in the quality of the use of time already in the school year, and the enormous costs involved in adding student contact hours, the more profitable focus should be on improving current time usage.

Pacing is a variable related to both time allocation and content focus. Stated most directly, "the more a teacher covers, the more students seem to learn" (Berliner, 1984, p. 55). This mandate for a brisk pace to instruction, however, must be qualified in several important ways. Leinhardt et al. (1982) noted the tension that must exist between a rapid pace to instruction whose goal is more complete coverage and allowing enough time for students to absorb and master the material. These authors stated that in at least one area of instruction, reading, the importance of pacing "washes out in the presence of curriculum overlap and time spent in direct reading" (p. 410). The issue with regard to pacing is achieving the balance required between movement through content and attainment of high levels of mastery.

The ways children are grouped can have an important effect on learning outcomes but the relationships seem to be rather complex. Within the classroom, grouping of students for instruction seems to have positive benefits when the following conditions are evident:

- Number and size of groups are dependent on student characteristics and content taught.
- Different groupings are used for different subjects.
- Frequent shifts among groups occur during the school year as well as between years.
- Groups are based on current levels of specific skills.
- Groups are established as a result of instruction.
- There is a combination of small group and whole class instruction.
- Groupings are responsive to instruction. (Mackenzie, 1983b).

Conversely, when grouping patterns are static, based on testing prior to instruction, held constant across subject areas, and grounded in perceptions about general ability, the effects can be negative.

Mackenzie (1983b) also reviewed grouping practices at the school level. In a discussion of the tracking of students in high schools he reported that the instructional environments experienced by "lower track students" compared to those of other students can differ sharply along such process variable dimensions as content, level of cognitive demands, time on instruction versus noninstructional activity, teacher enthusiasm, and quality of peer relationships (p. 46). An essential element in understanding the potential negative effects of static grouping patterns lies with these differences in instructional processes that are associated with various tracking patterns, whether tracks are within classrooms or across classrooms in schools.

Instructional support. Classroom instruction can be supported in ways that can positively affect student outcomes. Two variables of importance involve class size, and teacher inservice training. The importance of class size to student achievement has been a much-debated topic. In a comprehensive review of the research in this area, Glass, Cahan, Smith and Filby (1982) found that smaller classes are associated with higher student achievement. This seems to hold true as one drops from 40 students in a class to 20 and below. Both Mackenzie (1983b) and Leinhardt et al. (1982) note some important caveats to this trend, however. The relationship is hardly automatic. "Reeducations in class may have to be accompanied by productive innovations in classroom process in order to boost achievement" (Mackenzie, 1983b, p. 31). Smaller classes clearly can positively affect the ability of the teacher to employ more of the effective teaching strategies noted earlier, developing more powerful and intense interactions with students. However, size differences alone will not guarantee success.

An important component in supporting effective instruction in classrooms concerns the development of sound staff development of inservice programs (Berliner, 1984; Hunter, 1984; Mackenzie, 1983b; Rosenshine, 1983). In a sense, the findings on the importance of inservice programs for teachers brings full circle this brief portrait of effective classroom process variables that are emerging from recent research. We say this because the strength of the inservice finding is directly tied to whether such efforts are focused on teachers being trained in the effective classroom process procedures emerging from the literature. That is,

> when the (effective classroom process) research is used to develop training procedures for teachers, teachers can learn the recommended practices, and if they implement the teaching practices . . . they can affect in a positive way student classroom behavior and achievement. (Berliner, 1984, p. 74).

This concludes our brief review of instructional support variables found to be important for classroom instructional outcomes. The intriguing question in this area, of course, is how many of the effective schools variables belong in this category as well. We suspect that one could find many strong and positive relationships. Therein lies an important agenda for future research efforts.

Cautionary Notes

Like the findings on effective schools, those associated with effective classrooms and instructional processes should be viewed with several qualifications in mind. Perhaps two of the most significant concerns involve a potential narrowing of the curriculum that could result from an unbridled implementation of certain of the findings previously reported, and the relationships, as yet not well understood, among some of these variables and achievement increase other than basic skills (for example, higher order thinking skills, and social skills).

Teachers who analyze their curriculum and more certainly focus time and student instruction on core basic skill areas are likely to be more effective in stimulating learning outcomes. To the extent that this focused instruction is highly related to what students are tested on (whether the instruments are criterion-referenced or normative), achievement scores most likely will rise. The danger in this process comes when other important instructional goals are left out at the same time as the links among usage of time, focused basic skill goals, and assessment of student progress are tightened.

Effective classroom/teacher research has focused heavily on basic skills achievement as the central outcome measure for judging the worth of a given procedure or practice. This focus is quite justified given the importance of the goal and the ambiguity that existed in our knowledge about how to achieve success in this area.

What is not well understood, and what remains as an important area of future research, is the relationship of these effective practices to other valued student outcomes. For example, will higher order thinking skills be facilitated or actually inhibited if the current effective classroom process model is used? Intuitively, some of the recommended practices (e.g., smaller classes, flexible grouping) should not be harmful but rather similarly positive in effect. However, other findings raise questions. The heavy orientation toward teacher-directed instruction may not be amenable to the achievement of higher order thinking skills. Nevertheless, intuitions are not enough; educators need to know much more about such relationships.

Commentary on Effective Classroom Instruction

With cautionary notes aside but not out of mind, the growing convergence of research on effective classroom organization and instruction has made significant contributions to the knowledge of what works and what does not work for basic skills achievement. Like the effective schools research, a central message here is one of optimism and empowerment of educators. Like school environments, teaching processes can have an important effect on student outcomes. What was often known among educators at an intuitive, anecdotal level of experience has been increasingly codified in classrooms and the professional knowledge of teachers. It is along this dimension concerned with transferability that the effective classroom process literature is ahead of the effective schools research. In the latter instance, the case must still be made that the research results can be powerful tools for stimulating change in other school settings. The evidence of transferability seems to be much stronger for the research on effective classrooms.

What has emerged from this research inside the classroom walls is the image of the teacher actively, directly engaged in the teaching/learning process. Precious resources like time and curriculum content are allocated and used in increasingly efficient ways. Students learn more because they, in effect, have more opportunity to learn. They are rewarded for their efforts by success as they proceed in incremental steps through the curriculum. The goals are clear and both students and teachers share responsibility for meeting them.

What Are the Implications for Special Education?

We believe that the research reviewed in the preceding two sections has substantial implications for the special education of students classified as mildly mentally handicapped. These implications are grounded partly in the fact that the effectiveness literatures have focused on student outcomes shared to a significant degree by special educators (i.e., academic achievement). Further, the effectiveness research has developed concepts and procedures that, in most instances, may not be setting contingent. Indeed, some studies encompassed in the effective classroom research were conducted in special as well as regular education settings. This discussion of implications first focuses on the effective classroom processes literature. We then turn to implications that can be drawn from the effective school research. We close this section and the article with a few comments about future special education research and practice.

While there are still many unanswered questions, educators and researchers today know much more about how to productively organize schools and classroom instruction. As Berliner (1984) stated in the context of classroom processes research, the "glass is half full."

It is important to emphasize that this emergent knowledge base is not entirely new to special education educators and researchers. We have already noted that some of the original studies typically included in the effective classroom research have involved special education students either in special or mainstream settings (e.g., Leinhardt, Zigmond & Cooley, 1981). In addition, applied behavioral analysis research has produced a number of significant findings relevant to improving the academic performance of special education students (Strain & Kerr, 1981). Many of the articles in this issue are of a similar vein in identifying specific procedures that are important in influencing valued student outcomes.

The importance of the "new" formal knowledge (regardless of the specific research tradition) is that it provides details about how some of the powerful variables that affect achievement work. Perhaps as important, it provides a substantive, potentially generalizable, public knowledge base that can serve as a lever for and stimulant of educational reform. Intuitive knowledge alone would be hard pressed to provide such a lever. It must be remembered, for each educator or researcher who "knew" of an effective school or classroom, there were many who did not. And those who did not too often found the message that education has little impact in the presence of negative student and home background characteristics all too persuasive.

Traditional Concepts Must Be Challenged

What we have said thus far holds true for both regular and special education. The codified knowledge base being generated by research inside the classroom walls in many respects is germane to any instructional setting. What is especially important for the field of special education is the timing and focus of the classroom instructional research. We say this because the focus on specific treatments differs sharply from the way some researchers have investigated special education effectiveness over the years. Reviews and meta-analyses of what have come to be designated as special education "efficacy studies" have consistently reported little or no effects for students placed in special education settings (Carlberg & Kavale, 1980; Cegelka & Tyler, 1970; Glass, 1983; Kavale & Glass, 1982; Leinhardt & Pallay, 1982; Madden & Slavin, 1983; Semmel, Gottlieb, & Robinson, 1979; Strain & Kerr, 1981).

The efficacy reviews identify several problems with the special education research being reviewed. Some of these concerns parallel those we have noted in relation to the effective schools literature. A fundamental issue, one that directly pertains to this discussion, is that many of the efficacy studies reviewed have used settings as the primary treatment variable (Leinhardt & Pallay, 1982). In contrast, the effective classroom and applied behavioral analysis research focuses directly on variations in actual instructional processes experienced by students. With this more fine-grained focus, researchers have increasingly been able to identify powerful instructional procedures that can positively affect student outcomes.

Before we turn to a consideration of the effective schools research and its potential connection to and implications for special education, several caveats are in order. We have briefly reviewed some of the major concerns and issues earlier in this article. To the cautionary notes already mentioned, we add another, namely, that this literature generally does not consider special education classrooms in any visible way. This reflects the overall school level emphasis in this body of research. Classroom and within-classroom analyses are simply not the foci of these studies. Nevertheless, we feel that the central message that emanates from the effective schools research does relate to special education in important ways. What is that message? It is that instruction takes place in a larger social environment, the school, and that school level variables appear to have important roles to play in building a productive instructional climate.

Like the knowledge being generated by classroom level research, the general effective school research message is germane to both regular and special educators. What is particularly significant for special educators, however, is that this literature implicitly challenges the historical and functional "separateness" that often exists between mainstream and special education programs.

The separateness is expressed in many ways and at many levels in educational systems (e.g., administrative structures and procedures, resource generation and allocation mechanisms, personnel training and certification practices, curriculum, and communication patterns). There are powerful arguments for separateness (e.g., political power, professional expertise and status, and characteristics of the populations served (Leinhardt et al., 1982). However, in terms of the instructional process and how schools can be organized to be more effective, it seems clear that more closely integrated programming is likely to be far more productive than continuing the historical separateness. The same school environment that can affect regular classroom instruction will also have an impact on special classrooms in the same building.

The natural and artificial distinctions that exist between special and regular education at the classroom level have come under growing scrutiny in the context of mainstreaming large numbers of special needs students. The press for mainstreaming is forcing an examination of many of the current assumptions on both sides. The conversations that have begun offer an important vehicle for further exploring the utility of effective educational practices (regardless of setting) of the kinds discussed in the previous sections.

We have suggested that there is much in the effective classroom and applied behavioral analysis research that can be helpful to both special and regular educators. However, as far as we can tell, the school has not been considered in the mainstreaming context as a social/educational system in which special education instruction takes place. A recognition of the importance of the nested relationship of classroom instruction to the larger school environment is a fundamental message of the effective schools research. The connections are not yet certain, but the potential is there. Special classrooms and special education programs, for the students who are the focus of this discussion, are most often delivered in regular education school settings. The "inter-relatedness" of school variables to classroom instruction is just as relevant to special education classes, students, and programs as it is for regular education classes, students, and programs. The challenge then for both special and regular educators is to extend to the school, efforts already begun at the classroom level in the context of mainstreaming to diminish the separateness of regular and special education programming and to share in the increasing knowledge base about what constitutes effective instruction.

The basic implication, then, of the effective classroom and school literatures is that there is a growing knowledge base about how to effectively organize schools and instruction that is relevant to both special and regular educators and that there is a growing rationale for special and regular educational programming to become more integrated at the school level, at least in terms of the students who are the focus of this article. Special and regular educators have much to learn from each other.

New Ideas Must Be Tested

More fundamentally, in terms of special education as it is currently manifested in thousands of schools, classes, and programs, the effectiveness research may offer a potential basis for an important reconceptualization about how instructional services should be conceived and delivered. The reader will recall that one component of our review of the classroom processes literature dealt with instructional support. In this category we discussed results related to staff development programs and manipulations of class size. We further suggested that much that is supported by the effective schools research also logically fits in the category of support for instruction.

We submit that one way to think about special education would be as a powerful administrative tool that provides support for the instructional process. The emphasis in such a reconceptualization would be on garnering, at the school level, neutral resources such as time, personnel, data, and management expertise and, drawing upon a growing knowledge base about effective schooling instructional practices, match specific student skill deficits with powerful instructional environments and treatments.

How would such a reconceptualization of special education differ from present practice? A detailed discussion of possible differences is beyond the scope of this article. Several examples are offered as initial points for further discussion.

Special education as a tool of instructional leadership for "instructional support" would not be a treatment at all. Rather, special education would be a decision process (perhaps in the form of an instructional cabinet) led by the building's instructional leader responsible for matching a wide range of resources with a range of educational needs. One critical aspect here is that the process would be knowledge and data driven (knowledge about effective practices and data gathered on student performance and classroom procedures tried). The scope of intervention in the programmatically integrated setting that we envision would not be constrained to individual students, but also could encompass the instructional processes experienced by students.

The notion of assessing the quality of the instructional environment as part of identifying student needs is not as far-fetched as it might seem at first glance. Similar concepts are implicit in a report by the National Academy of Sciences (Heller, Holtzman, & Messick, 1982) when the authors stated that the "main purpose of assessment in education is to improve instruction and learning . . .

[and] a significant portion of children who experience difficulties in the classroom can be treated effectively through improved instruction (in the regular classroom)" (p. 72). This report also indicated that there is significant empirical evidence for a group of instructional practices that seem to benefit a variety of students classified as having academic difficulties. The practices the authors refer to are those emanating from the effective classroom processes research. The implication for these authors was that

> in planning instruction for the special child, primary attention should be directed to the specific features of the instructional treatments that have been identified as fostering academic progress in children with initial poor performance. (p. 88)

In our reconceptualization of special education, "instructional support activities" also might include the provision of intensive training to staff in schools that have significant numbers of students not reaching mastery in specific skills areas. The training would focus on instructional practices found to be effective in treating particular skill deficits. Again, this notion is not entirely new. Some of the concepts implicit in special education consultation models are quite similar (Idol-Maestas, 1984).

Setting, the way it is discussed in the macroefficacy studies, would be a relevant concept only to the extent that specific kinds of settings (e.g., a resource room) would have been found to be especially effective for the treatment of specific student needs. "Placement" as such would mean the linking of students to special services with the special relationship ending when specified goals are reached (Leinhardt et al., 1982; Meyen & Lehr, 1980). Labeling would focus on skills to be learned, whether it is the school management, the teacher, or the student that is the focus of assessment.

Again, the notion of setting and placement being contingent upon effective instructional practices, rather than categorical labeling of children, is not entirely new. These concepts are not too dissimilar from Lloyd (1984) when he argued that, given educators' present state of knowledge, it makes more sense to organize instruction on the basis of "skills students need to be taught" and relevant kinds of instruction to meet these needs, than on the basis of categorical labels (p. 13-14). Meyen and Lehr's (1980) discussion of the instructional implications of the concept of least restrictive environment has a similar tone when they argued for a particular treatment setting for short-term intensive instruction, while at the same time making significant modifications in the classroom where a special student would be mainstreamed.

These modifications would focus on training teachers in "techniques related to the intense instruction" (p. 7).

We realize this brief discussion leaves many unanswered questions of both a practical and philosophical nature. A reconceptualization of the type we have discussed must be cautious in not going beyond the current knowledge base about what are effective practices for specific learning outcomes. All of the qualifications about the effectiveness literatures we have noted pertain to their application with special needs students, teachers, and schools. Further, we recognize the important resource generation role played by the categorical labels that have structured special education services. Whether similar amounts of resources would be generated under a different conceptualization is open to serious question. These qualifications notwithstanding, we feel that the growing knowledge base about how to organize schools and classrooms for the benefit of student academic learning offers an important challenge and opportunity for regular and special educators interested in children with special needs. We submit that one use of this opportunity would be to change the notion of "special education" into "powerful, effective education." The "separateness" of regular and special education programs would be diminished in such circumstances. The delivery of effective instructional support to schools, teachers, and students would be the essential goal, and in the presence of a growing knowledge base, we have reason to be optimistic that such goals are achievable.

REFERENCES

Armor, D.J., Conry-Oseguera, P., Cox, M., King, N., McConnell, L., Pascal, A., Pauly, E., & Zellman, G. (1976). *Analysis of the school referred reading program in selected Los Angeles minority schools* (Report No. R-2007-LAUSD). Santa Monica: Rand Corporation.

Austin, G.R. (1979). Exemplary schools and the search for effectiveness. Educational Leadership, 37, 10-14.

Berliner, D.C. (1984). The half-full glass: A review of research on teaching. In P.L. Hosford (Ed.). *Using what we know about teaching* (pp. 51-77). Alexandria, VA: Association for Supervision and Curriculum Development.

Bloom, B.S. (1980). The new direction in educational research: Alterable variables. *Phi Delta Kappan, 61,* 382-385.

Brookover, W.B., & Lezotte, L.W. (1979). *Changes in school characteristics coincident with changes in student achievement*. East Lansing: Michigan State Univ., Institute for Research on Teaching.

Brookover, W.B., & Schneider, J.M. (1975). Academic environments and elementary school achievement. *Journal of Research and Development in Education, 9*(1), 82-91.

Brophy, J. (1983). Classroom organization and management. *Elementary School Journal, 83,* 265-286.

Carlberg, C., & Kavale, K. (1980). The efficacy of special versus regular class placement for exceptional children: A meta-analysis. *Journal of Special Education, 14,* 295-309.

Cegelka, W.J., & Tyler, J. (1970). The efficacy of special class placement for the mentally retarded in proper perspective. *Training School Bulletin, 66,* 33-66.

Cicirelli, V.G., Evans, J.W., & Shiller, J.S. (1970). The impact of Head Start: A reply to the report analysis. *Harvard Educational Review, 40,* 105-129.

Clark, D.L., Lotto, L.S., & McCarthy, M.M. (1980). Secondary source study of exceptionality in urban elementary schools. In *Why do some urban schools succeed?* (pp. 143-210). Bloomington, IN: Phi Delta Kappa.

Clark, T., & McCarthy, D.P. (1983). School improvement in New York City: The evolution of a project. *Educational Researcher, 12*(4), 17-23.

Coleman, J.S., Campbell, E.Q., Hobson, C.J., Mc-Partland, J.M., Mood, A.M., Weinfield, F.D., & York, R.L. (1966). *Equality of Educational opportunity.* Washington, DC: National Center for Education Statistics, Office of Education.

Cooley, W.W., & Leinhardt, G. (1980). The instructional dimensions study. *Educational Evaluation and Policy Analysis, 2*(1), 7-25.

Doss, D., & Holley, F. (1982). *A cause for national pause: Title I school wide projects* (ORE Publication No. 8155). Austin, TX: Austin Independent School District, Office of Research and Evaluation.

Edmonds, R. (1979). Programs of schools improvement: An overview. *Educational Leadership, 40*(3), 4-11.

Edmonds, R., & Frederiksen, J.R. (1978). *Search for effective schools: The identification and analysis of city schools that are instructionally effective for poor children.* Cambridge: Harvard University, Center for Urban Studies.

Frechtling, J. (1893, April). *Problems in evaluating school effectiveness: A shopping list of dilemmas.* Paper presented at the annual meeting of the American Educational Research Association, Montreal, Canada.

Gage, N.L. (1983). When does research on teaching yield implications for practice? *Elementary School Journal, 83,* 492-496.

Glaser, R. (1977). *Adoptive education: Individual diversity and learning.* New York: Holt, Rinehart, & Winston.

Glass, G.V. (1983). Effectiveness of special education. *Policy Studies Review, 2,* 65-78.

Glass, G.V., Cahan, L.S., Smith, M.L., & Filby, N.N. (1982). *School class size: Research and policy.* Beverly Hills, CA: Sage Publications.

Heller, K.A., Holtzman, W.H., & Messick, S. (1982). *Placing children in special education: A strategy for equity.* Washington, DC: National Academy Press.

Hunter, M. (1984). Knowing, teaching, and supervising. In P.L. Hosford (Ed.), *Using what we know about teaching* (pp. 169-192). Alexandria, VA: Association for Supervision and Curriculum Development.

Idol-Maestas, L. (1983). *Special educators consultation handbook.* Rockville, MD: Aspen Pbulications.

Kavale, K.A., & Glass, G.V. (1982). The efficacy of special education interventions and practices: A compendium of meta-analysis findings. *Focus on Exceptional Children, 15*(4), 1-14.

Leinhardt, G., Bickel, W.E., & Pallay, A. (1982). Unlabeled but still entitled: Toward more effective remediation. *Teachers College Record, 84*(2), 391-422.

Leinhardt, G., & Pallay, A. (1982). Restrictive educational settings: Exile or haven? *Review of Educational Research, 52,* 557-578.

Leinhardt, G., Zigmond, N., & Cooley, W.W. (1981). Reading instruction and its effects. *American Educational Research Journal, 18*(3), 343-362.

Lloyd, J.W. (1984). How shall we individualize instruction—or should we? *Remedial and Special Education, 5*(1), 7-15.

Mackenzie, D.E. (1983a). Research for school improvement: An appraisal of some recent trends. *Educational Researcher, 12*(4),5-17.

Mackenzie, D.E. (1983b). School effectiveness research: A synthesis and assessment. In P.C. Duttweiler (Ed.) *Educational productivity and school effectiveness.* Austin, TX: Southwest Educational Development Laboratory.

Madaus, G.F., Airasian, P.W., & Kellaghan, T. (1980). *A reassessment of the evidence: School effectiveness.* New York: McGraw-Hill Book Company.

Madden, N.A., & Slavin, R.E. (1983). Mainstreaming students wtih mild academic handicaps: Academic achievement and social outcomes. *Review of Educational Research, 53,* 519-569.

Meyen, E.L., & Lehr, D.H. (1980, March). Least restrictive environments: Instructional implications. *Focus on Exceptional Children, 12*(7), 1-8.

Odden, A., & Dougherty, U. (1982). *State programs of school improvement: A 50-state survey.* Denver, CO: Education Commission of the States.

Purkey, S.C., & Smith, M.S. (1983). Effective schools: *A review. Elementary School Journal, 83,* 427-452.

Reynolds, D. & Sullivan, M. (1981). The effects of

school: A radical faith restated. In Gillham, B. (Ed.), *Problem behavior in the secondary school.* London: Croom Helm.

Rosenshine, B.V. (1983). Teaching functions in instructional programs. *Elementary School Journal, 83,* 335-352.

Rowan, B., Bossert, S.T., & Dwyer, D.C. (1983). Research on effective schools: A cautionary note. *Educational Researcher, 12*(4), 24-31.

Rutter, M., Maughan, B., Morimore, P., Ouston, J., & Smith, A. (1979). *Fifteen thousand hours: Secondary schools and their effects on children.* Cambridge: Harvard University Press.

Semmel, M., Gottlieb, J., & Robinson, N. (1979). Mainstreaming: Perspectives on educating handicapped children in the public schools. In D. Berliner (Ed.), *Review of research in education* (Vol. 7). Washington, DC: American Educational Research Association.

Strain, P.S., & Kerr, M.M. (1981). *Mainstreaming of children in schools: Research and programmatic issues.* New York: Academic Press.

Trisman, D.A., Waller, M.I., & Wilder, G. (1976). *A descriptive and analytic study of compensatory reading programs: Final report, Vol. II.* Princeton, NJ: Educational Testing Service.

Venezky, R.L., & Winfield, L.F. (1979). *Schools that succeed beyond expectation in teaching* (Studies in Education Technical Report No. 1). Newark: University of Delaware.

Weber, G. (1971). *Inner-city children can be taught to read: Four successful schools.* Washington: Council for Basic Education.

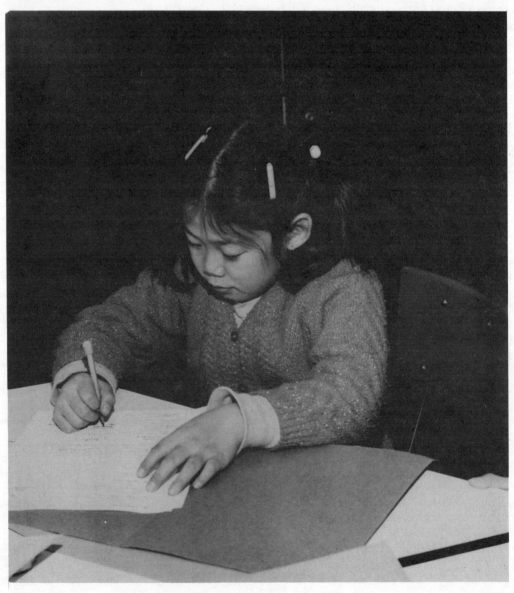

Paul A. Basso

Chapter 34

"SMRT-STEPS": Development of a Diagnostic-Prescriptive System in Reading to Improve Schools

Gary M. Kippel and Garlie A. Forehand*

Project Description

The primary objective of this project is to develop a system to provide school administrators and teachers with reading performance scores and information useful for improving the school instructional program. In order to accomplish this objective, we are developing a standardized measure of reading performance which can be readily administered and scored on a large scale and which accurately reflects multiple skills involved in reading. Subsequently, various school improvement plans will be reviewed to assess the potential linkage between school level diagnosis and prescription for enhancing school progress.

Consequently, when SMRT-STEPS (pronounced "smart steps") is completely validated it may be considered a school level diagnostic-prescriptive system. In effect, weaknesses requiring remediation will be identified. Subsequently, results from testing may "elicit" or assist in the selection of school improvement plans designed to improve the effectiveness of the instructional program in those grades for which they are available.

To expedite communication, the acronym "SMRT-STEPS" will be used to refer to the entire School Mastery of Reading Test System to Enhance Progress of Schools. The acronym "SMRT" will be used to refer primarily to the assessment component, School Mastery of Reading Test.

This project is being implemented by a consortium comprised of the New York City Board of Education and the Educational Testing Service of Princeton, New Jersey. In addition to providing a technically sound and useful system, financial savings will be realized because public schools will not have to pay royalties to a test publisher for the diagnostic part of the system.

A professional panel of New York City school administrators, teachers, reading experts and curriculum specialists has reviewed SMRT for appropriateness, usefulness and potential bias. In addition, professional panel members have provided judgments related to performance criteria. This panel will continue to be involved in the project in order to review and establish the relationship between assessment and school improvement materials, plans and programs.

The School Mastery of Reading Test

To enhance its relevance and usefulness for improving instruction, SMRT is being developed as an objective test of mastery of reading, rather than as a norm-referenced test. As such, SMRT is being designed to indicate the extent to which specific reading skills have been mastered, rather than to differentiate or discriminate between children. Consequently, resulting subtest scores will reflect mastery or competence and will provide a relatively sensitive measure of instruction. This is in contrast to norm-referenced scores such as grade equivalents, normal curve equivalents (NCE's) and percentiles which can be misleading and are susceptible to misinterpretation.

The currently available grade four research version of SMRT is divided into two 50 item parts administered with a brief intermission. SMRT is being developed as a "power" test with approximate time guidelines rather than as a "speed" test with specific time limits which must be strictly enforced. In most instances, approximately 34 minutes are required for administration of each of the two parts for a total testing time of approximately 68 minutes.

*Dr. Gary M. Kippel is Project Director and Assistant Director of Educational Research, Office of Educational Assessment: Board of Education of New York City. Dr. Garlie A. Forehand is Director of Research, Program Planning and Development, Educational Testing Service of Princeton, NJ.

The current 100 item research version of SMRT consists of four separately reported subtests including: Word Attack (18 items), Word Meaning (21 items), Literal Comprehension (31 items) and Reasoning Comprehension (27 items). Test items were categorized into subtests based upon the professional opinions of several curriculum, reading, research and teaching specialists. When scored, SMRT provides four subtest scores and one total test score. Three additional Word Recognition items appear at the beginning of the test to orient students to test directions, format and the separate answer sheet. In addition, they begin students on a positive note in that they are relatively easy items.

The SMRT booklet is not comprised of clearly defined subtests. Rather, items from the various subtests appear in both parts one and two. Furthermore, the actual tasks required of students change frequently. Directions for the most part are read to students.

The currently available research version of SMRT is designed to identify reading subtest areas in which either small instructional groups, intact classes or the entire grade four in particular schools are not achieving mastery. The short-term objective is to develop an instructionally useful grade four reading test. Subsequently, the development of a grade three School Mastery of Reading Test will be considered.

It is likely that SMRT will be most useful if it is administered at the beginning of the school year. When administered at that time, it can provide diagnostic information to assess needs and to help guide planning and instruction. To some extent, in addition, SMRT administered at the beginning of the school year may be predictive of test scores from the annual citywide reading testing program conducted near the end of the school year. This can be accomplished by developing appropriate regression equations (see for explanation, Pedhazur, 1982). It is noted, also, that a computerized SMRT item bank will be established. Furthermore, innovative uses of computer technology for test delivery, scoring and interpretation will be explored.

Field Test Administration

The current version of SMRT was administered to 889 fourth grade students in three elementary schools in each of three Community School Districts. Each participating school had been identified by the New York State Education Department's Comprehensive Assessment Report as "in need of improvement" based upon their previous year's grade three Degrees of Reading Power (DRP) test results.

Schools were requested to provide answer sheets for every student who was eligible for the annual citywide reading test, with the exception of those special education students for whom some testing variance (e.g., large print, extended time limits) was required and Limited English Proficient (LEP) students who were exempted from the annual citywide reading test. In order to minimize disruption of instruction, provision was not made for "make-up" testing of absentees. It is anticipated that, in the future, relevance of SMRT for special education and LEP students will be demonstrated.

To ensure test security, each test administration manual and test booklet was stamped with a unique identification number. Careful records were maintained of the identification numbers on both administration manuals and test booklets delivered to, and retrieved from, every school.

All test materials were delivered in strong cartons carefully sealed with white tape with the following message in red letters: "SECURE TEST MATERIALS—DO NOT OPEN." Cartons were delivered directly to the Principal's office and receipts were obtained. The sealed cartons were then locked in secure storage closets, usually in the Principal's office.

On the day of testing, program staff visited each school. These staff members retrieved the sealed cartons from locked closets and distributed test materials to participating classes. A careful accounting was maintained of the quantity and identification numbers of both administration manuals and test booklets delivered to, and subsequently retrieved from, each class.

Project staff monitored the test administration in each school. All tests were administered by fourth grade teachers using the test administration manuals prepared for that purpose. Appropriate "Testing—Do Not Disturb" signs were placed on the door of each class. Students read the test questions from their test booklet, then responded on the separate answer sheet provided for that purpose. After testing, teachers were asked to complete a one-page survey designed to assess their opinions of the test and testing procedures.

Students provided their answers on machine scannable general purpose National Computer Systems (NCS) answer sheets which were scanned on an NCS 7018 Optical Mark Reader with NCS Scanpak "Test Scoring Package" software. Scanned answers were stored on magnetic tape as a data file. Subsequently, answers were read and scored using an SPSS-X (1986) program which generated subtest and total test score results for individual students and aggregates. To ensure accuracy of results at all stages of scanning, scoring and statistical analyses, several manual and computerized quality control procedures were instituted.

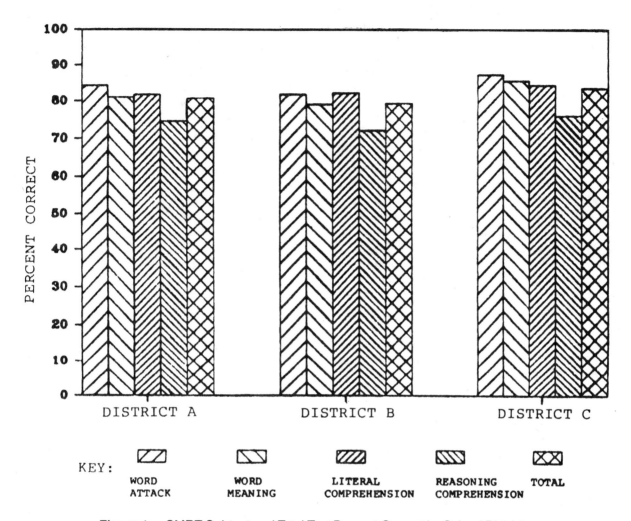

Figure 1. SMRT Subtest and Total Test Percent Correct by School District

Results from the Field Test

Percent of correct responses for four subtests and the total test is depicted or all three participating school districts in Figure 1. In addition to the district results, it is noted that reports which included additional individual student listings and summary statistics were generated by class and grade.

The overall mean total test score was 80.54 with a standard deviation of 13.49. The overall median total test score was 84 with an inter-quartile range of 16. In effect, these statistics reflect a negatively skewed distribution. In other words, this is a relatively easy test with a ''piling up of scores'' at the high end or the score distribution. Relatively high scores were expected for a curriculum-based test, such as SMRT, administered at the end of the school

year. It is likely that the relatively high scores reflect mastery of fourth grade curriculum taught during the school year. Furthermore, the relatively high Word Attack subtest performance may reflect the fact that strong emphasis is placed on Word Attack instruction in the early grades.

Figure 1 depicts relatively similar subtest profiles for all three participating school districts. In each school district, percent correct for the word attack subtest was either the highest (districts A and C) or one of the two equally high subtests (district B). For the entire sample, greatest mastery was demonstrated on the Word Attack subtest. In all three school districts, the lowest percent correct was obtained for the reasoning comprehension subtest. For the entire sample, least mastery was demonstrated on the Reasoning Comprehension subtest. For all three school districts, in addition, the percent correct for the total test reflecting overall mastery of reading (i.e., the last column of each school district profile in Figure 1) was very similar.

A norms table has been developed to provide norm-referenced interpretations of each subtest or total test raw score. Such norms provide relative rather than absolute performance. This norms table reflects overall group performance in that it was based upon all 889 student scores from the May 1986 field test and was promulgated to illustrate the manner in which "local" New York City norms might be developed and used. Any SMRT subtest or total test raw score can be converted into either a percentile or stanine by using this "raw score to percentile rank and stanine norms" table. It is anticipated that both Fall and Spring empirical norms would be instructionally useful.

Percentiles allow us to compare any student's performance at a given time with that of the overall group on a scale ranging from 1 to 99. On this scale, the fiftieth percentile, or median, might be considered "average." Stanine scores (i.e., a contraction of "standard nine") are normally distributed standard scores which range from one to nine. They have the convenience of being a single digit and are relatively easy to interpret. The stanine scale has a mean of five and a standard deviation of 1.96.

It is important to note that percentile scores are most appropriate for norm-referenced interpretations of test results. The primary intention is to develop SMRT as a test which reflects mastery or competence rather than as a norm-referenced test. Primary effort, therefore, is being placed on developing mastery scores. Percentiles may be used, subsequently, in a secondary or ancillary capacity to mastery scores.

Developing Mastery Scores and Establishing Performance Standards

Mastery scores reflect performance criteria or standards. Failure to achieve these "benchmarks" is usually interpreted as need for improvement and more or different instruction.

In order to establish SMRT mastery criteria, both empirical data and judgments of experts are being reviewed. Empirical data which have been obtained for this purpose include:

1. SMRT scores of fourth graders in the nine schools tested during the second and third weeks in May 1986,
2. For these same students, Degrees of Reading Power (DRP) test scores from a May 7, 1986 test administration, and

3. For these same students, also, Metropolitan Achievement Test (MAT) reading test scores from an April 21 and 22, 1986 MAT administration.

Actual performance on every SMRT item has been obtained for relatively low, moderate and high achieving groups of students as defined by their DRP and MAT test scores. This empirical data will be used along with the expert judgments provided by the Professional Panel. Panel members were asked to estimate the difficulty level of each item for each of the three hypothetical groups of students described below:

Group I: *Satisfactory readers.* Students in this group:
    a) read well enough to learn from fourth grade text material in reading and other subject areas,
    b) read well enough to follow instructions in workbooks, arithmetic problems, and other school work, and
    c) can be expected to continue to learn in the fifth grade.

Group II: *Minimally competent readers.* Students in this group:
    a) have developed sufficient reading skills that they can continue to learn to read, perhaps with special help,
    b) can be expected to have some difficulty with fourth grade text material, but can learn at a minimal level from such material, and
    c) can be expected to need continuing special help with basic reading skills in the fifth grade.

Group III: *Readers below minimum competence.* Students in this group:
    a) have not achieved some or all of the basic reading skills appropriate to fourth grade,
    b) cannot learn by reading fourth grade text material in reading and other subject areas, and
    c) cannot read sufficiently well to follow directions in workbooks and arithmetic problems.

Once reasonable performance expectations of items are established, standards for test objectives, item clusters, subtests, and/or the total test can be set by aggregating items. Both empirical and judgmental information will be reviewed carefully and alternative strategies for setting performance standards (see, for discussion: Livingston & Zieky, 1982) will be considered.

Validity and Reliability of the School Mastery of Reading Test

In order to demonstrate the validity of any test, we must provide evidence that the test measures that which we want it to measure (Kerlinger, 1973, p.457; Thorndike & Hagen, 1977, pp. 56-57). Evidence for the validity of SMRT comes from various sources. First, the strong relationship between SMRT and New York City reading and language arts curriculum was demonstrated both by project staff and by curriculum, language arts and reading specialists of the Division of Curriculum and Instruction of the New York City Board of Education. Second, teacher opinions of SMRT were elicited after they administered this test to their students. Among other favorable comments, the majority of teachers indicated that the reading difficulty level of test items was appropriate, the majority of items correspond favorably to fourth grade curriculum and the items are free of technical flaws and bias. Third, the Professional Panel of New York City teachers and supervisors provided ratings reflecting their opinions that SMRT would be of "above average usefulness," in general, and that it would be most useful for identifying remedial cases and for planning instruction for both individuals and groups.

Fourth, the relationship between SMRT and other measures of reading is being assessed. For example, the initial version of the group administered SMRT was validated using the individually administered Interactive Reading Assessment System (IRAS) developed by Robert and Kathryn Calfee. The IRAS instrument was based on a review of research and practice in the teaching of reading. It assesses a set of component skills which have generally been accepted as necessary for proficient reading. A very strong relationship was found between the initial version of SMRT and the IRAS.

The relationship between the School Mastery of Reading Test (SMRT) and both the Degrees of Reading Power (DRP) test and the Metropolitan Achievement Test (MAT) was examined. Total test scores were available on all three tests for 744 students. Correlation coefficients were calculated. The correlation between SMRT and the DRP was .791 and the correlation between SMRT and the MAT was .819. In summary, information from the abovementioned sources provides evidence that SMRT is a valid measure of reading competence.

Indices of reliability provide an indication of the extent to which a particular measurement is consistent and reproducible (Thorndike & Hagen, 1977, p.56). Reliability implies dependability, stability, consistency, predictability and accuracy (Kerlinger, 1973, p.442).

Coefficient alpha is the basic formula for determining the reliability based on internal consistency (Nunnally, 1978, p. 230). Coefficient alpha is the expected correlation of one test with an alternative form of the test, of the same length, when the two tests purport to measure the same thing (Nunnally, 1978, p.215). In order to obtain reliability estimates for SMRT, coefficient alpha was calculated and found to be .928 for the total test, and .861 and .881 for parts one and two of SMRT, respectively. These data provide support for the contention that SMRT can be used reliably.

National Assessment of Educational Progress and the School Mastery of Reading Test

National Assessment of Educational Progress (NAEP) is a program which has been developed to measure how effectively 9-, 13- and in-school 17-year-old American students can read (Messick, Beaton, & Lord, 1983). NAEP bases each assessment on a wide range of materials and asks questions requiring use of a variety of reading skills and strategies. Reading selections range from simple sentences expressing a single concept to complex articles about specialized topics in science or social studies. A scale raging from 0 through 500 has been developed. Various points on the scale have been provided criterion-referenced interpretations. Items have been calibrated using the three-parameter latent trait model (see, for discussion: Messick, Beaton, & Lord, 1983, pp. 43-55).

Incorporated within SMRT are 16 items obtained from the National Assessment of Educational Progress (NAEP). Selection of particular items was based upon item scale value, content, and format. The primary intent is to determine the feasibility of:

1. obtaining norm-referenced interpretations of SMRT results with respect to NAEP national norms,
2. demonstrating the extent to which SMRT results relate to NAEP absolute performance, and
3. establishing a cost-effective source of items by incorporating NAEP items within SMRT.

The intent is to use the NAEP items to determine the SMRT item parameters. First, it must be demonstrated that the test data fits the Latent Trait Model (see, for discussion: Hulin, Drasgow, and Parsons, 1983). Subsequently, SMRT item calibrations will be calculated. In effect, the overall goal is to establish a common SMRT-NAEP scale with a Latent Trait calibrated item pool. Consequently, new forms and levels of SMRT can be designed which will be based upon New York City curriculum and will, in some grades, yield NAEP norm-referenced information.

System to Enhance the Progress of Schools

A New York City curriculum-based test, such as SMRT, is needed to improve local school planning, decision-making and instruction. It is anticipated that SMRT will be particularly useful to Principals and others (including advisory and consultative bodies) charged with the responsibility of developing or selecting, and successfully implementing instructional programs to improve reading skills which have not been adequately mastered. Subsequently, different profiles or patterns of SMRT subtest scores may then be related to prescriptive choices of corrective actions (e.g., instructional materials, programs and strategies) which are most likely to improve school achievement in those skill areas of greatest need (see, for discussion: Becoming a nation of readers . . . 1984; United States Department of Education, 1986).

Reports of SMRT results will be designed in such a manner as to enhance the likelihood that they will be perceived and interpreted in a constructive and non-pejorative manner. The intent is to elicit non-punitive corrective action on the local school level. It should be noted that SMRT is not proposed for ranking schools or for invidious comparisons between schools. The clear intent is to enhance educational effectiveness and to encourage positive change in a non-threatening manner.

In summary and conclusion, SMRT-STEPS is designed to assist the school improvement process by providing cost-effective and instructionally useful school level diagnostic information based upon local school system curriculum and related to prescriptions for school improvement.

REFERENCES

Becoming a nation of readers: The report of the Commission on Reading (1984). Washington, D.C.: The National Institute of Education.

Hulin, C.L., Drasgow, F., & Parsons, C.K. (1983). *Item response theory: Application to psychological measurement*. Homewood, Illinois: Dow Jones-Irwin.

Kerliner, F.N. (1973). *Foundations of behavioral research* (2nd ed.). New York: Holt, Rinehart & Winston.

Livingston, S.A., & Zieky, M.J. (1982). *Passing scores: A manual for setting standards of performance on educational and occupational tests*. Princeton, New Jersey: Educational Testing Service.

Messick, S., Beaton, A., & Lord, F. (1983). *National Assessment of Educational Progress Reconsidered: A new design for a new era* (NAEP Report 83-1). Princeton, New Jersey: National Assessment of Educational Progress at Educational Testing Service.

Nunnally, J.C. (1978). *Psychometric theory* (2nd ed.). New York: McGraw-Hill.

Pedhazur, E.J. (1982). *Multiple regression in behavioral research: Explanation and prediction*. New York: Holt, Rinehart & Winston.

SPSS-X: User's Guide (2nd ed.). (1986). Chicago, Illinois: SPSS, Inc.

Thorndike, R.L., & Hagen, E.P. (1977). *Measurement and evaluation in psychology and education* (4th ed.). New York: John Wiley & Sons.

United States Department of Education (1986). *What works: Research about teaching and learning*. Washington, D.C.: Author.

Chapter 35
What We Know About Learning to Read
The Report of the Commission on Reading*

Which approach to phonics works better—explicit phonics or implicit phonics? Is it possible to write interesting and natural-sounding selections for young readers while at the same time constraining the vocabulary on the basis of letter-sound relationships? What are the pluses and minuses of "round robin reading"? Is ability grouping an effective strategy to use with the slow child? How well do tests assess reading ability?

Under the auspices of the National Academy of Education's Commission on Reading, the country's leading experts on reading and language development have addressed these and related topics. The result: Becoming a Nation of Readers, *a 147-page booklet that, in clear, readable style, synthesizes a diverse and rich body of scientific information into a systematic account of what we know about learning to read. The report was funded by the National Institute of Education, and the research team was chaired by Richard C. Anderson of the Center for the Study of Reading at the University of Illinois. We are pleased to be able to present excerpts from this ambitious and comprehensive study.*

—Editor

How Are We Doing?

How well do American children and youth read? How well do American schools teach reading? These are difficult questions to answer objectively. Partial answers can be gleaned from historical trends in achievement test data. Studies dating back to the middle of the 19th century usually have shown that succeeding generations of students perform better than earlier generations. In one study, for example, 31,000 students in grades 2-6 representative of the United States at large were given a reading test in 1957 and the scores were compared to those of

107,000 students who had taken the same test in 1937. After adjusting for the fact that the 1937 sample was older by 4 to 6 months, because fewer children were promoted to the next grade at that time, the investigator concluded that children in 1957 had a reading ability advanced a half year over children of the same age and intelligence 20 years before.

Recent trends in test scores are mixed. With respect to basic reading skill, as gauged by ability to comprehend everyday reading material, results from the National Assessment of Educational Progress confirm that slight gains continued to be made during the 1970s. The largest gains were made by black children living in large cities. Probably these gains are attributable to the increasing aspirations and confidence of blacks and improvements in the quality of instruction that black children receive.

On the other hand, scores on tests that gauge advanced reading skill, among other abilities, showed small but steady declines from the early 1960s until the late '70s, at which point they leveled off and started to climb slightly. Declines were sharpest on the SAT and ACT, which are taken by high school seniors hoping to enter selective colleges and universities, but there were also declines on advanced tests given to all kinds of students in junior and senior high school. Reasons offered to explain the test score decline include erosion of educational standards, increases in TV viewing, changes in the size of families and spacing of children, shifts in young people's motivations and life goals, and the fact that larger numbers of youth from less advantaged families have been staying in school and taking the tests.

Another approach to evaluating the level of reading proficiency attained in this country is to compare our achievement with achievement in other countries. A survey of reading performance in 15 countries completed just over a decade ago showed that American students

*Reprinted with permission from the Winter 1985 issue of the *American Educator,* the quarterly journal of the American Federation of Teachers.

were never in first or second place on any test, and that on most tests they ranked at or below the international average. A more recent comparison between the United States, Taiwan, and Japan showed a much wider spread of achievement among children in this country; many American children did well, but disproportionate numbers were among the poorest readers in the three countries. International comparisons are tricky, depending, for instance, on the numbers of children in each age group that remain in school in different countries and the assumption that test items translated into different languages are really equivalent. Still, the figures offer no grounds for complacency.

How Americans have compared in the past is less urgent than the question of whether current generations will be literate enough to meet the demands of the future. The world is moving into a technological-information age in which full participation in education, science, business, industry, and the professions requires increasing levels of literacy. What was a satisfactory level of literacy in 1950 probably will be marginal by the year 2000.

There is reason to be optimistic about the potential for the improvement of literacy in this country. From research supported by the National Institute of Education, and to some extent other government agencies and private foundations, the last decade has witnessed unprecedented advances in knowledge about the basic processes involved in reading, teaching, and learning. The knowledge is now available to make worthwhile improvements in reading throughout the United States. If the practices seen in the classrooms of the best teachers in the best schools could be introduced everywhere, the improvements would be dramatic.

Word Recognition and Beginning Reading

One of the cornerstones of skilled reading is fast, accurate word identification. Well into the 20th century almost all children in this country were started on the road to skilled word identification by teaching them the letters of the alphabet, the sounds the letters make, and, using this knowledge, how to sound out words. During the first third of this century, educators such as William S. Gray were responsible for turning Americans schools away from what they perceived to be the "heartless drudgery" of the traditional approach. In its place, Gray and others advocated the look-and-say approach. The thinking was that children would make more rapid progress in reading if they identified whole words at a glance, as adults seem to do.

The look-say approach gradually came to dominate the teaching of beginning reading. Nonetheless, educators continued to debate the best way to introduce chil-

dren to reading. Rudolph Flesch brought the debate forcibly to the public's attention in the mid-1950s with his book, *Why Johnny Can't Read,* in which he mounted a scathing attack against the look-say method and advocated a return to phonics. More influential in professional circles, though, was Jeanne Chall's now-classic book a decade later, *Learning to Read: The Great Debate.* Chall concluded on the basis of evidence available at the time that programs that included phonics as one component were superior to those that did not.

The question, then, is how should children be taught to read words? The answer given by most reading educators today is that phonics instruction is one of the essential ingredients. All the major published reading programs include material for teaching phonics to beginning readers. Thus, the issue is no longer, as it was several decades ago, whether children should be taught phonics. The issues now are specific ones of just how it should be done.

Classroom research shows that, on the average, children who are taught phonics get off to a better start in learning to read than children who are not taught phonics. The advantage is most apparent on tests of word identification, though children in programs in which phonics gets a heavy stress also do better on tests of sentence and story comprehension, particularly in the early grades.

Data on the long-term effects of phonics instruction are scanty. In one of the few longitudinal studies, children who had received intensive phonics instruction in kindergarten or first grade performed better in the third grade than a comparison group of children on both a word identification test and a comprehension test. By the sixth grade, the group that years earlier had received intensive phonics instruction still did better than the comparison group on a word identification test but the advantage in comprehension had vanished. The fact that an early phonics emphasis had less influence on comprehension as the years passed is probably attributable to the increasing importance of knowledge of the topic, vocabulary, and reasoning ability on advanced comprehension tests.

The picture that emerges from the research is that phonics facilitates word identification and that fast, accurate word identification is a necessary but not sufficient condition for comprehension. More will be said later about the need for comprehension instruction in tandem with phonics instruction.

The purpose of phonics is to teach children the alphabetic principle. The goal is for this to become an *operating principle* so that young readers consistently use information about the relationship between letters and sounds and letters and meanings to assist in the identification of known words and to independently figure out unfamiliar words. Research evidence tends to favor explicit phonics (over the implicit approach). However, the "ideal" phonics program would probably incorporate features from implicit phonics as well. The Commission believes that the approaches to phonics recommended in programs available today fall considerably short of the ideal, and we call for renewed efforts to improve the quality of instructional design, materials, and teaching strategies.

The right maxims for phonics are: Do it early. Keep it simple. Except in cases of diagnosed individual need, phonics instruction should have been completed by the end of the second grade.

Comprehension and Beginning Reading

The heart of reading instruction in American classrooms is the small group reading lesson in which the teacher works with some children while the rest complete assignments at their seats. This is the usual arrangement in first, second, and third grade, and sometimes beyond. The small group lesson provides the opportunity for instruction and practice on all aspects of reading. For the beginning reader, it is a major opportunity to acquire insights into comprehension and to link word identification and comprehension.

The typical teacher's major resource on how to conduct this lesson is the manual that is part of the commercial reading program the school district has purchased. The teacher's manual contains detailed suggestions for conducting every lesson, often in as much detail as the script for a play. Presented in bold type within the manual is the exact wording of statements that the teacher can make to students. For example, to begin a lesson the manual may suggest that the teacher say, "Today we're going to read a story about polar bears. Have any of you ever seen a polar bear in a zoo?" Further directions will then be given in plain type such as "Give children several moments to discuss polar bears. After that, read the introductory statement about the story."

Some school districts afford teachers the option of using any of a variety of materials and approaches to teach reading. More typical, though, is the district that requires the use of the basal reading program that it has purchased. Even these districts usually give teachers flexibility in whether or not they follow the teacher's manual word for word. Classroom observation and interviews with teachers suggest that, whether by choice or not, most teachers do rely on manuals. The teachers' manuals that accompany the best-selling commercial reading programs suggest lessons with three basic parts: preparation, reading, and discussion.

Preparation. In the preparation phase, the teacher is supposed to introduce the new words that will be encoun-

tered in the day's basal reader selection and make sure the children possess the background knowledge required to understand the story. The preparation phase is one place where an aspect of comprehension may be explicitly taught or, in the primary grades, where phonics may be taught. The preparation phase may conclude with the teacher's stating a purpose or asking a question to guide reading.

Systematic classroom observation reveals that preparation for reading is the phase of the small group lesson that is most often slighted, or even skipped altogether. Thus, as a rule, little focused attention is given to developing the background knowledge that will be required to understand the day's story. This is a topic on which teachers' manuals do include specific recommendations. When asked why they neither follow the recommendations in the manuals nor substitute instruction of their own design, teachers say they don't have the time.

Several studies indicate that using instructional time to build background knowledge pays dividends in reading comprehension. It must be warned, though, that there has been a rush of enthusiasm for this practice in professional circles. Teachers are receiving all manner of suggestions waving the banner of background knowledge, some of which may, indeed, be a waste of time. Teachers are being urged to engage children in activities and discussion that may range over too wide an array of topics.

Useful approaches to building background knowledge prior to a reading lesson focus on the concepts that will be central to understanding the upcoming story, concepts that children either do not possess or may not think of without prompting. The advice in teachers' manuals is often unfocused, as in the polar bear example at the beginning of this section. Unstructured preparation may wander away from the concepts of central importance.

The effect of preparation for reading on children's recall of a story was examined in a study which compared unfocused preparation with preparation that highlighted the central ideas of the story. The plot of the story involved a woman who wishes on a star, a raccoon who comes nightly to her doorstep to look for food, and some bandits. The raccoon's masked appearance frightens the bandits into dropping a bag of money, which the racoon picks up and eventually drops at the woman's doorstep on his nightly search for food. Finding the money, the woman attributes it to her wish on a star.

The suggested steps for preparation in the teacher's manual led to a discussion of raccoons as clever, playful animals. Yet to understand the story, children must grasp the ideas of coincidence and habit, since the raccoons' habitual behavior allows the coincidences to occur. Children who received preparation that concentrated on these ideas did much better in remembering the central ideas of the story than children prepared according to the suggestions in the teacher's manual.

Much of the research showing that it is essential for children to learn to construct meaning based on background knowledge, as well as information in the text, has been conducted recently. This probably explains the low priority this aspect of reading receives in most classrooms today. Teachers, principals, and reading supervisors are just now getting the opportunity to learn about the research and adjust their priorities.

Reading.   The second phase of a typical lesson is reading the day's selection. A basic issue is the proper role for silent and oral reading considering the children's age and ability. Frequent opportunities to read aloud make sense for the beginning reader. In the first place, oral reading makes a tie with the experience children have had of reading in their homes, nursery schools, and kindergartens as adults have read to them. Further, oral reading makes observable aspects of an otherwise unobservable process, providing teachers with a means for checking progress, diagnosing problems and focusing instruction. Not to be underestimated is the function oral reading serves in providing young children a way to share their emerging ability with their parents and others.

Nor should oral reading be discarded altogether once children are fairly skilled readers. Opportunities to read aloud and listen to others read aloud are features of the literate environment, whatever the reader's level. There is no substitute for a teacher who reads children good stories. It whets the appetite of children for reading, and provides a model of skillful oral reading. It is a practice that should continue throughout the grades. Choral reading of poetry and reading plays also contribute to oral reading skill and help keep oral traditions alive. However, as the reader moves beyond the initial stages of literacy, more time will be devoted to silent reading, since that is the form that skilled reading most often takes.

Current observations of American classrooms indicate that teachers do differentiate the amount of oral and silent reading according to the reader's level. A study of 600 reading-group sessions found that low-ability readers at the first-grade level read orally during about 90% of the time allocated to the lesson, while high-ability first-graders read aloud about 40% of the time. By Grade 5, low-ability groups spent somewhat over 50% of lesson time reading aloud whereas high-ability groups averaged less than 20%.

The way oral reading is handled in the typical classroom may not be optimum. Authorities recommend that children read a selection silently before they read it aloud. Research suggests that this practice improves oral reading fluency. However, classroom observations reveal that silent reading before oral reading is frequently omit-

ted, which is like being asked to perform a play without having read the script beforehand. Consequently, unless the children are already rather good readers, the reading is unnecessarily slow and halting, and the experience may be needlessly stressful for some children.

The value of oral reading depends in part on the way the teacher deals with mistakes. If a child makes a large number of mistakes, this usually means that the selection is too difficult and that the child ought to be moved to an easier one. Otherwise, a sensible rule of thumb is to ignore most mistakes unless the mistake disrupts the meaning of the text. Even professional oral readers, such as radio and TV announcers, frequently deviate from the text in small ways. When a teacher is compulsive about always correcting small mistakes, the child's train of thought will be interrupted.

Some teachers pay too much attention to correcting what they judge to be imperfections in the pronunciation of children, and thereby may interfere with comprehension. Overemphasis on standard pronunciation can be a serious problem when the child is not a native speaker of English or the child speaks a different dialect of English than the teacher. For instance, in one study a lesson was observed in which the children were reading a selection that contained the word *garbage*. Their white teacher interrupted a black child several times trying to get him to say /garrbage/ instead of /gahbage/.

When a child makes an oral reading mistake that changes the meaning, the best technique is to first wait and see whether the child can come up with the right word without help. If not, the teacher should direct the child's attention to clues about the word's pronunciation or meaning, depending upon the nature of the error. When the word has been correctly identified, the child should be encourage to reread the sentence. This helps to assure that the child assimilates the correction and can recover the meaning of the whole sentence. Research suggests that teachers who deal with oral reading errors in the manner that has just been outlined produce larger-than-average gains in reading achievement. Teachers who routinely supply the correct word, or permit other children in the group to call out the correct word, get children in the habit of waiting passively for help.

When children read orally, it is most often in a format called "round robin reading." Each child in a reading group takes a turn reading aloud several lines or a page of the story. An issue in round robin reading is equal distribution of turns for reading among the children. When a teacher always calls on volunteers, it has been shown that assertive children get more than their share of turns. This is undesirable because there is evidence that the child reading aloud and directly receiving instruction from the teacher is getting more from the lesson than the children who are following along. A simple method for equalizing opportunity is to move around the group giving each child a turn in order. This method has produced good results in several studies.

A problem with round robin reading is that the quality of practice is often poor. This problem is acute in the low-ability group where children hear only other poor readers stumbling over words. This problem can be lessened by having the children read the selection silently before-hand.

Even under the best of circumstances, round robin reading is not ideal for developing fluency and compre-hension. An alternative technique that has proved suc-cessful in small-scale tryouts is to have children repeat-edly read the same selections until an acceptable standard of fluency is attained. This can be done in several ways. Small groups can read along with an adult or they can follow a tape-recorded version; they can practice silently and then read aloud to the teacher; pairs of children can take turns reading aloud to one another. Poor readers who engage in repeated reading show marked improve-ment in speed, accuracy, and expression during oral read-ing of new selections and, more important, improvement in comprehension during silent reading. Repeated read-ing deserves consideration as an alternative to the con-ventional practice of having children read aloud new ma-terial every day. No one would expect a novice pianist to sight read a new selection every day, but that is exactly what is expected of the beginning reader.

In addition to oral reading, children of every age and ability ought to be doing more extended silent reading. The amount of time children spend reading silently in school is associated with year-to-year gains in reading achievement. Even young readers benefit from opportu-nities for silent reading. For instance, increased silent reading for beginners is one of the features of a very successful program for low-income Hawaiian children who are otherwise at risk for educational failure.

To summarize, classroom time spent on either oral or silent reading is time well spent. Even beginning readers should do more silent reading. They should usually read silently before they are asked to read aloud. Getting the most from the customary practice of round robin oral reading requires the teacher to distribute turns equally among the children, skillfully handle mistakes, and focus attention on meaning. But alternatives to round robin reading of new material, such as repeated reading, ap-pear to hold more promise for promoting reading fluency and comprehension.

Discussion. Following the reading of a selection, the final phase of a typical reading lesson is discussion. In the primary grades, there are brief discussions after each section of the selection and a longer discussion when the whole story has been completed. In the intermediate grades, the interspersed discussion periods are not usu-ally present. The discussion phase is a place where the teacher may provide direct instruction in some aspect of reading comprehension, using the day's selection for il-lustration. In the primary grades, this is the point where phonics instruction is usually provided. The last thing the teacher does is explain the seatwork assignment and make sure the children understand what they are sup-posed to do before they return to their seats.

A clear finding from research of the past decade is that young readers, and poor readers of every age, do not consistently see relationships between what they are read-ing and what they already know. Research also estab-lishes that questions asked during the discussion phase of a lesson are a useful tool for helping children see relation-ships. Questions that lead children to integrate informa-tion about the central points of a selection with their prior knowledge significantly enhance reading compre-hension.

Classroom research indicates that teachers make heavy use of manuals when leading discussions. Manuals include a large number of questions for each story, and most of them are asked during a typical lesson. While research verifies that asking well-crafted questions can be an important means of promoting comprehension, anal-ysis of the questions in manuals reveals many that are poorly crafted—too general, leading the children's thinking afield; or trivial, focusing their thinking on un-important details.

Questions are a means of conveying to students the points they should be attempting to understand as they read future selections as well as a means for checking to see that they have understood the selection they have just read. Thus, questions following a story should probe the major elements of the plot. If the story has a moral, discussion should bring out this deeper meaning.

No piece of advice about questioning has been re-peated more often than the proscription, "Don't ask to many detail questions." For instance, if a story were to say that Sally was wearing a red dress, teachers may be warned against asking about the color of her dress. This advice is incomplete, however. The question is perfectly sensible if the color of Sally's dress figures in the plot. A more complete statement about questions is that, as a general rule, they should be formulated to motivate chil-dren's higher-level thinking. When questions about de-tails are asked, usually they should be links in a chain of questions that lead to an inference about a hard-to-un-derstand part of the passage or an understanding of the selection as a whole.

While questions during the preparation and discus-sion phases of a reading lesson are important, these do not substitute for active, direct instruction. In direct in-struction, the teacher explains, models, demonstrates, and illustrates reading skills and strategies that students ought to be using. There is evidence that direct instruction produces gains in reading achievement beyond those that are obtained with only less direct means such as questions.

The emphasis during reading lessons should be on understanding and appreciating the content of the story.

Lessons in which the children do little else but take turns reading the story, and the teacher does little else but correct reading errors, are ineffective. Teachers should periodically ask students questions that lead them to understand the critical points of the story. As needed, the teacher should explain points that students have confused or demonstrate skills that students should be using.

Van Bucher

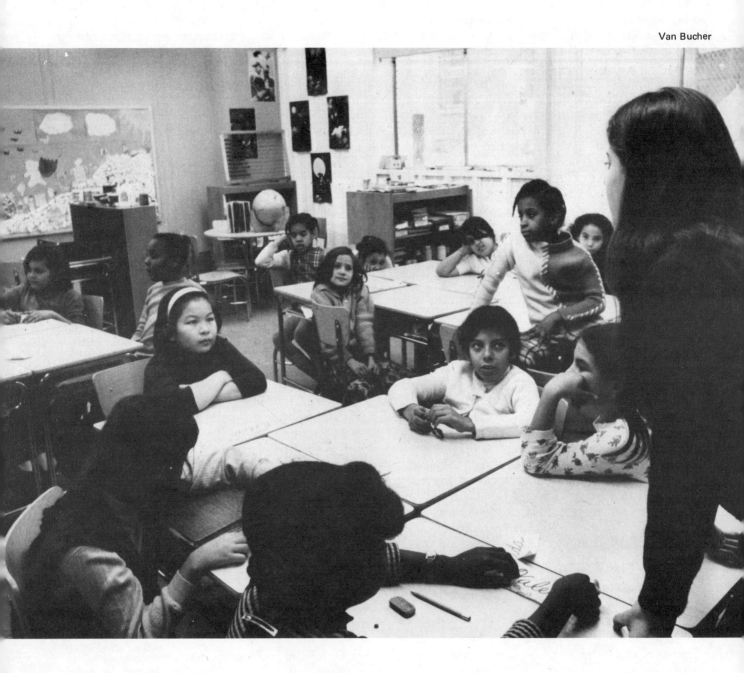

Chapter 36
The Disappearing Child
Neil Postman*

Children have virtually disappeared from the media, especially from television. I do not mean, of course, that people who are young in years cannot be seen. I mean that when they are shown, they are depicted as miniature adults in the manner of 13th and 14th century paintings. We might call this condition the Gary Coleman Phenomenon, by which I mean that an attentive viewer of situation comedies, soap operas, or any other popular TV format will notice that the children on such shows do not differ significantly in their interests, language, dress, or sexuality from the adults on the same shows.

The "Adultification" of Childhood

Having said this, I must concede that the popular arts have rarely depicted children in an authentic manner. We have only to think of some of the great child stars of films such as Shirley Temple, Jackie Coogan, Jackie Cooper, Margaret O'Brien, and the harmless ruffians of the Our Gang comedies, to realize that cinema representations of the character and sensibility of the young have been far from realistic. But one could find in them, nonetheless, an ideal, a *conception* of childhood. These children dressed differently from adults, talked differently, saw problems from a different perspective, had a different status, were more vulnerable. Even in the early days of television, on such programs as *Leave It to Beaver* and *Father Knows Best,* one could find children who were, if not realistically portrayed, at least different from adults. But most of this is now gone, or at least rapidly going.

Perhaps the best way to grasp what has happened here is to imagine what *The Shirley Temple Show* would be like were it a television series today, assuming of course that Miss Temple were the same age now as she was when she made her memorable films. (She began her career at age four but made most of her successful films between the ages of six and ten.) Is it imaginable except as parody that Shirley Temple would sing—let us say, as a theme song—"On the Good Ship Lollipop"? If she would sing at all, her millieu would be rock music, that is, music as much associated with adult sensibility as with that of youth. (See Studio 54 and other adult discos.) On today's network television there simply is no such thing as a child's song. It is a dead species, which tells as much about what I am discussing here as anything I can think of. In any case, a ten-year-old Shirley Temple would probably require a boyfriend with whom she would be more than occasionally entangled in a simulated lover's quarrel. She would certainly have to abandon "little girls'" dresses and hairstyles for something approximating adult fashion. Her language would consist of a string of knowing wisecracks, including a liberal display of sexual innuendo. In short, *The Shirley Temple Show* would not—could not—be about a child, adorable or otherwise. Too many in the audience would find such a conception either fanciful or unrecognizable, especially the youthful audience.

Of course, the disappearance from television of our traditional model of childhood is to be observed most vividly in commercials. I have already spoken of the wide use of 11- and 12-year-old girls as erotic objects (the Brooke Shields Phenomenon), but it is necessary to mention one extraordinary commercial for Jordache jeans in which both schoolgirls and schoolboys—most of them prepubescent—are represented as being driven silly by their undisciplined libidos, which are further inflamed by the wearing of designer jeans. The commercial concludes by showing that their teacher wears the same jeans. What can this mean other than that no distinction need be made between children and adults in either their sexuality or the means by which it is stimulated?

*Dr. Neil Postman is Professor of Media Ecology, New York University, NY. This article, which appeared in the March, 1983 issue of *Educational Leadership,* is excerpted from his book, *The Disappearance of Childhood* (New York: Delacorte Press, 1982). Reprinted with permission of the Association for Supervision and Curriculum Development and the author. Copyright © 1983 by the Association for Supervision and Curriculum Development.

But beyond this, and just as significant, is the fact that children, with or without hyperactive libidos, are commonly and unashamedly used as actors in commercial dramas. In one evening's viewing I counted nine different products for which a child served as a pitchman. These included sausages, real estate, toothpaste, insurance, a detergent, and a restaurant chain. American television viewers apparently do not think it either unusual or disagreeable that children should instruct them in the glories of corporate America, perhaps because as children are admitted to more and more aspects of adult life, it would seem arbitrary to exclude them from one of the most important: selling. In any case, we have here a new meaning to the prophecy that a child shall lead them.

The "adultification" of children on television is closely paralleled in films. Such movies as different as *Carrie, The Exorcist, Pretty Baby, Paper Moon, The Omen, The Blue Lagoon, Little Darlings, Endless Love, and A Little Romance* have in common a conception of the child who is in social orientation, language, and interests no different from adults. A particularly illuminating way in which to see the shift in child film imagery that has taken place in recent years is to compare the Little Rascals movies of the 1930s with the 1976 film *Bugsy Malone,* a satire in which children play the roles of adult characters from gangster movies. Most of the humor in the Little Rascals films derived its point from the sheer incongruity of children emulating adult behavior. Although *Bugsy Malone* uses children as a metaphor for adults, there is very little sense of incongruity in their role playing. After all, what is absurd about a twelve-year old using "adult" language, dressing in adult clothes, showing an adult interest in sex, singing adult songs? The point is that the Little Rascals films were clearly comedy. *Bugsy Malone* comes close to documentary.

Most of the widely discussed changes in children's literature have been in the same direction as those of the modern media. The work of Judy Blume has been emulated by many other writers who, like Ms. Blume, have grasped the idea that "adolescent literature" is best received when it simulates in theme and language adult literature, and, in particular, when its characters are presented as miniature adults. Of course, I do not wish to give the impression that there are currently no examples in children's literature (or, for that matter, in television or movies) of children who are emphatically different from adults. But I do mean to suggest that we are now undergoing a very rapid reorientation in our popular arts in regard to the image of children. One might put the matter, somewhat crudely, in this way: Our culture is not big enough for both Judy Blume and Walt Disney. One of them will have to go, and as the Disney empire's falling receipts show, it is the Disney conception of what a child is and needs that is disappearing.[1] We are in the process of exorcising a 200-year-old image of the young as child and replacing it with the imagery of the young as adult.

Although this is exactly what Ms. Blume, our modern film makers, and TV writers are doing, no moral or social demerit may be charged against them. Whatever else one may say in criticism of our popular arts, they cannot be accused of indifference to social reality. The shuffling black, the acquisitive Jew, even (to some extent) the obedient and passive wife, have disappeared from view, not because they are insufficiently interesting as material but because they are unacceptable to audiences. In a similar way, Shirley Temple is replaced by Brooke Shields because the audience requires a certain correspondence between the imagery of it popular arts and social reality as it is experience. The question of the extent to which, say, television reflects social reality is a complex one, for there are times when it lags slightly behind, times when it anticipates changes, times when it is precisely on target. But it can never afford to be off the mark by too great a margin or it ceases to be a popular art. This is the sense in which we might say that television is our most democratic institution. Programs display what people understand and want or they are canceled. Most people no longer understand and want the traditional, idealized model of the chill because that model cannot be supported by their experience or imagination.

The "Childified" Adult

The same is true of the traditional model of an adult. If one looks closely at the content of TV, one can find a fairly precise documentation not only of the rise of the "adultified" child but also of the rise of the "childified" adult. Television is as clear about this as almost anything else (although, without question, the best representation of the childlike adult is in the film *Being There,* which is, in fact, about the process I am describing). Laverne, Shirley, Archie, the crew of the Love Boat, the company of Three, Fonzie, Barney Miller's detectives, Rockford, Kojak, and the entire population of Fantasy Island can hardly be said to be adult characters, even after one has made allowances for the traditions of the formats in which they appear. With a few exceptions, adults on television do not take their work seriously (if they work at all), they do not nurture children, they have no politics, practice no religion, represent no tradition, have no foresight or serious plans, have no extended conversations, and in no circumstances allude to anything that is not familiar to an eight-year-old person.

Although students of mine who are dedicated TV watchers have urged me to modify the following statement, I can find only one fictional character regularly seen on commercial television, Felix Unger of *The Odd Couple,* who is depicted as having an adult's appetite for serious music and whose language suggests that he has, at one time in his life, actually read a book. Indeed, it is quite noticeable that the majority of adults on TV shows are depicted as functionally illiterate, not only in the sense that the content of book learning is absent from what they appear to know but also because of the absence of even the faintest signs of a contemplative habit of mind. *(The Odd Couple,* now seen only in reruns, ironically offers in Felix Unger not only an example of a literate person but a striking anomaly in his partner, Oscar Madison—a professional writer who is illiterate.)

A great deal has been written about the inanity of popular TV programs. But I am not here discussing that judgment. My point is that the model of an adult that is most often used on TV is that of the child, and that this pattern can be seen on almost every type of program. On game shows, for example, contestants are selected with great care to ensure that their tolerance for humiliation (by a simulated adult, the "emcee") is inexhaustible, their emotions instantly arousable, their interest in things a consuming passion. Indeed, a game show is a parody of sorts of a classroom in which childlike contestants are duly rewarded for obedience and precociousness but are otherwise subjected to all the indignities that are traditionally the schoolchild's burden. The absence of adult characters on soap operas, to take another example, is so marked that as of this writing a syndicated "teenage" version of a soap opera, called *Young Lives,* has been embarked upon as if to document the idea that the world of the young is no different from the world of the adult. Here television is going one step further than the movies: *Young Lives* is *Bugsy Malone* without satire.

The Merging of Nonchild with Nonadult

All of this is happening in part because TV tries to reflect prevailing values and styles. And in our current situation the values and styles of the child and those of the adult have tended to merge. One does not have to be a sociologist of the familiar to have noticed all of the following:

The children's clothing industry has undergone vast changes in the past decade, so that what was once unambiguously recognized as "children's" clothing has virtually disappeared. Twelve-year-old boys now wear three-piece suits to birthday parties, and 60-year-old men wear jeans to birthday parties. Eleven-year-old girls wear high heels, and what was once a clear marker of youthful informality and energy, sneakers, now allegedly signifies the same for adults. The miniskirt, which was the most embarrassing example of adults mimicking a children's style of dress, is for the moment moribund, but in its place one can see on the streets of New York and San Francisco grown women wearing little white socks and imitation Mary Janes. The point is that we are now un-

dergoing a reversal of a trend, begun in the 16th century, of identifying children through their manner of dress. As the concept of childhood diminishes, the symbolic markers of childhood diminish with it.

This process can be seen to occur not only in clothing but in eating habits as well. Junk food, once suited only to the undiscriminating palates and iron stomachs of the young, is now common fare for adults. This can be inferred from the commercials for McDonald's and Burger King, which make no age distinctions in their appeals. It can also be directly observed by simply attending to the distribution of children and adults who patronize such places. It would appear that adults consume at least as much junk food as do children.[2] This is no trivial point; it seems that many have forgotten when adults were supposed to have higher standards than children in their conception for what is and is not edible. Indeed, it was a mark of movement toward adulthood when a youngster showed an inclination to reject the kind of fare that gives the junk-food industry its name. I believe we can say rather firmly that this marker of the transition to adulthood is now completely obliterated.

There is no more obvious symptom of the merging of children's and adults' values and styles than what is happening with children's games, which is to say, they are disappearing. While I have found no studies that document the decline of unsupervised street games, their absence is noticeable enough and, in any case, can be inferred from the astonishing rise of such institutions as Little League baseball and Pee Wee football. Except for the inner city, where games are still under the control of the youths who play them, the games of American youth have become increasingly official, mock-professional, and extremely serious. According to the Little League Baseball Association, whose headquarters are in Williamsport, Pennsylvania, Little League baseball is the largest youth sports program in the world. More than 1400 charters have been issued, over two and a half million youngsters participate, from ages six to eighteen. The structure of the organization is modeled on that of major league baseball, the character of the games themselves on the emotional style of big league sports: there is no fooling around, no peculiar rules invented to suit the moment, no protection from the judgments of spectators.

The idea that children's games are not the business of adults has clearly been rejected by Americans, who are insisting that even at age six, children play their games without spontaneity, under careful supervision, and at an intense competitive level. That many adults do not grasp the significance of this redefinition of children's play is revealed by a story that appeared in *The New York Times,* July 17, 1981. The occasion was a soccer tournament in Ontario, Canada, involving 4,000 children from ten nations. In one game between ten-year-old boys from East Brunswick, New Jersey, and Burlington, Ontario, a brawl took place "after fathers had argued on the sidelines, players had traded charges of rough play and foul language, and one man from Burlington made a vulgar gesture." The brawl was highlighted by a confrontation between the mothers of two players, one of whom kicked the other. Of course, much of this is standard stuff and has been duplicated many times by adults at "official" baseball and football games. (I have myself witnessed several 40-year-old men unmercifully "riding" an eleven-year-old shortstop because he had made two errors in one inning.) But what is of most significance is the remark made by one of the mothers after the brawl, In trying to put the matter in perspective, she was quoted as saying, "It [the brawl] was just 30 seconds out of a beautiful tournament. The next night our boys lost, but it was a beautiful game. Parents were applauding kids from both teams. Overall, it was a beautiful experience." But the point is, What are the parents doing there in the first place? Why are 4,000 children involved in a tournament? Why is East Brunswick, New Jersey, playing Burlington, Ontario? What are these children being trained for? The answer to all these questions it that children's play has become an adult preoccupation, it has become professionalized, it is no longer a world separate from the world of adults.

The entry of children into professional and world-class amateur sports is, of course, related to all of this. The 1979 Wimbledon tennis tournament, for example, was marked by the extraordinary performance of Tracy Austin, then not yet 16, the youngest player in the history of the tournament. In 1980, a 15-year-old player made her appearance. In 1981, a 14-year-old. An astonished John Newcombe, an old-time Wimbledon champion, expressed the view that in the near future twelve-year-old players may take the center court. But in this respect tennis lags behind others sports. Twelve-year-old swimmers, skaters, and gymnasts of world class ability are commonplace. Why is this happening? The most obvious answer is that better coaching and training techniques have made it possible for children to attain adult-level competence. But the questions remain: Why should adults encourage this possibility? Why would anyone wish to deny children the freedom, informality, and joy of spontaneous play? Why submit children to the rigors of professional-style training, concentration, tension, media hype? The answer is the same as before: The traditional assumptions about the uniqueness of children are fast fading. What we have here is the emergence of the idea that play is not to be done for the sake of doing it but for some external purpose, such as renown, money, physical conditioning, upward mobility, national pride. For

adults, play is serious business. A childhood disappears, so does the child's view of play.

This same tendency toward the merging of child and adult perspectives can be observed in their tastes in entertainment. To take an obvious example: The 1980 Nielsen Report on Television reveals that adults (defined as people over the age of 18) rated the following as among their 15 most favored syndicated programs: *Family Feud, The Muppet Show, Hee Haw, M*A*S*H, Dance Fever, Happy Days Again,* and *Sha Na Na.* These programs were also listed among the top 15 most favored by those between the ages of 12 and 17. And they also made the favored list of those between the ages of two and eleven! As for (the then) current shows, the male adult group indicated that *Taxi, Mork & Mindy, M*A*S*H, Three's Company, ABC Sunday Night Movie,* and *The Dukes of Hazzard* were among their favorites. The 12-to-17 age group included the same shows.[3] In the 1981 Nielsen Report, adult males favored six syndicated programs (out of ten) that were the same as those favored by the 12-to-17 age group, and four (out of ten) that were the same as those favored by the 12-to-17 age group, and four (out of ten) that were the same as the 2-to-11 age group.[4]

Such figures are painful to contemplate but are entirely consistent with the observation that what now amuses the child also amuses the adult. As I write, *Superman II, For Your Eyes Only, Raiders of the Lost Ark,* and *Tarzan, the Ape Man* are attracting customers of all ages in almost unprecedented numbers. Twenty-five years ago, such films, which are essentially animated comic strips, would have been regarded as children's entertainment. Not as charming, innocent, or creative as, say, *Snow White and the Seven Dwarfs* but nonetheless clearly for a youthful audience. Today, no such distinctions need to be made. Neither is it necessary to distinguish between adult and youthful taste in music, as anyone who has visited an adult discotheque can attest. It is still probably true that the 10-year-old-to-17-year-old group is more knowledgable about the names and styles of rock groups than are those over the age of 25, but as the declining market for both classical and popular "adult" music suggests, adults can no longer claim that their taste in music represents a higher level of sensitivity than teen-age music.[5]

The Decline of Adult Authority

As clothing, food, games, and entertainment move toward a homogeneity of style, so does language. It is extremely difficult to document this change except by repairing to anecdotes or by asking readers to refer to their own experience. We do know, of course, that the capacity of the young to achieve "grade level" competence in reading and writing is declining.[6] And we also know that their ability to reason and to make valid inferences is declining as well.[7] Such evidence is usually offered to document the general decline of literacy in the young. But it may also be brought forward to imply a decline of interest in language among adults; that is to say, after one has discussed the role of the media in producing a lowered state of language competence in the young, there is still room to discuss the indifference of parents, teachers, and other influential adults to the importance of language. We may even be permitted the assumption that adult control over language does not in most cases significantly surpass children's control over language. On television, on radio, in films, in commercial transactions, on the streets, even in the classroom, one does not notice that adults use language with more variety, depth, or precision than do children. In fact, it is a sort of documentation of this that there has emerged a small industry of books and newspaper columns that advise adults on how to talk as adults.

One may even go so far as to speculate that the language of the young is exerting more influence on adults than the other way around. Although the tendency to insert the work *like* after every four words still remains a distinctive adolescent pattern, in many other respects adults have found teen-age language attractive enough to incorporate in their own speech. I have recorded many instances of people over the age of 35, and from every social class, uttering, without irony, such phrases as "I am into jogging," "Where are you coming from?" (to mean "What is your point of view?"), "Get off my case," and other teen-age locutions. I must leave it to readers to decide if this tendency is confirmed by their own experience. However, of one thing, I believe, we may be sure: Those adult language secrets to which we give the name "dirty words" are now not only fully known to the young (which may always have been the case) but are used by them as freely as they are by adults. Not only on the soccer field in Ontario but in all public places—ball parks, movie theaters, school yards, classrooms, department stores, restaurants—one can hear such words used comfortably and profusely even by children as young as six years old. This fact is significant because it is an example of the erosion of a traditional distinction between children and adults. It is also significant because it represents a loss in the concept of manners. Indeed, as language, clothing, taste, eating habits, and so on, become increasingly homogenized, there is a corresponding decline in both the practice and meaning of civilité, which is rooted in the idea of social hierarchy.[8] In our present situation, adulthood has lost much of its authority and aura, and the idea of deference to one who is older has become ridiculous. That such a decline is in process can

be inferred from the general disregard for rules and rituals of public assembly: the increase in what are called "discipline problems" in school, the necessity of expanded security at public events, the intrusion of the loudest possible radio music on public space, the rarity of conventional expressions of courtesy such as "thank you" and "please."

The Innocent Child, a Contradiction of Terms

All of the foregoing observations and inferences are, I believe, indicators of both the decline of childhood and a corresponding diminution in the character of adulthood. But there is also available a set of hard facts pointing to the same conclusion. For example, in the year 1950, in all of America, only 170 persons under the age of 15 were arrested for what the FBI calls serious crimes: murder, forcible rape, robbery, and aggravated assault. This number represented .0004 percent of the under-15 population of America. In that same year, 94,784 persons 15 years and older were arrested for serious crimes, representing .0860 percent of the population 15 years and older. This means that in 1950, adults (defined here as those over and including 15 years of age) committed serious crimes at a rate 215 times that of the rate of child crime. By 1960, adults committed serious crimes at a rate 8 times that of child crime; by 1979, the rate was 5.5 times. Does this mean that adult crime is declining? Not quite. In fact, adult crime is increasing, so that in 1979 more than 400,000 adults were arrested for serious crimes, representing .2340 percent of the adult population. This means that between 1950 and 1979, the rate of adult crime increased threefold. The fast-closing difference between the rates of adult and child crime is almost wholly accounted for by a staggering rise in child crime. Between 1950 and 1979, the rate of serious crimes committed by children increased 11,000 percent! The rate of nonserious child crimes (for example, burglary, larceny, and auto theft) increased 8,300 percent.[9]

If America can be said to be drowning in a tidal wave of crime, then the wave has mostly been generated by our children. Crime, like most everything else, is no longer an exclusively adult activity, and readers do not need statistics to confirm this. Almost daily the press tells of arrests being made of children who, like those playing tennis at Wimbledon, are getting younger and younger. In New York City a nine-year-old boy tried to hold up a bank. In July 1981, police in Westchester County, New York, charged four boys with sexual assault of a seven-year-old girl. The alleged rapists were a 13-year-old, two 11-year-olds, and a 9-year-old, the latter being the youngest person ever to be accused of first-degree rape in Westchester County.[10]

Ten- to 13-year-olds are involved in adult crime as never before. Indeed, the frequency of serious child crime has pushed youth crime codes to their limits. The first American juvenile court was established in 1899 in Illinois. The idea could come to its end before the century is out as legislators throughout the country hurriedly try to revise criminal laws so that youthful offenders can be treated as adults. In California a study group formed by the attorney general has recommended sending juveniles convicted of first-degree murder to prison rather than to the California Youth Authority. It has also recommended that violent offenders 16 years old and younger be tried as adults, within the court's discretion.[11] In Vermont the arrest of two teen-agers in connection with the rape, torture, and killing of a 12-year-old girl has driven the state legislature to propose hardening the juvenile codes.[12] In New York, children between the ages of 13 and 15 who are charged with serious crimes can now be tried in adult courts and, if convicted, can receive long prison terms. In Florida, Louisiana, New Jersey, South Carolina, and Tennessee, laws have been changed to make it easier to transfer children between the ages of 13 and 15 to adult criminal courts if the crime is serious enough. In Illinois, New Mexico, Oregon, and Utah, the privacy that usually surrounds the trials of juveniles has been eliminated: newspaper reporters may now regularly attend the proceeedings.[13]

This unprecedented change in both the frequency and brutality of child crime, as well as the legislative response to it, is no doubt attributable to multiple causes but none more cogent, I think, than that our concept of childhood is rapidly slipping from our grasp. Our children live in a society whose psychological and social contexts do not stress the differences between adults and children. As the adult world opens itself in every conceivable way to children, they will inevitably emulate adult criminal activity.

They will also participate in such activity as victims. Paralleling the assault on social orders *by* children is the assault by adults *on* children. According to the National Center on Child Abuse and Neglect, there were 711,142 reported cases of child abuse in 1979. Assuming that a fair amount of child battering goes unreported, we may guess that well over two million instances of child abuse occurred that year. What can this mean other than that the special status, image, and aura of the child has been drastically diminished? It is only half an explanation to say that children are beaten up because they are small. The other half finds that they are beaten up because they are not perceived as children. To the extent that children are viewed as unrealized, vulnerable, not in possession of a full measure of intellectual and emotional control, normal adults do not beat them as a response to conflict. Unless we assume that in all cases the adult attackers are psychopaths, we may conclude that at least part of the

answer here is that many adults now have a different conception of what sort of a person a child is, a conception not unlike that which prevailed in the 14th century: that they are miniature adults.

This perception of children as miniature adults is reinforced by several trends besides criminal activity. For example, the increased level of sexual activity among children has been fairly well documented. Data presented by Catherine Chilman indicate that for young white females the rise has been especially sharp since the late 1960s.[14] Studies by Melvin Zelnick and John Kantner of The Johns Hopkins University conclude that the prevalence of sexual activity among never-married teen-age women, among all races, increased by 30 percent between 1971 and 1976, so that by age 19, 55 percent have had sexual intercourse.[15] We may safely assume that media have played an important role in the drive to erase differences between child and adult sexuality. Television, in particular, not only keeps the entire population in a condition of high sexual excitement but stresses a kind of egalitarianism of sexual fulfillment; sex is transformed from a dark and profound adult mystery to a product that is available to everyone—let us say, like mouthwash or underarm deodorant.

One of the consequences of this has been a rise in teen-age pregnancy. Births to teen-agers constituted 19 percent of all the births in America in 1975, an increase of 2 percent over the figure in 1966. But if one focuses on the childbearing rate among those of age 15 to 17, one finds that *this is the only age group whose rate of childbearing increased in those years, and it increased 21.7 percent.*[16]

Another, and grimmer, consequence of adult-like sexual activity among children has been a steady increase in the extent to which youth are afflicted with venereal disease. Between 1956 and 1979, the percentage of 10-to-14 year olds suffering from gonorrhea increased almost threefold, from 17.7 per 100,000 population to 50.4. Roughly the same increase is found in the 15-to-19-year-old group (from 415.7 per 100,000 to 1,211.4). The traditional restraints against youthful sexual activity cannot have great force in a society that does not, in fact, make a binding distinction between childhood and adulthood. And the same principle applies in the case of the consumption of drugs. For example, the National Institute on Alcohol Abuse and Alcoholism concludes that a substantial number of 15-year-olds drink "considerable amounts." In one study of the drinking habits of 10th-to-12th-graders, almost three times as many males indicated they were "heavier" drinkers (meaning they drink at least once a week and consume large amounts when they drink) than those who indicated they were "infrequent" drinkers (meaning they drink once a month at most and then in small amounts). Alcoholism, once considered an exclusively adult affliction, now looms as a reality for our new population of miniature adults. Of other drugs, such as marijuana, cocaine, and heroin, the evidence is conclusive: American youth consume as much of it as do adults.[17]

Such figures as these are unmistakable signs of the rise of the "adultified" child, but there are similar trends suggestive of the rise of the "childified" adult. For example, the emergence of the "old persons' home" as a major social institution in American bespeaks of a reluctance on the part of young adults to assume a full measure of responsibility for their parents. Caring for the elderly and integrating them into family life are apparently perceived as an intolerable burden and have rapidly diminished as adult imperatives. Perhaps more significant is the fact that the present generation of young adults is marrying at a dramatically lower rate and having fewer children than their parents' generation. Moreover, their marriages are not as durable. According to the National Center for Health Statistics, parents are getting divorced at twice the rate they did 20 years ago, and more children than ever before are involved in marital dissolution: 1.18 million in 1979 as compared to 562,000 in 1963. Although we must assume multiple causality for such a trend, including what Christopher Lasch calls the rise of the narcissistic personality, we may fairly claim that it indicates a precipitous falling off in the commitment of adults to the nurturing of children. The strongest argument against divorce has always been its psychological effect on children. It is now clear that more adults than ever do not regard this argument to be as compelling as their own need for psychological well-being. Perhaps we might even say that, increasingly, American adults want to be parents of children less than they want to be children themselves. In any case, children have responded to this new mood by, among other things, running away in droves. According to the FBI, 165,000 children were taken into custody by police in 1979. It is assumed that at least three times that number went undetected.

Rationalizing the Disappearance of Childhood

In the face of all this one would expect the rise of a "philosophy" of sorts to justify the loss of childhood. Perhaps there is a principle governing social life that requires people to search for a way to affirm that which is inevitable. In any case, such a philosophy has, indeed, emerged, and we may take it as evidence of the reality it addresses. I refer here to what is sometimes called the Children's Rights Movement. This is a confusing designation, because under its banner are huddled two conceptions of childhood that are, in fact, opposed to each other. One of them, which I do *not* have in mind in these remarks, believes that childhood is desirable although fragile, and wishes to protect children from neglect and

abuse. This view argues, for example, for the intervention of public authority when parental responsibility fails. This conception of childhood dates back to the 19th century and is simply a widening of the perspective that led to child labor laws, juvenile crime codes, and other humane protections. *The New York Times* has referred to those who stand up for this idea as "child savers."

The other conception of "child's right" rejects adult supervision and control of children and provides a "philosophy" to justify the dissolution of childhood. It argues that the social category "children" is in itself an oppressive idea and that everything must be done to free the young from its restrictions. This view is, in fact, a much older one than the first, for its origins may be found in the Dark and Middle Ages when there were no "children" in the modern sense of the word.

As is frequently the case in such matters, we have here a "reactionary" position being advanced by those who think of themselves as "radicals." In any case, these are people who might be called "child liberators." Among the earliest of them was Ivan Illich, the brilliant social critic, whose influential book *Deschooling Society* (1971) argued against compulsory schooling not only on the grounds that schools were unimprovable but, even more, that compulsory schooling effectively bars the young from fully participating in the life of the community; that is, prevents them from being adults. Illich redefined the relationship of children to school by insisting that what most people see as a benevolent and nurturing institution is instead an unwarranted intrusion in the life and learning of a certain segment of the population. The force of Illich's argument derives from the fact that information is now so widely distributed, available from so many sources, and codified in ways that do not require sophisticated literacy that the school has lost much of its meaning as the fountainhead of learning. Moreover, as the distinction between childhood and adulthood becomes less marked, as children less and less have to *earn* adulthood, as less and less is there anything for them to *become,* the compulsory nature of schooling begins to appear arbitrary.

This impression is intensified by the fact that educators have become confused about what they ought to be doing with children in school. Such ideas that one ought to be educated for the greater glory of God or Country, or even for the purpose of beating the Russians, lack both serious arguments and advocates, and many educators are willing to settle for what Marx himself would have emphatically rejected: education for entry into the marketplace. This being the case, a knowledge of history, literature, and art, which once was the mark of an educated adult, recedes in importance. Moreover, it is not as well established as many think that schooling makes an important difference in one's future earning power.

Thus, the entire edifice of our educational structure is laced with dangerous cracks, and those who would demolish the structure altogether are by no means misinformed. Indeed, there is a sense in which their proposals are redundant. As childhood disappears, so must schools. Illich does not have to write a book about it so much as merely wait.

All of this is the theme of John Holt's *Escape from Childhood*. In this and other books he argues for the liberation of the child from the constraints of a 300-year-old tradition of bondage. His arguments are broadened—that is, taken to their logical conclusion—in Richard Farson's extraordinary book, *Birthrights* (1974). Farson argues that the child's right to information, to his or her own choice of education, to sexual freedom, to economic and political power, even to the right to choose his or her own home environment, must be restored at once. "We are not likely to err," he says, "in the direction of too much freedom."[18] Farson, who is not unaware of the history of childhood, evidently finds the 14th and 15th centuries a suitable model for the ways in which the young ought to be integrated into society. He believes, among other things, that the principal objection to incest is that people are made to feel unreasonably guilty about practicing it; that all sexual behavior should be decriminalized, including sex between adults and children; that arrangements need to be made to permit children to live wherever and with whom they wish, including "homes" governed by themselves; and that children must be given the right to vote "because adults do not have their interests at heart and do not vote in their behalf."[19]

Such a child's rights movement as this may be said to be a case of claiming that the disease is the cure. Expressed more neutrally, what this sort of advocacy represents, as noted, is an attempt to provide a rationalization for what appears to be an irreversible cultural tendency. Farson, in other words, is not the enemy of childhood. American culture is. But it is not a forthright enemy, in the sense that one might say, for example, that America is against communism. American culture does not *intend* to be against childhood. In fact, the language we use to talk about children still carries within it many of the assumptions about childhood that were established in the 18th and 19th centuries. Just as our language about war preserves the idea of a 19th-century war, when, in fact, such an idea today is preposterous, our language about children does not match our present social reality. For in a hundred years of redesigning how we communicate, what we communicate, and what we need to be in order to share in it all, we have reached the point of not needing children, just as we have reached the point (although we dare not admit it) of not needing the elderly. What makes Farson's proposals so horrifying is that without irony or regret he reveals the future.

FOOTNOTES

1. For documentation and analysis of the decline of the Disney empire, see "Wishing Upon a Falling Star at Disney," *The New York Times Magazine,* November 16, 1980.

2. McDonald's insists on keeping private its figures as to how much of its food different age groups consume. The best I could get from them is the statement that young adults with small children are the largest group among those who patronize McDonald's. The categories that McDonald's inventories are small children, "tweens," teens, young adults, and seniors.

3. These figures are from *Nielsen Report on Television 1980.*

4. *Nielsen Report on Television 1981.* Both this report and the 1980 report are available upon request to A.C. Nielsen Company, Nielsen Plaza, Northbrook, IL 60062.

5. According to RCA, the largest producer of classical music recordings, in the early 1960s the company released approximately eight new recordings a month. Today, that figure is down to four. A spokesman for RCA claims this situation is similar for every other company in the business. RCA also concedes that there has been a steady decline in the share of the market of both classical music and sophisticated popular music. Today, classical music, opera, and chamber music account for about 7 percent of all sales. The rest is mostly rock, country, and jazz.

6. Among the many studies documenting this decline is one conducted by the California Department of Education in 1979. Seniors tested under the California Assessment Program continued to perform (as they had in 1978) 16 percentage points below what the testing industry says is the national average for reading.

7. In a report released in 1981, the National Assessment of Educational Progress revealed that the inferential reasoning of 13-year-olds declined throughout the period of the 1970s.

8. For an excellent historical analysis of these relationships, see Richard Sennett's *The Fall of Public Man* (New York: Random House, Vintage Books, 1978).

9. These figures were compiled by using the 1950 and 1970 Uniform Crime Report (published by the FBI) and the 1950 and 1970 census.

10. See the New York *Daily News,* July 17, 1981, page 5.

11. See the United Press International report of June 22, 1981.

12. See the New York *Daily News,* July 17, 1981, page 5.

13. For a comprehensive review of the changing attitudes toward child crime, see *The New York Times,* July 24, 1981.

14. Cited in Melvin Zelnik and John Kantner's "Sexual and Contraceptive Experience of Young Unmarried Women in the United States, 1976 and 1971." *Family Planning Perspectives* 9 (March/April 1977): 55-58.

15. See Zelnik and Kantner, above.

16. See Stephanie Ventura's "Teenage Childbearing: United States, 1966-75," *The Monthly Vital Statistics Report,* a publication of the National Center for Health Statistics.

17. See "Student Drug Use in America, 1975-1980," prepared by Lloyd Johnson, Jerald Bachman, and Patrick O'Malley of the University of Michigan Institute for Social Research. It is available from the National Institute on Drug Abuse, Rockville, MD 20857.

18. Richard Farson, *Birthrights* (New York: Macmillan, 1974), p. 153.

19. Farson, p. 179.

REFERENCES

Holt, John. *Escape from Childhood.* New York: Ballantine Books, 1976.

Illich, Joseph. "Child Rearing in Seventeenth Century England and America." In *The History of Childhood.* Edited by Lloyd de Mause. New York: The Psychohistory Press, 1974.

Lasch, Christopher. *Haven in a Heartless World: The Family Besieged.* New York: Basic Books, 1977.

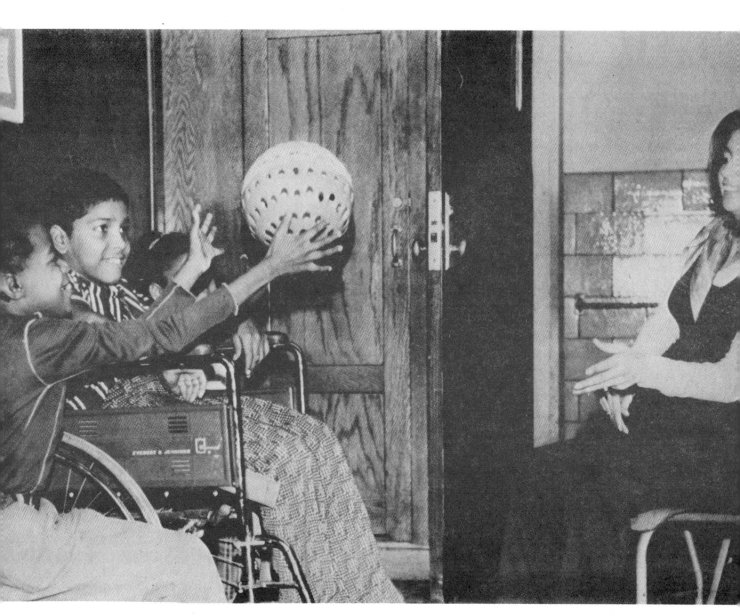

Samuel Teicher

Chapter 37

Mainstreaming: A New Solution to an Old Problem, or a New Problem?

Barbara Ruth Peltzman*

Court decisions and state and federal legislation have laid the groundwork for a legal responsibility on the part of the school systems to provide free public education in the "least restrictive environment" for all handicapped children. *(Education Digest,* November, 1976, p.6)

One of these pieces of legislation is the Education of All Handicapped Children Act, Public Law 94-142. It is the result of a new civil rights movement, which is, according to Frederick Weintraub and Alan Abeson (1974) "a quiet revolution" for the right of all handicapped children to be educated in an environment which allows full development of academic and creative potential regardless of physical or other handicapping conditions. Greer in Hechinger (1976) states that

> The education of exceptional children is no longer perceived as a matter of charity—or even as a wise practice of an enlightened society determined to make the fullest uses of its assets. It is now a matter of their rights as citizens to the same sort of education as other children. This new status of special education is really the latest expression of the civil rights movements of the '60's.

The least restrictive environment has been interpreted to mean that handicapped children are to be educated in regular classrooms with non-handicapped children. This principle of least restrictive environment is stated in section 612-5 of Public Law 94-142.

> The states are required to establish procedures to assure that to the maximum extent appropriate, handicapped children . . . are educated with children who are not handicapped, and that special classes, separate schooling, or other removal from the regular educational environment occurs only when the nature or severity of the handicap is such that education in regular classes with the use of supplementary aids and services cannot be achieved satisfactorily . . . (p.9).

The principle of the least restrictive environment has been translated into a form of administrative organiza-

tion known as mainstreaming. According to Byron Brenton (1974):

> In essence, mainstreaming means moving handicapped children from their segregated status in special education classrooms and integrating them with 'normal' children in regular classrooms (p. 18).

Mainstreaming is one form of implementation of Public Law 94-142. It grows out of the belief that handicapped children should not be locked away from the mainstream of society. While PL 94-142 does not mandate mainstreaming, the language of section 612-5 makes mainstreaming the means by which the provisions of the law can most effectively be carried out. Mainstreaming, according to an editorial in *Education Digest* in November, 1976, aims at providing for handicapped children with "the most appropriate and effective educational experience which will enable them to become self-reliant adults. It is thought preferable to educate children the least distance away from the mainstream of society. . . ."(p.6). Mainstreaming is intended to create greater interaction between handicapped and non-handicapped children. As with every new movement people take sides for and against it. Thus, mainstreaming has its advocates and opponents among teachers, parents, and administrators.

Those who favor mainstreaming offer various rationales for its adoption. These advocates state that handicapped children achieve better academically and socially when they are not isolated from their non-handicapped peers. However, Martin Kaufman (1974) states that "some studies support this notion while others do not. The results are equivocal. . . ." Sheldon and Sherman (1974) state that "at the present time there . . . seems to be no conclusive evidence that children assigned to special classes benefit more or less than children assigned to

*Dr. Barbara Ruth Peltzman is an Assistant Professor at St. John's University, Staten Island, NY.

regular classes. . . . If . . . children can be educated as well in regular classes . . . it would seem preferred in terms of the 'least restrictive' method and in reducing labels attached by special classroom. . . . This implies that the educational goals should be accomplished in a way which limits an individual's freedom and liberty least." As a supporter of mainstreaming, Roberts (1975) states:

> The most important reason for mainstreaming is that the self-contained special education classrooms have not worked best for most mildly handicapped children. There has been a great deal of speculation about why. . . . Whatever the reason, recent studies have shown that, in general, the mildly handicapped children in self-contained special education classes compare unfavorably with similar children left in regular classes. Most educators have concluded that the benefits of segregating exceptional children from their peers are doubtful and that this should be done only as a last resort.

Advocates go further in stating that mainstreaming helps handicapped children become better adjusted to the real world when they leave school. Waleski (1965) states that "it is important that the school world resemble the real or adult world as closely as possible, so that the children can adapt to living in an environment that they will not always be able to control." Mainstreaming advocates further state that, according to Brenton (1974), exposure to handicapped children will help normal children understand individual differences in people and will diminish the stereotyping of the handicapped. Thus, the non-handicapped children will be able to work and play in an environment in which it is natural to give and accept help when necessary. Children will not fear or suspect others who are different from themselves. Waleski (1965) states that "by giving aid when needed, the normal child can learn to understand and accept differences and also learn when to give help and when to withhold it." In this way, the advocates of mainstreaming feel that children learn that at times all people need help and at times everyone wants to "go it alone."

Children will become more sensitive to the feelings and needs of others as well as to their own feelings and needs. Roberts (1975) states that "if mainstreaming . . . is viewed as a challenge and a chance to help handicapped children and non-handicapped children learn together, understand each other, value each other, mainstreaming can be an exciting and rewarding experience for all students and their teacher."

Those who favor mainstreaming state that it has the potential for far reaching changes in society. Robins (1975) states that "the long range benefits of mainstreaming are enormous. It eliminates the effects of isolating and segregating handicapped students for their

school years and later returning them to the community. Mainstreaming offers these children a more normal learning and social environment. As adults, non-handicapped and handicapped people work, play, and live together in the same community; for children we should expect no less."

Mainstreaming can help create a new social order in which the handicapped sub-culture created by separate special classes is eliminated and a new respect for differences develops. Both handicapped and non-handicapped people benefit. Carpenter (1975) states: "separateness on the basis of difference is stigmatizing. Learning and playing together in spite of differences, develops an appreciation of human individuality. . . . " Weintraub and Abeson (1974) believe that mainstreaming will have two important effects on society:

> At the minimum it will make educational opportunity a reality for all handicapped children. At the maximum it will make our schools heal their learning environments for all children.

The advocates of mainstreaming have presented sound arguments for its adoption, but what about concrete evidence? There are several programs currently in effect that provide concrete illustrations of the success of mainstreaming. These programs include children who are hearing impaired, visually impaired, learning disabled, mentally retarded, and physically impaired. One such program is known as the Holcomb Plan developed in Newark, Delaware. It provides a model for mainstreaming deaf and hard of hearing children. The program centers around total communication, an approach, which according to Vernon and Athey (1977) "uses sign language and finger spelling in combination with speech training, lipreading, and amplification (hearing aids). "It was decided that the deaf and hard of hearing should be placed with their hearing peers because traditional programs for the deaf created social isolation which resulted in inadequate development of communication skills. Vernon and Athey (1977) comment on the Holcomb Plan:

> Research shows that total communication results in better achievement and better personal adjustment than do other fragmented methods. In the Holcomb Plan hearing impaired children are carefully selected. In each regular class containing one or more of these children, an interpreter-tutor translates what the teacher and students say in sign language. . . . The child knows who is talking and what is being said.

The teachers in Newark received orientation to deafness and an in-service course in sign language. The hearing impaired children to be mainstreamed are carefully selected on an individualized basis and there are strong support services for teachers and pupils. Many hearing children requested instruction in sign language in order to communicate with new friends. Vernon and Athey (1977) state:

> Signing skill becomes a status symbol and many hearing children become eager to learn it. Because of the varying interests and abilities of children, not all choose to learn sign language. The degree of involvement is left to each child.

It is felt that the Holcomb Plan is successful because it has begun slowly and used all its resources carefully. Vernon and Athey (1977) state that the Holcomb Plan is a success because

> Newark's attitude is an enlightened one encompassed in cooperation and flexibility. By careful experimentation on a small scale, and through the use of the total communication method, Newark's educators are providing optimal learning experiences for both hearing impaired and hearing children.

The physically impaired are also benefiting from a mainstreaming plan. Handicapped children at Harry S. Truman High School in the Bronx spend 75% of their time in regular classes. One such 15 year old boy moves about in his wheelchair to a specially designed homeroom for orthopedically handicapped youths. He spends the first period each day in the homeroom on the ground floor and is helped up to his classes by an aide. Hechinger (1976) states "Several times a day he returns to the special homeroom for the teachers help in making up lapses in his notetaking caused by partial paralysis. . . . " This program at Truman is seen as, according to Hechinger (1976), "the beginning of the end of the dual system of education for 'normal' and handicapped children."

Learning disabled students are mainstreamed at the Learning Center at Acton-Boxborough Regional High School in Acton, Massachusetts. Manopoli (1976) states that "the goal of those who work in the Center is to be helpful to the teachers in working with the learning disabled and to assist the students themselves in their independent efforts to meet the requirements of the classroom. . . . " There are 50 students attending the center on a voluntary basis during unassigned periods. Various kinds of help is available to the students and those who work in the center, according to Manopoli (1976), "help subject matter teachers structure alternative approaches to exams and assignments. Many teachers allow us to give oral exams or to read test questions to them. With the consent of the classroom teachers, we develop modified assignments for students who are unable to meet the regular curriculum standards . . . we sometimes work in the regular classroom with whoever needs help." The program is successful because of cooperation and mutual

understanding on the part of the Center personnel and the classroom teachers. Manopoli (1976) believes that the success also grows out of the visibility of the Center personnel in the classroom.

> Special-needs students see us working with others and realize that they are not the only ones who need assistance. Classroom teachers see us as people interested in making their courses work for all students. . . . With the enthusiastic support of the faculty and administration at our school, the special-needs student is definitely meeting success in the classroom.

The Resource Room program allows mildly handicapped children to remain in regular classes while receiving help in a small group setting once or twice a day. Teachers report that help of this kind in reading and math skills is invaluable. The children spend most of their time in the regular classroom setting thus establishing friendships and experiencing a wide variety of activities with non-handicapped peers. These are just a few of the many successful programs in which mainstreaming is the key.

Although these programs strongly support mainstreaming, there are other examples which do not. Hechinger (1976) states that "Many observers warn that such "heartwarming" illustrations ignore the wide variations of the children to be served and the difference between integrating one or two handicapped children and adding a substantial number of youngsters with a diversity of problems to the ordinary already harassed teacher."

Some handicapped children are better able to adjust to mainstreaming because their intelligence and motivation enable them to work to overcome their disability. When these children are given modified classroom equipment and additional out-of-classroom help they become an asset to any class. However, there are children whose disabilities stand in the way of successful mainstreaming. Hechinger (1976) states that

> Some handicaps are more receptive to mainstreaming than others . . . [however] children with varying degrees of retardation . . . may benefit from being integrated into non-intellectual activities, such as sports, shop, and other non-verbal subjects. But their sense of defeat and frustration might be heightened rather than diminished in intellectual competition with non-handicapped peers. . . . Children with serious emotional problems may not only disrupt ordinary educational procedures, but also arouse anger and antagonism in their classmates.

There are other forms of handicaps which, according to Shanker (1977), create many problems for educators. These include:

> Hydrocephalic children who were born with holes in their hearts, who turn blue periodically and have water on the

brain and tubes in their heads which drain the excess water. When the tubes do not work properly, they must be reshunted by a nurse in the school. Many schools do not have a nurse. Children with bones so brittle that if they are touched the wrong way, their bones break. Children with separations in their spines who are paralyzed from the waist down; these children are on crutches. Children who are amputees and double amputees. Cerebral palsied children, some are severely impaired, others who function well in an academic setting. Children who still need to be taught toilet training, self-feeding and so forth. Autistic children, mildly retarded children, children with learning disabilities, and the emotionally disturbed, including children who are schizophrenic and autistic. . . .

If integrating children with such disabilities means greater danger for them, then perhaps it is better to let these children remain in special classes. There are many questions which are raised by the mainstreaming movement. Among them are those posed by Shanker (1977):

Should handicapped be taught by teachers who have not had special training? . . . Will handicapped children be better off in a mixed class with 25, 30 or 35 students than in smaller groups of students with specially trained teachers, therapists, psychologists and others? Will non-handicapped children in the class lose out because of the inordinate amount of time and energy which will have to be devoted to those with special needs? . . . There are no quick and easy answers to these questions. . . .

It is felt that many questions and objections will be raised when mainstreaming gets underway in full force in New York State. Parents' groups and special education teachers in other states have already voiced their opinions. Brenton (1974) states that

Some special education teachers and administrators are not keen on it [mainstreaming]. They fear that the gains made on behalf of handicapped children will be wiped out and they are not happy about the drastic changes their own professional approaches will have to undergo.

Special education teachers and administrators cite the lack of special training to deal with the handicapped as a reason why mainstreaming will not work. An editorial in *Education Digest* (1976) examines the question of teacher preparation for dealing with the special child.

Mainstreaming is intended to maximize interaction with non-handicapped students. It is understandable that the transition may produce special hazards and misgivings for all parties, including the teacher. . . . Without significant reconciliation of needs and capabilities through retraining and provision for supportive services to regular classroom teachers many fear that mainstreaming will result not only in deteriorated education for handicapped, but will bring less effective education for all students. . . . Although regular classroom teachers may have some training in the education of the handicapped many will not have the expertise to prescribe learning experiences for all of them. . . . The retraining of every public school teacher is quite improbable and . . . very expensive. . . . [Therefore] mainstreaming may produce adverse results unless there is a major effort to help teachers cope in the daily classroom.

Parents of disabled children fear that mainstreaming will destroy everything they have worked for and that the financial crises faced by the school systems throughout the country will severely affect the education of special children. Brenton (1974) states

Some parents of handicapped children dislike the concept of mainstreaming—the reason . . . is that they worked hard to get their boys and girls special education and they're afraid that now their children will be dumped into regular classrooms without supportive services, or that if the services are available at first they will vanish the moment city and state budgets are cut.

Parents and teachers of the handicapped have another fear about mainstreaming. They fear that mainstreaming will be seen by certain sectors of the educational community as a means of making money. Just as the new math and open education were seen as "the thing" to talk about, write about, and to put into action and then to be written off as not working, it is feared that mainstreaming will go the same route. Brenton (1974) notes:

Another . . . risk concerned with mainstreaming is that it will eventually become too popular—that it will be seen as a cure-all.

Hechinger (1976) states that

Essentially sympathetic commentators nevertheless express concern lest, in the way of so many American educational panaceas, mainstreaming will abolish special education classes altogether, not on the basis of sound pedagogical policy, but in response to irresistible ideological pressure.

Thus, we see that there are major objections to mainstreaming. The advocates and opponents of mainstreaming provide evidence to support their arguments. There is also a third camp which is not opposed to mainstreaming, but is not as enthusiastic as the advocates. This group is composed of conservative, cautious individuals who take a careful look at the situation and dislike the "hurry-up-let's-do-it-now" philosophy. According to Hechinger (1976):

Advocates of caution insist that they do not want to stop the beneficial trend toward returning as many handicapped youngsters as possible to regular classes for all or part of the time. What they do want to stop, or at least slow down, is the bandwagon of instant change and the confusion between civil rights and the right kind of education for every child.

There is supportive evidence for both points of view. Advocates of mainstreaming make a strong case with examples of successful programs throughout the country. Opponents also provide strong supportive evidence citing failures and problems created by mainstreaming. However, there are circumstances and unforseen problems which arise when any innovation is put into practice on a large scale. Hechinger (1976) states that

> Mass education tends to aggravate the problem faced only in small scale projects. The difficulties are, moreover multiplied in direct proportion to the often inadequate preparation of the teachers asked to respond to the new situation and the equally inadequate facilities of the ordinary school.

The body of literature called change theory attempts to deal with ways of helping people accept innovations and of examining conditions which make an innovation a success or failure. The work of Gross, Giaquinta, and Bernstein (1971) points out that a new program may appear successful in theory, but in practice many factors contribute to success. Among the factors necessary is the role of the school and district administrators. Administrative support and guidance and the fact that teachers do not operate in a vacuum cannot be overlooked. The teacher operates in the context of an administrative system. The actions of administrators can have a critical baring on the implementation of an innovation, most notably in establishing and maintaining the conditions that will facilitate staff implementation of the innovation. Administrators have an obligation to the teachers to:

1. take the steps necessary to provide a clear picture of new role requirements;
2. adjust organizational arrangements to make them compatible with the innovation;
3. provide necessary retraining experience required if the capabilities for coping with the difficulties in *implementing the innovation* are to develop;
4. provide the resources necessary to carry out the innovation;
5. provide the appropriate rewards and supports to maintain the staff's willingness to make implementation efforts overtime.

Gross, Giacquinta, and Bernstein make a point of emphasizing retraining for coping with the difficulties associated with an innovation. What kinds of new skills will teachers need to deal with handicapped children in the regular classroom? *Education Digest* (1976) states that

The most immediate training needs for classroom teachers include the development of: understanding how a handicap affects learning, skill in recognizing handicaps, prescriptive teaching, skill in behavior management techniques, understanding of an ability to respond to the emotional needs of handicapped children.

It is important to acknowledge the necessity of providing adequate preparation for teachers and schools to accept handicapped children. A smooth transition to a new situation depends upon preparation of personnel and facilities. Attitudes must be examined and in many cases brought out into the open. Not every teacher will be able to accept a handicapped child into the classroom. Therefore, it is important to treat every teacher as an individual and not demand that every teacher accept handicapped children. This would defeat the purpose of mainstreaming. Those who do accept the special child must have help in dealing with the new situation. Just as Gross, Giacquinta, and Bernstein identified the importance of administrative leadership in making an innovation work, *Education Digest* (1976) has made seven (7) recommendations for nation-wide guidance in dealing with the impact of mainstreaming. It is felt by this author that it would be wise to follow the seven recommendations to insure success for both children and teachers. The seven points are:

1. The programs must be closely monitored to ensure educational services for the handicapped without diminishing the educational opportunities of others . . . study mainstreaming and its alternatives and strictly define the conditions under which mainstreaming will be permitted (child's needs, class size, supportive services, preparation of staff, procedural safeguards).
2. Financial support for in-service training of the regular teacher which emphasize skills acquisition and leadership development.
3. Training of administrative and special education personnel to work with regular teachers. All three groups should be trained together to break barriers and facilitate coordination.
4. Pre-service training programs should be aware of curriculums for personnel to work with handicapped children.
5. The National Institute of Education should investigate types of widespread delivery systems for in-service training.
6. All relevant Federal sources should be coordinated to provide teachers and school systems with materials, information and consultation which will increase their capacity to service handicapped children.

7. As a force for rapid change in teacher preparation, state certification requirements are invaluable.

It is recommended that the Office of Education or the National Institute of Education sponsor regional conferences which aim at the examination and rapid revision of certification requirements to include training in the education of handicapped children. . . .

Thus we see that coordination and cooperation are necessary to provide quality education for all children. Careful management and slow implementation of mainstreaming programs will provide a basis for evaluation of its success or failure. An innovation must be given time to "live." Change theory cites 5 years as the life-time required for an innovation to prove itself. Any less time and it is very difficult to evaluate success or failure adequately. An innovation must be allowed to grow and develop overtime to prove its worth. We in the educational community need to go slowly and watch mainstreaming over the years before we pronounce it a success or failure. We need to ask critical questions about the effects of mainstreaming on the handicapped and non-handicapped child and on the teacher.

The advocates and opponents of mainstreaming cite evidence to support their points of view. We need to examine all the evidence carefully in order to make decisions based on data and not on emotional reactions. Every child is entitled to quality education regardless of his or her handicaps. Educators must think of the child as an individual and not make mass decisions. Mainstreaming may be the answer for one child and not for others. Mainstreaming can become a beneficial practice if handled conscientiously.

REFERENCES

Brenton, Myron. Mainstreaming the Handicapped. *Today's Education,* March-April, 1974, 20-25.

Carpenter, Robert. Get Everyone Involved when You Mainstream Your Child. *Instructor Magazine,* 85(1) August-September, 1975, 181-188.

Culver, Carmen, and Hoban, Gary (editors). *The Power To Change: Issues for the Innovative Educator.* New York: McGraw-Hill, 1973.

Education Digest. The Challenge of Mainstreaming. 42(3), November, 1976, 6-9.

Fiske, Edward. Special Education is Now a Matter of Civil Rights. *New York Times-Spring Survey of Education,* April 25, 1976, p. 1.

Gickling, Edward E., and Theobold, John T. Mainstreaming: Affect or Effect. *Journal of Special Education,* 9(3), March, 1975, 317-328.

Gross, Neal, Giacquinta, Joseph B., and Bernstein, Marilyn. *Implementing Organizational Innovations.* New York: Basic Books, 1971.

Hechinger, Fred M. Bringing the Handicapped into the Mainstream. *New York Times-Spring Survey of Education,* April 25, 1976, p. 15.

Manopoli, John, et al. Teachers' Experiences in Massachusetts. *Today's Education,* 65(2), March-April, 1976, 23-27.

NYSUT Looks at Special Education Law. Testimony of Thomas Y. Hobart. *New York Teacher,* 18(29), May 22, 1977, 2-5.

Roberts, Bonnie. Making it into "Mainstreaming." *Teacher Magazine,* 93(4), December, 1975, 37-39.

Sarason, Seymour B. *The Culture of the School and the Problem of Change.* Boston: Allyn and Bacon, 1971.

Shanker, Albert. Help Ahead for Handicapped, New Law Also Creates Some Problems. *New York Times,* March 20, 1977.

Sheldon, Jan, and Sherman, James. The Right to Educate the Retarded. *Journal of Education,* 156(3), August, 1974, 24-48.

Vernon, McCay, and Athey, Judy. The Holcomb Plan. *Instructor Magazine,* 86(5), January, 1977, 136-137.

Waleski, Dorothy. The Physically Handicapped in the Regular Classroom. *Education Digest,* 30(8), April, 1965, 38-41.

Wechsler, Henry, Suarez, Amorita, McFadden, Mary. Teachers' Attitudes Toward the Education of Physically Handicapped Children: Implications for the Implementation of Massachusetts Chapter 766. *Journal of Education,* 157(1), February, 1975, 17-24.

Weintraub, Frederick, J., and Abeson, Alan. New Education Policies for the Handicapped: The Quiet Revolution. *Phi Delta Kappan,* 55(8), April, 1974, 526-569.

SUGGESTED READINGS

Alson, Mary Lou. He's Blind-He's in our Class-Everybody's Learning. *Instructor Magazine,* 87(2), September, 1977, 222-224.

Birch, Jack W. *Mainstreaming: Educable Mentally Retarded Children in Regular Classes.* University of Minnesota: Leadership Training Institute/ Special Education, 1974.

Board of Education of the City of N.Y. *Educating Visually Handicapped Pupils.* New York: 1967.

Board of Education of the City of N.Y. *Educating the Physically Handicapped.* New York: 1971.

Peltzman, Barbara R. Josh, a Disabled Reader and How He was Helped: A case study. *Instructor Magazine,* 86(6), February, 1977, 151-153.

St. John, Walter, and Child, Charles. Paul-Justin Two

Case Stories. *Instructor Magazine,* 85(6), February, 1976, 114-117.

Solomon, Edward L. N.Y. City's Prototype School for

Educating the Handicapped. *Phi Delta Kappan,* 59(1), September, 1977, 7-10.

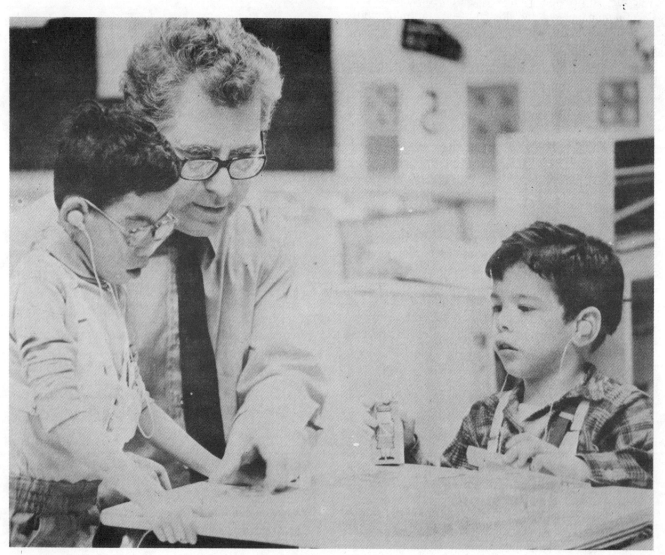

Samuel Teicher

Chapter 38
Sharpening Our Focus on Learning Disability

Richard A. Schere*

The largest percentage of children with mental handicaps are those who are classified as having learning disabilities. A national analysis of the handicaps of school children by state indicates that the learning disability category accounts for 42% of the handicapped population (Hallahan, Keller and Ball, 1986). However, just what a learning disability is has been hard to discern. Congress defined specific learning disability as a disorder "in one or more of the basic psychological processes involved in understanding or in using language, spoken or written, which may manifest itself in an imperfect ability to listen, think, speak, read, write, spell, or do mathematical calculations." Congress' definition excluded such conditions as visual, hearing, and motor handicap, mental retardation, emotional disturbance, and environmental, cultural, or economic disadvantage. It included such conditions as perceptual handicap, brain injury, minimal brain dysfunction, dyslexia, and developmental aphasia. (*Federal Register*, 1977, p. 65083).

This "definition of consensus" (Bryan and Bryan, 1975, p. 3) was seen by most professionals as very vague and extremely hard to operationalize. A study by a task force of Division 33 of the American Psychological Association culminated in an operational definition of learning disability as "an academic deficit accompanied by a disorder in one or more of the basic psychological processes involved in understanding or using language—spoken or written—in a child whose intellectual, emotional, and/or physical status allows for participation in a traditional academic curriculum" (Schere, Richardson and Bialer, 1980, p. 9). This definition excluded physiology as a major component because learning disability was viewed as an effect that had multiple causes. Each critical element in this definition, (1) academic achievement deficit, (2) basic psychological processes, and (3) exclusion factors, was operationally defined and specific strategies for measuring each element were proposed.

Academic achievement deficit was defined as being at fifty percent of grade expectation in a specific academic area (e.g. reading, arithmetic). Grade expectation was determined by "time in school."

In order to measure basic psychological processes, the following recommendations were made:

1. Skill deficiencies will be "suspected" when a child's failure on at least three sub-tests of diagnostic achievement tests appear related to a common skill area found within an accepted psychoneurological model (e.g. visual motor integration, auditory discrimination, visual memory at the abstract presentation level).
2. "Suspected" skill deficiencies will be "confirmed" when a direct measure of the skill area places its level one or more standard deviations below the mean for children of that age. (Schere, pp. 9-17).

One of the difficulties with the classification of learning disabilities has been that many states had little experience with this handicap until the Federal legislation of 1975. Despite the coining of the term (Kirk, 1963) many states such as New York never before had classes for the learning disabled. Rather, such children were placed in health conservation classes with presumably incurable minimal brain dysfunctions. With each passing year, more and more experience with learning disabled youngsters has created new questions for professionals to consider:

1. In light of the interaction between left and right hemisphere processes needed for successful academic achievement, should the construct of learning disability focus so completely on spoken and written language?
2. Are not the many studies that attempt to identify patterns in such measures as the Wechsler Intelligence scales (for purposes of differentiating learning

*Dr. Richard A. Schere is Professor of School Psychology, Brooklyn College, CUNY, and Director of the Kennedy Learning Clinic.

disabled persons from persons with other handicaps) at fault because they do not consider the many different kinds of learning disabilities?

The essence of a learning disability is a disordered or weakly developed skill that directly hinders achievement in learning tasks that are dependent on that particular skill. They need not be left hemisphere language skills. A child who has difficulty visually imaging concrete concepts in his right hemisphere may have academic difficulty in such school tasks as problem solving and/or following directions.

Recent clinical experience has brought into light another problem that pertains to the interaction between left and right hemisphere processes and illustrates that there are many kinds of learning disability. Youngsters, many of whom are quite intelligent, have great learning difficulty when one very strong hemisphere must interface with a significant weaker hemisphere. In this case the weaker hemisphere need not be below average. Rather, it must be significantly weaker than the stronger hemisphere. This characteristic is most easily measured by a significant difference between the verbal portion and the performance portion in the Wechsler intelligence scales. However, one must be careful, since research has established that there are many causes for significant verbal-performance differences. Sattler (1974, p. 199) has indicated that significant differences between verbal and performance overall scores can be: (1) an expression of interests, (2) an expression of cognitive style, (3) an expression of psychopathology (such as emotional disturbance or brain damage), (4) deficiencies (or strengths) in processing information, (5) deficiencies (or strengths) in certain modes and expression, (6) deficiencies (or strengths) in working under conditions of pressure (such as time constraints on the performance scale), or (7) sensory deficits.

It is suggested that when verbal skills (left hemisphere) are significantly stronger or weaker than non-verbal, visual-motor (performance scale-right hemisphere) skills, even if none of the weaker skills are below average, a problem often occurs that is best perceived as a *disorder of cognitive rhythm.* The effect of such disorder is somewhat like running a race with a weight on one ankle.

Some youngsters have "thought out" their sentence even though, because of weaker visual-motor skill, they are writing only the second letter of the third word. Other youngsters may have the "gestalt" of what they wish to express, but, because of weaker verbal processing skills, can't find the words they need quickly enough. Such youngsters experience great frustration when working at traditional learning tasks. Many view themselves as "lazy." They are often considered "underachievers." If you know a bright youngster who has dropped out of high school, he may be a youngster with a disturbed cognitive rhythm.

Research needs to be designed to study disorders of cognitive rhythm and other specific forms of learning disability. For some, the inability to function fluidly in cognitive process creates a learning disability that is handicapping. Others struggle through their disability because they are intelligent, but they must work harder, longer, and with a greater tension than most others of equal ability. Such youngsters need to be identified, appreciated, encouraged, and assisted.

BIBLIOGRAPHY

Bryan T. and Bryan J. *Understanding Learning Disabilities.* New York: Alfred, 1975.

Federal Register, Vol. 42, No. 250, Thursday, December 29, 1977.

Hallahan, D.P., Keller C.E. & Ball, D.W. "A Comparison of the Prevalence Rate Variability from State to State for each category of Special Education." *Remedial and Special Education,* Vol. 7, No. 2 March/April, 1986, pp. 8-14.

Kirk, S.A. *Behavioral Diagnosis and Remediation of Learning Disabilities: Proceedings of the First Annual Meeting of the Conference on Exploration into the Problems of the Perceptually Handicapped child,* 1963.

Sattler, J.M. *Assessment of Children's Intelligence* Philadelphia: W.B. Saunders, 1974.

Schere, R., Richardson, E., and Bialer, I. "Toward Operationalizing a Psychoeducational Definition of Learning Disabilities," *Journal of Abnormal Child Psychology,* Vol. 8, No. 1, 1980, pp. 5-20.

Chapter 39

All-Day Kindergarten for All: Early Childhood Education in New York City

Charlotte Frank and Marjorie McAllister*

In September 1983, the largest urban school system in the United Sates embarked on an ambitious venture in early childhood education—providing all-day kindergarten programs for about 50,000 five-year-old children. What motivated New York City's actions? What steps did the central administration take to provide staff development for the many teachers and supervisors who would be involved in the new program? How were curricula developed and disseminated? What plans are being made to extend the educational gains of the all-day kindergarten program through the early childhood years?

A Bit of Kindergarten History

In New York City, State aid for kindergarten began in the 1940s. At that time, kindergarten programs were half-day due to both limited funding and current thinking which supported the belief that children should be at home with their mothers or other family caregivers the remainder of the time.

In 1982–83, 46,000 youngsters were enrolled in half-day kindergarten programs while 8,500 children were enrolled in all-day kindergartens. (New York City is comprised of 32 community school districts. Each of these community school districts allocates funds according to district priorities. Funds for the all-day kindergarten programs which served these 8,500 children came from Federal and other funding sources.)

As current research regarding contemporary society and changes in the family structure emerged, it became increasingly obvious that some modifications in the educational system had to be made to respond to new needs.

- Greater numbers of educators were challenging the belief that five-year-old children did not have the physical stamina or the emotional maturity to participate in a full-day educational program in a public school environment.
- Increasing numbers of children were coming from households where both parents worked full time.
- Many of the city's youngest children lived in one-parent households.
- Large numbers of young children were "latch-key" children—children who had very little or virtually no supervision when they returned home from school.
- Many neighborhoods throughout the city could not provide safe and supervised after-school education and/or recreation.
- An alarming number of young children tended to remain indoors, alone, with the TV as babysitter.

Cognizant of these trends, the New York City Board of Education recognized the tremendous educational potential of an all-day kindergarten program. Increased time in a well-supervised educational environment would provide additional opportunities to build essential cognitive, social, and motor skills. Children could be encouraged to think, reason, learn, and play in a language-rich setting surrounded by their peers. In 1983–84, 55,000 children participated in the new citywide all-day kindergarten program. Currently, there are approximately 60,000 children attending all-day kindergarten classes, with programs in every New York City community school district.

*Charlotte Frank is Executive Director and Marjorie McAllister is Director of Early Childhood Education, Division of Curriculum and Instruction, New York City Board of Education.

Curriculum Development

In expanding the all-day kindergarten program, staff development was essential to prepare school and district personnel for a lengthened kindergarten day that would require many additional classes often staffed by teachers who, though licensed, had never taught kindergarten before. To assist staff, a new teacher's guide, *Getting Started in the All-Day Kindergarten* (1983), was developed under the direction of the Board's Division of Curriculum and Instruction and was distributed to all kindergarten teachers and elementary school principals. Evaluation data for 1983-84 indicated that 96 percent of those kindergarten teachers interviewed reported having used the new manual and almost all found it to be useful.[1] A major reason for the success of this 354-page curriculum can be attributed to its "grass roots" development. Curriculum writers for this project were selected from among New York City's most innovative and experienced kindergarten and early childhood teachers and supervisors.

Some children come to all-day kindergarten from pre-kindergarten, Head Start, or day care programs, while others come with no prior group experiences. In addition, children have varying language and home backgrounds. In New York City children speak as many as 60 languages other than English.[2] In developing the teacher's guide, a primary goal was to offer strategies for meeting the needs of children with such diverse experiences. The guide was written with the understanding that five-year-olds grow and learn developmentally. It incorporates practical suggestions for activities and first-hand experiences using concrete materials. Through experiential learning, the child is stimulated to think, ask questions, and solve problems. In order to develop these abilities, the teacher's guide describes an integrated approach in which all curriculum areas are taught within the context of themes. Beginning reading, writing, mathematics, and reasoning skills are developed as children explore these themes. Large group instruction is suggested and small group activities at learning centers are especially emphasized.

Staff Development

In August 1983, four experienced staff members from each of the 32 community school districts participated in a one-week training program offered at central headquarters. This training enabled these "turnkey trainers" to then plan and conduct practical, method-oriented staff development activities for the kindergarten teachers in their respective districts. District training took place the first week of school when children attended school for only a half-day. Approximately 900 new and experi-

enced teachers and their supervisors participated in staff development workshops organized either by the Division of Curriculum and Instruction or the community school districts. Because ongoing support is essential, additional staff development workshops were offered during the school year on topics of general concern such as classroom management, mathematics and science learning centers, and parent involvement.

Parent Involvement

Parents are encouraged to participate in the all-day kindergarten program through individual and group conferences with teachers and through hands-on workshops. They are also invited to visit classrooms during the school day to share their skills and experiences with children. Informal observation indicates that this parent participation generates positive attitudes towards learning and expands children's knowledge.

Evaluation

Assessing the impact for this major change in early childhood education in New York City required careful planning. The evaluation design called for classroom observations, analysis of the reactions of teachers and principals, and the collection of information about children's backgrounds and prior group experiences. Achievement data was collected utilizing the *Brigance K&1 Screen* (Brigance, 1982) as a pre- and post-test. Data from New York City's *Language Assessment Battery* (LAB)[3] was available for limited English proficient children. In total, 2,327 kindergarten children were included in the study. Information was collected on such variables as home language, place of birth, preschool experiences, attendance, class mobility, sex, and entry-level achievement.

The formal evaluation report indicates certain significant findings:[4]

1. Although children in both all- and half-day classes made substantial and significant gains between the pre- and post-test for both the *Brigance K&1 Screen* and the *Language Abilities Test,* the performance of the full-day children, including those with limited English proficiency, surpassed that of the half-day children; i.e., the all-day achievement level was significantly higher than for the half-day sample.

2. Low achieving, all-day kindergarten children demonstrated higher average post-test achievement scores than their half-day counterparts. It appears that the lengthened school day provided additional opportunities to acquire new skills.

3. Although the relationship is small, the higher the mobility rate the lower the post-test score. Also, chil-

dren with good attendance records tended to score higher than did children who were absent more frequently.

First and Second Grade: Assuring Continued Gains

The all-day kindergarteners of last year are now in first grade. To maintain and extend the gains they made, the school-based staff development program for 1984-85 included a variety of workshops and the preparation of a new, 366-page first-grade curriculum guide, *"Now We Are Six": A Guide to Teaching First Grade* (1984). Once again, effective teachers and supervisors served as curriculum writers and staff developers.

This guide continues the thematic approach to learning which was emphasized in kindergarten. To provide guidance for new and inexperienced teachers, this manual includes additional information on topics such as planning and organizing the classroom environment, and developing literacy. The scope and sequence for the curriculum areas included in *"Now We Are Six"* integrates the educational requirements of the New York State Education Department and the New York City Board of Education.

The teacher's guide for second grade is currently under development and continues to support a thematic approach to learning. The curriculum guide and staff development efforts again emphasize the importance of interactive teaching, participatory learning, language facility, and the development of reasoning skills.

Problems Along the Way

Plans for the All-Day Kindergarten Program began in May for implementation in September. It was a massive task, and much was accomplished in a short time. However, problems and concerns arose that required both short- and long-range solutions:

- In several districts, there was not enough space in the home school to accommodate all the children who ultimately registered for the All-Day Kindergarten Program.
- Since nearly 900 new classes were organized, vendors had difficulty in supplying equipment and materials in a timely fashion. The sheer volume of the purchase orders also required a great deal of processing time on the part of both the district and central administrations.
- Funds to provide for paraprofessional assistants were generally not available. Certain districts were able to assign paraprofessionals; other districts were not.
- While all classes were staffed with licensed teachers, many did not have specific training and experience in early childhood education.

All of these problems are of the utmost concern to our administrators, supervisors, and teachers; and we are taking specific steps to address them. Our curriculum guides and professional staff development programs are making a major contribution by giving teachers and supervisors the tools necessary to provide quality instruction. Problems involving space restriction are being solved through class reorganization, busing, and assigning or constructing new classroom space. Recognizing the importance of paraprofessional assistance in a comprehensive all-day kindergarten program, central and district administrators are making a concerted effort to provide this support. The commitment by central district, and school staff and the City Council of New York City to improve the early childhood program has been demonstrated by a remarkable dedication to creatively solving problems as they arise.

The Vision for the Future

The New York City public schools have embarked on exciting new programs in early childhood education that are designed to reduce the number of children retained in Promotional Policy Gates classes[5] and ultimately reduce the high school dropout rate. The expanded kindergarten program is based on research and experience indicating that the needs of a diverse student population can be met through early intervention programs. In all-day classes, five- and six-year-olds can expand their language competencies and develop the concepts and reasoning skills that will enable increased academic achievement. The formative and summative data collected on the progress of these children will assist in implementing, modifying and expanding programs where success has been demonstrated. Our current efforts in the first and second grade reflect our commitment to improving the quality of the entire early childhood education program in our public schools by including planned experiences that build on the concepts and skills learned during the previous years. As one early childhood teacher so aptly expressed, "Children should begin school in September in a classroom that feels familiar and not like a foreign country."

The task is not yet finished. Not only will curriculum and staff development continue, but also evaluation of the programs' effectiveness. The data from current evaluations will help shape the early childhood programs for the 1980s and 1990s. Understanding the implications of today's experiences will help us successfully meet tomorrow's challenges.

FOOTNOTES

1. *All-Day Kindergarten Programs 1983-1984 Preliminary Findings,* Office of Educational Assessment, New York City Public Schools, October, 1984.

2.   Data summarized from reports submitted for 1983-84 by community school districts and high schools for the New York State Comprehensive Plan for Compensatory Programs.

3.   The *Language Assessment Battery* (LAB), which measures listening and speaking skills in English, was developed by the New York City Board of Education. It is used to determine eligibility for services in bilingual education or English as a second language.

4.   *All-Day Kindergarten Program 1983-1984: Effects on Student Growth,* Office of Educational Assessment, New York City Public Schools, January, 1985.

5.   The Promotional Policy Gates Program was initiated in 1981 in New York City for students in the fourth and seventh grades whose achievement in reading was not at the level required for success in the next higher grade. In 1984-85, achievement is being measured by the *California Achievement Test* and, for limited English proficient students, by the English-*Language Assessment Battery*.

REFERENCES

Boehm, Ann E. *Boehm Test of Basic Concepts,* preschool edition (experimental version), Forms Q and R. Cleveland, OH: The Psychological Corporation, n.d.

Brigance, Albert H. *Brigance K&I Screen.* North Billerica, MA: Curriculum Associates, Inc., 1982.

Division of Curriculum and Instruction, *Getting Started in the All-Day Kindergarten.* Brooklyn, NY: New York City Board of Education, 1983.

Division of Curriculum and Instruction, *"Now We Are Six": A Guide to Teaching First Grade.* Brooklyn, NY: New York City Board of Education, 1984.

Lazar, I., Darlington, R., Murray H., Royce, J. and Snipper, A. *Lasting Effects of Early Education.* Monographs of the Society for Research in Child Development, 47 (1-2, Serial No. 194), 1982.

Office of Educational Evaluation, *An Evaluation of the 1982-83 Experimental Full-Day Prekindergarten Program.* Brooklyn, NY: New York City Board of Education, October, 1983.

Weikart, D.P., Bond, J.T., & McNeil, J.T. *The Ypsilanti Perry Preschool Project:* Preschool Years and Longitudinal Results Through Fourth Grade, Monographs of the High/Scope Educational Research Foundation, 3. Ypsilanti, MI: High/Scope Press, 1978.

Weikart, D.P., Deloria, D., Lawser, S., & Wiegerink, R., *Longitudinal Results of the Ypsilanti Perry Preschool Project,* Monographs of the High/Scope Educational Research Foundation, 1. Ypsilanti, MI: High/Scope Press, 1970.

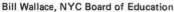

Bill Wallace, NYC Board of Education

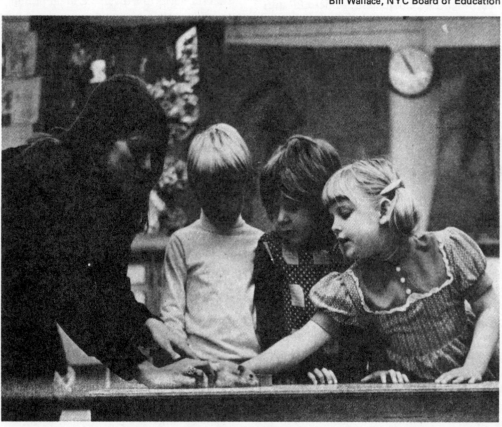

Chapter 40
A New Perspective on Math and Science Education
Iris C. Rotberg*

Most of the reports on education that have been receiving such widespread attention are quite grim, particularly in their conclusions about the state of mathematics and science education in U.S. public schools. Although *A Nation at Risk* acknowledges the success of our schools in graduating nearly 75% of our young people from high school and enrolling nearly in college, it nevertheless concludes, "Our once unchallenged preeminence in commerce, industry, science, and technological innovation is being overtaken by competitors throughout the world."[1]

Not all observers of education have been so pessimistic. But most have agreed that mathematics and science education in the U.S. are deficient in at least five respects:

1. The U.S. system of education is not producing trained scientists, mathematicians, engineers, and computer scientists in numbers sufficient to meet economic and military needs.
2. The problems will become even more severe in the next decade, when technological advances will increase the need for highly trained personnel in these fields.
3. U.S. students are less well trained, as measured by their test scores, than are their peers in other industrialized countries.
4. U.S. students today are less well trained than were their predecessors.
5. These problems result from a general laxity in educational standards and from a shortage of qualified science and mathematics teachers.

I will discuss here the extent to which these conclusions are supported by research findings. I will then describe the tradeoffs in curriculum, school finance, and social opportunity that should be considered before implementing solutions to these perceived problems.

Research Findings

1. *Is the U.S. system of education producing adequate numbers of trained scientists, mathematicians, engineers, and computer scientists to meet economic and military needs?* Consider some recent findings of the Bureau of Labor Statistics (BLS) and other organizations.[2] These figures show that the current supply of scientists and mathematicians is adequate, except in a few subfields of physical and biological science. Indeed, projections indicate that by 1990 the number of new science and mathematics graduates at all degree levels will *exceed* the number able to find jobs in those fields.

The projections also show an overall balance between supply and demand for engineers for the rest of the 1980s. The shortage of engineers that has received so much public attention in the past few years has been limited to a few specialties—electronics, computer design, and petroleum engineering—and certainly does not justify massive efforts to change basic curricula. There may be a shortage of engineers with doctorates who are willing to join university faculties. But this shortage is caused not by any inadequacies of the educational system but simply by a lack of financial incentive for young engineers, who are well-paid by industry, to accept lower-paid university positions. The BLS sums it up this way:

> During the 1980s, the United State will be turning out about twice as many bachelor's degree graduates in engineering as in the 1960s, a decade of rapid economic growth, high defense spending, and a space program that put an astronaut on the moon.[3]

The fact is that we will not need more engineers than we are now turning out. While the current demand for trained computer scientists does exceed the supply, the

*Dr. Iris C. Rotberg is Program Director, National Science Foundation. Reprinted with the permission of the author and *Phi Delta Kappan*, June, 1984.

number of students receiving computer science degrees is increasing so rapidly that by the end of the 1980s even these shortages should be over.[4]

In general, labor market projections show that the educational system is in fact producing adequate numbers of scientists, mathematicians, and engineers. Shortages that do exist are likely to be short-term, and there will be surpluses in many fields.

The BLS suggests that some of the exaggerated predictions of shortages stem from the methodology used in surveying the projected business and military demand.[5] Corporations typically overestimate both overall industrial growth and their share of the market. Each defense industry apparently assumes that it *will* receive a disproportionate share of the contracts it bids on. This multiplies the overall requirements of the industry many times, because only one award will actually be made. The result is a large overestimate of the need for technical staff. Other evidence suggests that corporations report shortages of highly trained personnel when they cannot attract the best graduates at the salaries they would prefer to pay. Under such circumstances, managers too quickly conclude—almost as a defensive gesture—that the fault lies in the dearth of qualified applicants.

2. *Will technological advances in the next decade rapidly accelerate the demand for highly trained scientific and computer personnel?* No one can predict with certainty what these advances or their effects will be. But projections suggest that some computer and engineering fields will be among the *fastest-growing* occupations. However, contrary to popular belief, the greatest *number* of new jobs will not be created in these fields. Most new jobs will be in low-skilled occupations that require quite low levels of scientific and mathematical knowledge.[6] This projection is consistent with the findings of a recent study of college graduates in the mid-Seventies, which showed that almost half were employed in jobs that did not require college training. These graduates were doing jobs in which at least 70% of their colleagues doing the same job had not attended college.[7]

Not one of the 19 occupations expected to produce the largest numbers of new jobs in the 13-year period between 1982 and 1985 will be in a high-technology area. Recent estimates show 779,000 new openings for building custodians, 744,000 new openings for cashiers, 719,000 new openings for secretaries, and 696,000 new openings for office clerks—but only 217,000 new openings for computer systems analysts, 205,000 new openings for computer programmers, 584,000 new openings for engineers, and 418,000 new openings for engineering and science technicians.[8] Probably more surprising is the prediction that the number of new kindergarten and elementary teaching positions (511,000) will be greater than the number of positions for computer systems analysts

and for computer programmers *combined*—and not substantially lower than the total number of new openings for engineers.

Compare these numbers with the results of a survey of freshmen entering college in 1983: 3.1% of these students planned to become elementary school teachers; 10.8% planned to become engineers; 8.5% planned to become computer programmers or analysts.[9] Interest in computer fields among college-bound seniors taking the SAT is more than three times greater today than in 1979 and more than six times greater than in 1975.[10]

Just as important, it is not at all certain that the technological innovations of the next 10 to 20 years will require higher levels of skill.[11] Some economists argue that high technology is more likely to reduce the skill requirements of jobs than to increase them and that the supply of technically trained personnel will outstrip the demand for their skills. This conclusion is contrary to the popular assumption that we can expect shortages of qualified scientists and engineers.

Computers offer one example of potential reduction in skill requirements.[12] Before recent advances in computer technology, programmers and operators needed many complex skills to use computers. Now the creative and skilled work is done by systems analysts, packaged programs are readily available, and programming and operating a computer have become routine tasks. The drop in prices of home computers also argues against the ever-increasing need for a high-cost labor force to develop and produce these machines.

I do not mean to suggest by all of this evidence that our society will not need significant numbers of highly trained scientists, engineers, and computer specialists. We clearly need such specialists. However, reports of shortages, poor training, and the proportion of total employment accounted for by these fields have been greatly exaggerated.

3. *Are U.S. students less well trained in science and mathematics (as measured by achievement test scores) than their peers in other industrialized countries?* I doubt it. The *average* high school student enrolled in the U.S. scores lower in international comparisons than the *average* high school student enrolled in other industrialized countries. But these comparisons do not compare equal proportions of the high school age groups. In Europe, academic schooling for those between ages 16 and 18, while perhaps not elitist, certainly does not attempt to serve virtually the entire age group. Only about 20% of the high-school-age children in Europe attend upper-secondary school—the highest-achieving 20%. About 80% of that age group in the U.S. attend high school. Consequently, international studies of achievement often compare the average score of more than three-fourths of the age group in the U.S. with the average score of the top

9% in West Germany, the top 13% in the Netherlands, or only the top 45% in Sweden.

However, when the same proportions of relevant age groups are compared, the results are quite different. Top U.S. students score at about the same level in mathematics as comparable groups in many other industrialized countries, though they still score lower than their peers in Sweden, Japan, and Israel. Top U.S. students also score at about the same levels in science as students in other industrialized countries—better than students in France, Belgium, and Italy; not as well as students in New Zealand, England, and Australia.[13] I could go on, but it is sufficient to note that, when equal proportions of age groups are compared, the results do not reflect badly on the U.S. system of education. This is especially true in light of the fact that U.S. schools not only provide an education of high quality for the brightest students but, unlike their counterparts abroad, must do so in a school environment that includes virtually the entire age group, often working together in the same classroom.

4. *Are U.S. students today less well trained in science and mathematics (as measured by test scores) than were their predecessors?* The achievement test scores of students who are likely to major in science or mathematics have remained high in these areas. Declines are more evident in tests that assess the basic scientific and mathematical knowledge of the general population.

Scores on College Board science achievement tests in biology, physics, and chemistry, taken by the top students among the college-bound population; are as high as or higher than they were in the early 1970s. The same is true of mathematics achievement test scores.[14] In addition, scores on College Board Advanced Placement tests in science and mathematics were at least as high in 1983 as they were in 1973, despite increased numbers of students taking the tests.[15] Achievement test scores on the Graduate Record Examinations (GRE) show mixed results over the past nine years. Mathematics scores have gone up; physics scores have gone down; engineering scores have remained steady.[16]

The widely reported declines in test scores are based on tests administered to a broad cross section of the population. Even here results are mixed. The National Assessment of Educational Progress (NAEP), which assesses representative samples of elementary and secondary students, shows that 9-year-olds have scored at about the same level in science since the 1972-73 science assessment, while scores for 13- and 17-year-olds have declined.[17] During roughly the same period, mathematics scores have stayed about the same for 9-year-olds, improved for 13-year-olds, and declined for 17-year-olds.[18]

The scores of college-bound students on the American College Testing (ACT) Program natural science examination (a broader cross section of students than those who take the College Board achievement tests) have remained approximately the same since the mid-1970s.[19] Mathematics scores for college-bound students on both the ACT exam and the Scholastic Aptitude Test (SAT) declined from the late 1960s to the mid-1970s, when they began to level off. ACT math scores show some evidence of continuing decline, while SAT math scores have remained essentially the same for the past six years.[20] Finally, scores of graduate school applicants on the quantitative portion of the GRE are higher now than they were in the early 1970s.[21]

When interpreting the results of all of these tests, it is most important to remember that changes in the populations taking the test have a great deal to do with changes in the scores. The ACT Program notes that "small changes in average scores can result from a variety of factors, the most notable being changes in the demographic characteristics of the students taking the tests."[22] An advisory panel on SAT scores noted that as much as three-fourths of the decline in scores between 1963 and 1970 can be attributed to changes in the numbers and socioeconomic characteristics of students taking the test, and one-fourth of the decline after 1970 can be accounted for by continuing demographic shifts.[23] Moreover, these changes have nothing to do with the quality of education, and changes in test scores that can be attributed to population changes are certainly unreliable measures of the quality of education.

5. *Is there a general laxity of educational standards and a shortage of qualified science and mathematics teachers?* The actual data show that recent reports exaggerate or inadequately define both problems.

Contrary to public perception, high school students took more mathematics in 1980 than they did in 1972 and about the same amount of science.[24] Among college-bound students who took the SAT, the amount of academic coursework has *increased* over the past six years, with the largest increases occurring in mathematics and the physical sciences. There has also been greater enrollment in advanced, accelerated, and honors courses.[25]

Turning to the supply of qualified teachers, the well-publicized shortage of secondary school mathematics and science teachers has not reached serious proportions nationwide. Severe shortages may exist in certain parts of the U.S., but adequate data are not available to assess the extent of the problem. The shortages are expected to become more serious in the future because of increased high school graduation requirements and decreased enrollment in teacher education programs in mathematics and science. However, these factors will be offset somewhat by declining secondary school enrollments.[26]

Before enacting any proposed remedies for the projected shortages of science and mathematics teachers, such as extra pay or loan forgiveness programs, policy makers should consider several factors. First, teacher shortages are not limited to math and science. There are also shortages in special education and in vocational/technical fields.[27] Second, reported teacher shortages result at least partly from factors other than the unavailability of qualified math and science teachers. Budgetary constraints and an oversupply of teachers in other fields compound the problem of measuring the extent of the shortage of math and science teachers. For example, out-of-field teaching, which is used as one measure of teacher shortages, often reflects the placement of surplus teachers of other subjects who cannot be laid off because of their seniority. (Many school systems are expected to respond in this way to increased graduation requirements in mathematics and science.[28]) Indeed, out-of-field teaching occurs even in fields with teacher surpluses, when declining enrollments force schools to staff their classrooms with the most senior teachers. A North Carolina study, for example, found that out-of-field teaching in English occurred 60% as often as it did in math.[29]

Third, shortages of math and science teachers do not necessarily mean that these teachers can readily find jobs. For example, the state of Kentucky offered financial incentives for persons to enter teacher training programs in mathematics and science and then found that few available teaching positions existed for the first graduates.[30] And in April 1983—the month in which the National Commission on Excellence in Education released its report, noting "particularly severe" shortages of mathematics and science teachers—the Chicago press reported that the Chicago Board of Education had made substantial reductions in the number of math and science teachers during the past several years. Indeed, Chicago had a surplus of math and science teachers. Many of these teachers were working as substitutes and not necessarily in their fields of expertise.[31] More often than not, such problems arise as a result of financial strain on states and school districts. It is not so much that the teachers aren't needed as that the districts can't afford to hire them.

Other Considerations

The foregoing discussion suggests that recent reports tend to overstate or inadequately define the problems in mathematics and science education. Not unexpectedly, some of the proposed reforms derive from questionable assumptions about the nature of the problem and pay little attention to the overall implications for public policy.

An example may be useful. Many of the reports base their recommendations on the assumption—quite unsupported by research—that the U.S. educational system is not producing adequate numbers of highly qualified scientists, engineers, mathematicians, and computer specialists. These reports stress increasing requirements, so that all students must take more algebra, physics, or chemistry. However, the problem is quite different: the population in general is not well-informed about basic scientific issues or about how to perform simple mathematical applications, such as problem solving. The problem is *not* the number or quality of those trained to be scientists. The emphasis of the reports on increasing requirements for traditional science and math courses does little to improve the education of the large majority of students who might benefit more from curricula that are not designed along narrow disciplinary lines.

Bill Aldridge, executive director of the National Science Teachers Association, put it this way:

> High school science and math courses present content that largely duplicates content offered in college courses. These high school courses offer little more than preparation for that next course which the vast majority of students will never take. Present proposals to increase graduation requirements in science and math will force all students either to take these courses or drop out of school.[32]

Traditional courses often amount to little more than the students repeating chemical terms and formulas without understanding what they are learning or how it is relevant to the world around them. The result, which most of us know from our own experience or from that of our children, is that most students memorize a lot of material. But they cannot place it in context, understand the fields from which the material is derived, or explain how it is used. What they memorize is usually forgotten within a short time. Perhaps it would be more productive for students to understand scientific methodology and scientific issues that impinge on public policy, rather than to attempt to learn everything that is known about physics in one school year.

As Lee Shulman noted, "Forcing students to take the same chemistry or algebra II they have been avoiding for the last 20 years is no answer."[33] Irving Spitzberg, general secretary of the American Association of University Professors, summed it up this way: "Requiring courses does not guarantee learning in courses."[34] The French essayist Montaigne, in 1580, best reflected my concerns:

> But as the steps that we take walking in a gallery may tire us less than if they were taken on a fixed journey, so our lessons, occurring as if it were accidentally, without being bound to time or place, and mingling with all our other actions, will glide past unnoticed.[35]

In addition to proposing reforms that may not be based on solid evidence or a careful analysis of the problem, the reports generally overlook the implications of their recommendations for other parts of the curriculum. With notable exceptions, such as Ernest Boyer's study,[36] problems in mathematics and science education have received more attention than problems in other fields.

But other areas of the curriculum are in need of improvement at least as much as mathematics and science. SAT scores, for example, have shown *greater* declines in verbal than in math scores.[37] ACT social studies scores have declined, while science results are at least as high as they were in previous years.[38] Although the NAEP scores did not show a decline in the basic reading skills of 17-year-olds between 1970 and 1980, they did show a decline in students' ability to draw inferences from the material they read.[39] The quality of students' writing leaves much to be desired, and recent observers suggest that a simple writing requirement is more critically needed than improved science and mathematics instruction.[40] A number of engineering schools are now revising their curricula to include broader liberal arts courses.[41] Moreover, recent surveys of academic officials found that the humanities are losing many of the highest-achieving students to the sciences and engineering.[42]

In a widely reprinted article based on his recent conversations with high school and college students in the Los Angeles area, Benjamin Stein put the "problem" we face in some perspective.[43]

[A] student at (the University of Southern California) did not have any clear idea when World War II was fought. She believed it was some time this century. . . . She also had no clear notion of what had begun the war for the United States. ("Pearl Harbor? Was that when the United States dropped the atom bomb on Hiroshima?") Even more astounding, she was not sure which side Russia was on and whether Germany was on our side or against us. . . .

A few (students) have known how many U.S. senators California has, but none has known how many Nevada or Oregon has. ("Really? Even though they're so small?") . . .

Of the teenagers with whom I work, none had ever heard of Vladimir Ilyich Lenin. Only one could identify Joseph Stalin. (My favorite answer—"He was President just before Roosevelt.") . . .

None (of the students) could name even one of the first 10 Amendments to the Constitution or connect them with the Bill of Rights. . . .

Only a few could articulate in any way at all why life in a free country is different from life in an un-free country. . . .

I have mixed up episodes of ignorance of facts with ignorance of concepts because it seems to me that there is a connection. If a student has no idea when World War II

was and who the combatants were and what they fought over, that same human being is likely to be ignorant of just what this society stands for. If a young woman has never heard of the Bill for Rights, that young woman is unlikely to understand why this is a uniquely privileged nation with uniquely privileged citizens. . . .

There are other considerations in determining whether or how education reforms should be implemented. Few of the recent studies of education consider the financial or social costs of their recommendations and the trade-offs that would be required.[44] But money spent on a minor problem often uses resources that might better be spent on other, more pressing requirements. Similarly, reforms that do not consider implications for all parts of the society are likely to raise more problems than they solve. Two illustrations suggest the kinds of issues that need to be addressed.

Harold Howe estimates that the total cost of recommendations in recent education reports would be $20 billion to $30 billion in new funds *each year.*[45] To put this figure in perspective, the total federal expenditure for elementary, secondary, and higher education programs in fiscal year 1983, including student aid at the college level, was $15.4 billion. But aside from their prohibitive cost, each of the recommendations in the reform reports is fraught with controversy. How would meritorious teaching be measured? Who would decide? How would the recommendations be financed and from which sectors of our society? The recent education reports pay little attention to these issues.

Although some of these reports give a passing nod to the impressive role of the U.S. educational system in increasing social opportunity, they do not discuss the implications of such recommendations as stricter course and graduation requirements. For example, how will requiring algebra II or physics affect dropout rates, tracking, or the future employment prospects of students who fail? We cannot pretend any more to be a classless society, but we certainly do not wish to create an educational system that will put unnecessary roadblocks in the path of those who begin life with the fewest advantages. As a society, we are not content to educate only the top 10% to run the nation or its business. Moreover, there is no evidence that the brightest students are at a disadvantage in fulfilling their academic potential.

The recent discussion of education reform, prompted in part by romantic notions about future technology, has not been conducive to a careful consideration of the implications of the proposed changes. We must define precisely the problems we wish to solve and consider the broad implications of our solutions. Or else, in our rush to meet the putative demands of the future, we may neglect the students and issues most in need of attention.

FOOTNOTES

1. National Commission on Excellence in Education, *A Nation at Risk: The Imperative for Educational Reform* (Washington, D.C.: U.S. Department of Education, 1983), p. 5.

2. See, for example, Douglas Braddock, "The Job Market for Engineers: Recent Conditions and Future Prospects," *Occupational Outlook Quarterly,* Summer 1983, pp. 2-8; National Science Foundation and U.S. Department of Education, *Science and Engineering Education for the 1980's and Beyond* (Washington, D.C.: U.S. Department of Education, 1980), pp. 15-34; George T. Silvestri et al., "Occupational Employment Projections Through 1995," *Monthly Labor Review,* November 1983, pp. 37-49; Wilson K. Talley, "National Needs for Science and Technology Literacy—the Army as a Case Study," *Teacher Shortage in Science and Mathematics* (Washington, D.C.: National Institute of Education, 1983), pp. 5-8; and Betty M. Vetter, *Opportunities in Science and Engineering* (Washington, D.C.: Scientific Manpower Commission, 1982).

3. Braddock, p. 8.

4. For estimates of probable career choices, see Alexander W. Astin, *The American Freshman: National Norms for Fall 1983* (Los Angeles: American Council on Education and University of California at Los Angeles, 1983).

5. Braddock, p. 6.

6. Richard W. Riche et al., "High Technology Today and Tomorrow: Small Slice of Employment," *Monthly Labor Review,* November 1983, pp. 50-58.

7. Thomas J. More, "The Job Gap," *Chicago Sun-Times,* 18 September 1983, p. 4.

8. Silvestri, pp. 38, 45.

9. Astin, p. 48.

10. *National College-Bound Seniors, 1983,* Admissions Testing Program of the College Entrance Examination Board, 1983.

11. Henry M. Levin and Russell W. Rumberger, *The Educational Implication of High Technology* (Stanford, Calif.: Institute for Research on Educational Finance and Governance, Stanford University, 1983).

12. Ibid., pp. 9-11.

13. See Torsten Husén, "Are Standards in U.S. Schools Really Lagging Behind Those in Other Countries?," *Phi Delta Kappan,* March 1983, pp. 455-61.

14. These findings are based on data prepared by the Admissions Testing Program of the College Board for 1972-1973 and 1981-82, using corrected achievement test scores that are placed on the same scale and therefore are comparable. Test scores increased in mathematics 1 and 2, in biology, and in chemistry over the nine-year period; scores in physics declined by one point. The number of test-takers declined in mathematics 1, biology, and chemistry and increased in mathematics 2 and physics.

15. These findings are based on data for 1973 and for 1983, prepared by the Advanced Placement Program of the College Board.

16. *Graduate Record Examination (GRE) Regular On-Time Candidate Mean Scores,* 1972-1973 and 1981-1982 (Princeton, N.J.: Educational Testing Service, 1973 and 1982). The data are difficult to interpret because of changing populations, changes in program policy, and the fact that the sample may not be nationally representative. For example, the average score on the computer science test was 625 in 1976, the first year the test was given; in 1982, with three times as many test-takers, the average score was 602.

17. Barbara J. Holmes et al., *Reading, Science, and Mathematics Trends: A Closer Look* (Denver: National Assessment of Educational Progress, Education Commission of the States, 1982); and Stacey J. Hueftle, Steven J. Rakow, and Wayne W. Welch, *Images of Science: A Summary of Results from the 1981-82 National Assessment in Science* (Minneapolis: Science Assessment and Research Project, University of Minnesota, June 1983). For an analysis of trends in achievement, as reflected in the NAEP data, see Archie E. Lapointe, "The Good News About American Education," *Phi Delta Kappan,* June, 1984, p. 663.

18. *Third National Mathematics Assessment: Results, Trends, and Issues* (Denver: Education Commission of the States, April 1983).

19. American College Testing Program, News Release, September 1983.

20. *National College-Bound Seniors, 1983,* p. 4.

21. *Graduate Record Examination (GRE) Regular On-Time Candidate Mean Scores,* 1972-1973 and 1981-1982.

22. American College Testing Program, News Release, September 1983.

23. Lyle V. Jones, "Achievement Test Scores in Mathematics and Science," *Science,* 24 July 1981, pp. 412-16.

24. "NCES Study Examines Changes in Coursework of High School Seniors," *Statistical Bulletin,* National Center for Education Statistics, Washington, D.C., 3 August 1981.

25. *National College-Bound Seniors, 1983,* p. 6.

26. Sol H. Pelavin, Elizabeth R. Reisner, and Gerry Hendrickson, *Analysis of the National Availability of Mathematics and Science Teachers* (Washington, D.C.: Education Analysis Center for Educational Quality and Equality, 1983).

27. *Teacher Supply and Demand in Public Schools, 1981-82,* NEA Research Memo (Washington, D.C.: National Education Association, 1983).

28. Bill G. Aldridge and Karen L. Johnston, "Scientists and the Crisis in Science Education," draft paper, 23 January 1984.

29. Daniel Koretz, *Science and Mathematics Education: Issues in Shaping a Federal Initiative,* draft report (Washington, D.C.: Congressional Budget Office, 11 March 1983).

30. Aldridge and Johnston, p. 6.

31. George N. Schmidt, "Science Teaching in Chicago: Survival of the Fattest," *Reader,* 29 April 1983, Sect. I, p. 8.

32. Aldridge and Johnston, p. 15.

33. *Teacher Shortage in Science and Mathematics,* p. 7.

34. Jerry G. Gaff, *General Education Today* (San Francisco: Jossy-Bass, 1983), p. 115.

35. *Montaigne Essays,* J.M. Cohen, trans. (New York: Penguin, 1982), p. 72.

36. Ernest L. Boyer, *High School: A Report on Secondary Education in America* (New York: Harper & Row, 1983).

37. *National College-Bound Seniors, 1983,* p. 4.

38. Koretz, p. 8.

39. Lapoine, p. 666.

40. Gene I. Maeroff, "Teaching of Writing Gets New Push," *New York Times Education Winter Survey,* 8 January 1984, p. 1.

41. Gaff, p. 28.

42. Jean Evangelauf, "Top Students Move to Science Studies, Leave Humanities," *Chronicle of Higher Education,* 22 February 1984, pp. 1, 11.

43. Benjamin J. Stein, "Valley Girls View the World," *Public Opinion,* August/September 1983, pp. 18-19.

44. For a more detailed discussion of the implications of

the various proposals, see Harold Howe II, "Education Moves to Center Stage: An Overview of Recent Studies," *Phi Delta Kappan,* November 1983, pp. 167-72; and Paul E. Peterson, "Did the Education Reports Say Anything?," *Brookings Review,* Winter 1983, pp. 3-11.

45.   Howe, p. 170.

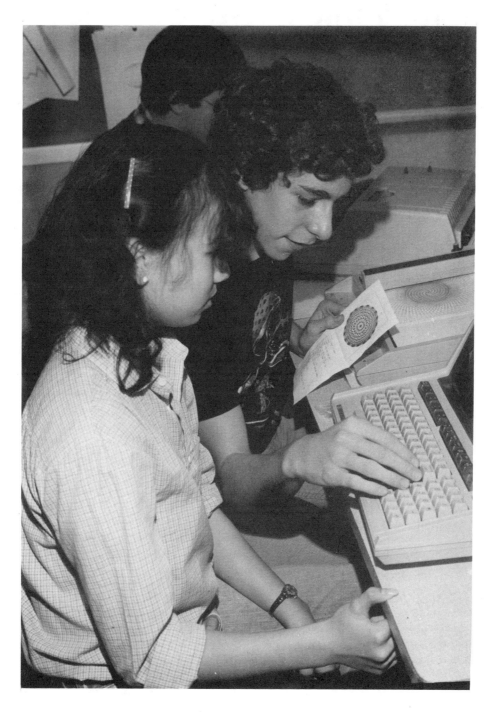

Paul A. Basso

Chapter 41
Computers in Education Today–and Some Possible Futures
Alfred Bork*

One remarkable feature of education at all levels in the past few years has been the increasing importance of computers in the instructional process. All indicators suggest that the presence and influence of the computer in education will continue to grow. Yet the uses to which the computer is now being put are sometimes disquieting, and many uncertainties exist about the future of this new technology in education.

Many individuals are totally supportive of computers in education; others are totally opposed to them. My aim is to present a balanced picture of the current situation with regard to computers in education and, based on that picture, to sketch several possible but very different futures. Many of the points that I will make here have been explored in more detail in my other writings.[1]

The Situation Today

The current situation of computers in education can best be discussed under three broad headings. Arranged from least to most important, they are: (1) the hardware now available in schools, (2) the instructional materials currently available for use with computers, and (3) the classroom situation with regard to computers.

Hardware

Estimates vary, but by April 1984 U.S. schools had approximately 350,000 computers available to students in grades 1 through 12—an average of about four computers per school. In the past few years, the number of computers in the schools has roughly *doubled* each year.

The rapid increase in the amount of raw computer power accessible to students occurred even when schools were in poor financial condition and when federal funding of education was on the wane. In many cases, parents demanded that the schools make computers available to their youngsters. It is not clear how long we can expect the exponential increase in the availability of computers to continue, but we ought to consider rapid growth a distinct possibility, at least for several more years.

It is more difficult to determine how many computers are available to students in colleges and universities. However, if we count both computers that the students own and those belonging to the colleges and universities, we can say with some confidence that students' access to computers continues to grow in high education.

Perhaps the most interesting trend in hardware at this level is the move toward one personal computer per student. At Drexel University, for example, freshmen entering in the fall of 1984 were required to purchase Apple Macintosh computers. Other universities have acquired vast numbers of computers through corporate gifts (such as those given by IBM to the Massachusetts Institute of Technology, the University of Texas at Austin, and the University of California, Berkeley) or as part of special projects (such as the advanced computer system system at Carnegie-Mellon University).

Two factors make it impossible to firmly predict the rate at which schools will acquire computers in coming years. First, we must bear in mind that the doubling in the number of school-owned computers in the recent past occurred *despite the fact that virtually no decent educational software existed for use with these machines.* Should such software become available in the future, its existence would certainly affect both the rate of computer acquisition by the schools and the duration of the purchasing interval.

The second factor is the increase in computer power now available. Newer machines offer more memory, greater speed, and better graphics. How will these new

*Dr. Alfred Bork is a professor of information and Computer Science and Director of the Educational Technology Center at the University of California, Irvine. Another version of this article appeared in the October, 1984 issue of *T.H.E. Journal,* published by Information Synergy, Inc. Reprinted with permission of the author and *Phi Delta Kappan,* December, 1984.

and better machines influence the development of educational software? And how will the higher cost of these new and better machines influence the rate at which schools purchase them? Without answers to these and similar questions, it is impossible to predict the rate of computer acquisition by the schools in coming years.

Educational Software

The situation with regard to the production and distribution of educational computer programs is less favorable. The *amount* of software—particularly commercially produced programs—available for use at all grade levels and in all content areas has increased greatly. But the *quality* of this software has remained consistently low. Thus, while the sheer numbers of machines in the schools and the power of each machine have increased dramatically, the quality of educational software has not kept pace.

We know how to produce decent computer-based learning materials. But that knowledge has largely gone unused. Most of the programs now available are not the products of a careful design process, and very few of them have undergone careful evaluation.

Dozens of companies have begun to produce and distribute such software in recent years. For example, many of the major textbook publishing companies have established electronic publishing subsidiaries that offer catalogues of computer-based learning materials. Computer manufacturers are also becoming increasingly involved in software production, which they see as a promising new market as well as a means of strengthening their hardware sales.

Many new companies, focused specifically on the production or distribution of educational software, have also arisen. Some such companies resemble book stores; they do not publish computer materials themselves, but their catalogues list software available from a wide variety of sources.

In addition to the learning modules that are commercially available, some educational software is available directly from the developers. Many of these programs will eventually become commercial products.

Clearly, the amount of educational software is rapidly increasing, but this increase is difficult to measure exactly. Nor is there much point in trying, since the average quality of available software is so low. Some observers have asserted that certain brands of computers are widely used in schools because they afford a vast array of software. This assertion seems to spring from a notion that large quantities of educational garbage are superior to small quantities.

The factors that characterize poorly designed educational software include:

- failure to make use of the interactive capabilities of the computer;
- failure to make use of the capabilities of the computer to individualize instruction;
- use of extremely weak forms of interaction, such as multiple-choice questions;
- too-heavy reliance on text;
- too-heavy reliance on pictures, when these pictures play no important role in helping students learn the material;
- treatment of the computer screen as though it were a book page;
- use of material that is entertaining or attractive but that is only vaguely educational;
- content that does not fit anywhere in the curriculum;
- focus on games that have no educational merit;
- use of long sets of instructions at the beginning of programs that are difficult to follow—even for teachers—and difficult to recall;
- heavy dependence on auxiliary print materials;
- presentation of segments of content that are not placed in context; and
- use of materials that fail to hold students' attention.

It is difficult to determine how much money software companies as a group are putting into curriculum development and instructional design. I suspect that the total sum is small, given the abundance of educational software on the market. Indeed, most of the larger companies have tended up to now to locate already-existing software and then to distribute it under their own labels. Notice how very different this process is from that used by textbook publishing companies in the development of a new book or series.

Some bright spots exist, however. Several large computer companies are now spending sizable sums for curriculum development; IBM's recent sponsorship of John Henry Martin's Writing to Read Program is a good example.

Federal involvement in the development of computer-based learning materials waned dramatically during the early years of the Reagan Administration. Federal support for the development of educational software is now growing again, but the outlook for the future is uncertain. Private foundations have put very little money into projects of this nature. However, some funding is now available from the states.

Some computer vendors are supporting the development of educational software, but most apparently fail to realize the close relationship between the availability of good software and the rate of hardware sales. In the future, school officials and the general public will buy certain brands of computers because of the ready availability of a wide variety of compatible software that is carefully prepared and effective.

Although few high-quality computer-based learning modules exist today, we know a variety of strategies for developing such materials. The Educational Technology Center at the University of California, Irvine, and some researchers elsewhere have focused in particular on the *process* that yields sizable amounts of these high-quality learning materials.[2]

The hallmarks of that process are the use of development teams, reliance on a careful procedure for development of the new material (including both formative and summative evaluation), and sufficient funding to carry out that procedure. Every useful computer-based learning material begins, I would argue, with a clear pedagogical purpose. Approaches to development that begin with the computer may produce some jazzy materials, but these materials are not likely to be very effective in the classroom.

The development of computer-based learning materials has been a tale of false directions. The development of authoring languages, for example, has been an enormous waste of large sums—perhaps billions of dollars, by now—that could have paid instead for the development of useful learning modules. Virtually no software of educational consequence has been developed with the use of any of the authoring systems or languages. (Tutor has been an exception, possibly because of the almost infinite amounts of money that Control Data Corporation was willing to spend on development.)

Many companies, recognizing that the schools are big business, are concentrating more on the distribution of software than on its development. And this trend seems likely to become even more pronounced in coming years

The issue of *why* currently available educational software is so poor is an interesting one that deserves far more attention than I can give it here. Many specialists in computer science blame the poor quality of available software on the current state of the hardware. They spread the myth that computers can never be used successfully for learning until educational software can make use of the techniques of artificial intelligence (which require computers far more powerful than the personal computers of today). I disagree. Many interesting examples of computer-based learning materials already exist, intended for use with current hardware. Although we can expect computers to continue to improve, it is wrong to believe that developers cannot create effective educational materials until available computers are able to support artificial intelligence software.

The Classroom Situation

Despite the growing presence of computers in U.S. schools and colleges, computer-based learning remains a *very small fraction* of the total instructional system. Even in those university courses that make the most extensive use of computers, this new technology occupies no more than half of the students' total learning time. And very few such courses are available. In fact, I would be surprised to discover that the computer occupies more than 1% of the total time devoted to instruction in the U.S.

Most learning in this nation is still taking place through the passive learning modes that have been dominant for hundreds of years: books and lectures. This is not surprising, considering the lack of high-quality educational software. The typical teacher is dependent on existing instructional materials. We like to believe that K-12 and college teachers develop their own courses, and this does happen occasionally—but only occasionally. Moreover, most teachers have little knowledge of how to use the computer. Current training programs for teachers leave much to be desired.

The vast majority of introductory courses at the university level follow a standard and prosaic format that includes large lecture sections and assigned readings in a few required textbooks. Most faculty members are content with this format; after all, as undergraduates they themselves enrolled and performed well in these very same courses. During the intervening years, very few of these faculty members have ever developed appreciable amounts of instructional materials. Most of them do not even know how to go about the task. In addition, they lack the necessary resources, and they work within a reward system that does not encourage this kind of activity.

Possible Futures

Given the current situation with regard to computers in education (which I have tried to portray realistically), what can we expect for the future?

- Clearly, the number of computers in schools and colleges—and thus students' access to computers—will continue to increase. Some observers are already predicting that more than a million computers will be in place in U.S. schools within the next two or three years.

- We can also expect commercial companies to step up their efforts to sell computers to schools and to produce and distribute—or to stimulate the production and distribution of—increasing quantities of computer-based learning materials.

- Computers will continue to evolve and improve, and their price will continue to come down. Their graphics capability will increase, and more of them will offer choices in type fonts and sizes. We can expect larger screens and better resolution of the images on those screens. In the not-too-distant future, videodisc technology will come into wider use. We can also expect such features as voice—and even brainwave—input to become practical as well.

- It seems likely, too, that many of the severe problems that U.S. education is now experiencing will continue. For example, the shortage of mathematics and science teachers will not be alleviated in the near future by any measure, no matter how dramatic.

Although these trends can be predicted with some assurance, the ways in which computers will affect education in the future are far less certain. Allow me to sketch briefly two general scenarios—one negative, one positive—for the future of computers in education.

A Dismal Future

One possibility for the future is that we simply continue with business as usual. Should we choose this path, schools and universities will continue to decline. Commercial forces will increasingly come to dominate the development of computer-based curricula, just as they dominate the development of book-based curricula today. And they will continue to distribute low-quality educational software to schools and universities.

As the number of computers in the schools increases, the audience for this low-quality software will grow. Teachers and administrators will have little opportunity to learn to identify good software because so much of it will be bad. So they will be "satisfied" with low-quality learning modules.

Most courses at all levels will be centered on books and lectures. Computer-based materials will be supplementary. Teacher training programs will continue to ignore this new technology, and the interactive capabilities of the computer will never be adequately realized.

In this unpleasant view of the future, the quality of schooling at all levels—both public and private—will continue to decline. The educational problems that plague us now will remain unsolved. Parental pressures for changes in education will grow, but these pressures will often lead to measures, such as the voucher system, that will not improve education but merely transform it into a private concern. Large corporations will view the voucher system as an invitation to participate in the "education market," and they will establish there own schools and colleges.

The achievement of U.S. students will continue to drop. Low-quality educational software will probably even accelerate this trend. But large American corporations will discover that they can find well-trained workers simply by moving their operations overseas; thus they will be minimally concerned about the declining quality of U.S. education

Although the scenario I have just painted may seem excessively negative, it could come to pass. I do not present it as a scare tactic, but as a very real possibility.

A Bright Future

In this scenario, which begins in 1984 or possibly a few years hence, powerful leaders in politics and business agree that the U.S. system of education must be reformed if the nation is to maintain its world position and if it is to provide the best possible education for *all* citizens. One major outcome of this new wave of education reform will be the large-scale development of curricular materials that make the computer an integral part of learning from first grade through college.

Such extensive curriculum development will not take place overnight. It will require instead a decade-long national commitment. During each of those 10 years, 1% of the total budget for U.S. education will be spent on curriculum development. Commercial forces will also contribute their resources to this massive national effort.

The development of new curricula lies at the heart of any effort to use the computer to improve U.S. education. The new computer-based learning materials must incorporate a wide range of learning theories and approaches. Several groups of developers will produce learning modules in each content area, to insure that the educational system becomes more diverse and pluralistic than it ever was during the era of dependence on textbooks. (The textbook-dependent courses of the Eighties tend to be extremely similar, even though the books have been written by different authors and come from different publishers.)

The new courseware will lead to changes in the organization of schools and to new and more dignified roles for teachers. Many activities that currently take place in the school will shift to the home, the public library, and other environments, since computer-based learning can take place almost anywhere. But some activities can best be done in groups, and those will continue to take place in the school.

The literature contains several sketches of possible school systems of the future that use the computer effectively. George Leonard has provided two of the more interesting of these.[3] The schools that Leonard proposed in *Education and Ecstasy* (1968) and those he proposed in a 1984 article for *Esquire* differ somewhat, but they also have many interesting features in common.

For example, in both of Leonard's sketches the computer is the major delivery device—in many cases, the *only* delivery device—for instruction. The schools in both sketches focus on educating the whole child; thus affective education and physical education are integral parts of the curriculum. The teachers play a major role in affective education. And the schools in both sketches rely on a computerized course management system to maintain a complete record of each student's progress.

In his 1968 sketch, Leonard placed the computer in complete charge of determining students' learning activities. In the 1984 sketch, Leonard proposed a more versatile management system in which the computer presents study options to the student; the computer and the student then agree on the student's academic responsibilities for a particular day. Other humans may also have a say in this decision.

In the 1968 sketch, all learning activities took place in school (although most of them *could* have taken place in other settings as well). In the 1984 sketch, by contrast, a student who has completed the minimum requirements can choose to spend the remaining time working at school, at home, or somewhere else.

Both of the schools that Leonard presented use mastery learning (a fact he stressed more in the 1984 sketch than in his earlier one). Mastery learning requires that a student stay with a given learning task until he or she can perform it with nearly 100% accuracy.

I do not mean to imply that Leonard's sketches are the only positive futures possible for education in the computer age. But Leonard has put a great deal of careful thought into these sketches, and they deserve wide reading. Many of the features that Leonard describes seem to me likely to characterize almost any school of the future that uses computers effectively as tools for learning. And that is what schools must ultimately do.

FOOTNOTES

1. See, for example, Alfred Bork, *Learning with Computers* (Bedford, Mass.: Digital Press, 1981); and idem, *Personal Computers for Education* (New York: Harper & Row, January 1985).
2. Alfred Bork, "Production Systems for Computer-Based Learning," in Decker F. Walker and Robert D. Hess, eds., *Instructional Software: Principles and Perspectives for Design and Use* (Belmont, Calif.: Wadsworth, 1984).
3. George Leonard, *Education and Ecstasy* (New York: Delacorte, 1968); and idem, "The Great School Reform Hoax," *Esquire,* April 1984, pp. 47-56.

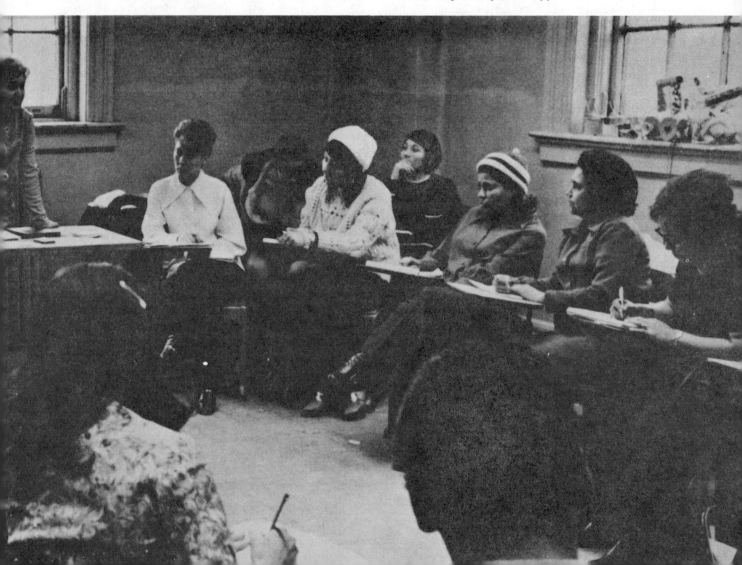

Chapter 42
Partnerships Unlimited–An Alliance of Home and School

Irene S Pyszkowski*

At the present time we are witnessing an increased effort on the part of parents and community alike to play a more significant role in the education that will affect their children. Unlike the past when education was regarded as the sole province of professional educators, today parents and the public-at-large all feel entitled and capable of making their voices heard in an evolving educational system. Educators need to recognize this growing trend in parental participation and community volunteerism. They need to learn to deal with it in such a manner as to maximize the benefits for our schools and our children.

Parental participation in schools and classrooms is hardly a novel concept. Before traditional schooling—as we know it—existed, education was largely the responsibility of the home and church. The teaching of basic literacy as well as vocational skills took place in the home or in other institutions created for purposes other than education, such as churches (Fiske 1958).

Parents have been active in Parent/Teacher Organizations and have served on school committees for quite some time. Lately efforts on the part of parents to become a more effective force in school affairs have been more aggressive. Within the past decade—parental pressure for more significant involvement in the schools has increased across the nation (Johnston & Slotnik 1985). This growing trend of involvement in the schools poses a question for school administrators and teachers alike. How do you channel this force to achieve positive results and harmonious relationships? The answer appears to be in the formation of partnerships with schools and communities.

Legal Basis for the Partnership Component

The rationale for parental partnerships involvement as a component in the educational process has been supported by various title programs funded by the federal government. Head Start, which has been funded continually since 1965 is a good example of a program that mandates active parent participation. Head Start parents are involved in four ways:

1. Participation in decision making.
2. Participation in classroom activities.
3. Participation in parent-oriented affairs.
4. Participation in home activities with their children.
(Lille John & Associates 1976).

Moreover the Elementary & Secondary Education Act requires that federally funded programs such as Title I include parents in their planning (Berger 1981). The Title I program requires that parents be included as advisory board members before funding is initiated.

Public Law 94-142 Education of All Handicapped Children Act strongly relies on parent participation in the design of the Individualized Educational Program (IEP). Involving parents in decisions about their handicapped children's education has a legal base under Public Law 94-142 (Spodek, Saracho & Lee 1984). This law mandates that educators consult with parents in formulating a mutually appropriate instructional program for their child. Parents must also serve as members of advisory committees which set policy and make decisions for the education of the handicapped. This new role assigned to parents under P.L. 94-142 underscores the importance of the parent component in the decision making process.

In areas where decentralization has occurred, parents and community residents are provided an opportunity to play key roles in school affairs. Local community school boards having jurisdiction over local school affairs have replaced a far-reaching and sometimes unwieldly central board. Members of these community school boards are duly elected by the community to vote on local school issues, appoint superintendents, hire other school personnel and have an ultimate voice in local school matters.

*Dr. Irene S. Pyszkowski is an Associate Professor, Division of Education, Notre Dame College, St. John's University, NY.

A major purpose of decentralization is to bring the parent into closer relationships with the schools—(N.Y.C. Bd. of Ed. 1971).

Influences of Parents

Before any program of parental participation can be initiated the faculty must agree that parental involvement has merit. Professional personnel initiating a program of parental involvement should become familiar with and respect the value system of parents (Kroth & Scholl 1978). Parents bring to the school attitudes developed through their lifetime experiences with schools. Their strengths and weaknesses vary as greatly as those of their children. Some parents become over-involved in school affairs while some parents stay away completely. But no matter what the diversity, all parents have one common concern and that is to do what is best for their children.

Involving parents in meaningful roles in education is a demanding and time-consuming responsibility. Administrators and other school personnel must be willing to make a commitment of time and energy to a parent-involvement program. Principals and teachers, aware of the frustrations and difficulties inherent in parent partnership programs, often shy away from such undertakings and/or respond with hostility. However, evidence has shown that advantages accrued from opening lines of communication with parents benefit everyone—teachers, administrators, parents, and pupils (Beale 1985).

Parental influences have a major impact on a child's development. Family experiences shape and mold the child before formal education commences. Educators may wish to denigrate learning that occurs at home but the fact is that parents can and do assume a role as partners in the educational process. Overtly or covertly some parents are accused of being indifferent and uncaring but the potential for assuming a more supportive role in their children's education is there, if it is properly activated and rendered more effective.

Popular polls and media articles have clearly shown that parents wish to be included in their children's education. Beginning with infancy, parents diligently seek ways to play a more important role in educating their children. Research findings in the U.S. Department of Education publication *What Works* states that parents are their children's first and most influential teachers (Bennett 1986).

Teachers who are not prepared for the presence of auxiliary personnel in the classroom do not realize the benefits of such an arrangement. They view offers of help by non-teaching professional staff and volunteer assistants as threatening and an intrusion on their professional status. But consider some of the advantages of a program of interaction between parents and teachers.

Parents can provide assistance in a vast array of non-instructional activities such as taking attendance, setting up audio-visual materials, checking homework and collecting money. This help frees the teacher to devote more time to students and instruction. Volunteers can also assist in extra-curricular activities such as field trips, clubs and class parties. Parents have proven their expertise in handling these functions through their experiences in serving as leaders in groups such as Boy Scouts, Girl Scouts and 4-H Clubs.

Classroom assistants can be trained to handle small reading groups. Listening to a small group read or practice word lists by an assistant enables the teacher to devote more time to individualized activities with other students. Some parents have special skills or experiences which they can share with the class. A father who practices dentistry e.g. can be enlisted to come to class to discuss dental hygiene and instruct the class on the proper use of dental aids. Programs that involve parents in the schools can play a major role in creating a desirable context for teaching and learning (Comer 1986).

Surveying the Needs

If a program to involve parents more significantly is developed, then it must be made acceptable to all participating members of the education community. Once the commitment is made, ways to integrate home and school must be explored. A highly useful approach is to conduct a survey, assessing the needs of the parents, the community and the school. A needs assessment study will reveal the areas of greatest concern. The following is a summary of the means available for gathering information, opinions and facts relevant to home-school partnerships.

1. Questionnaires circulated in the local community to survey the needs, interests and concerns of parents.
2. Personal interviews, on a one-to-one basis, with parents to elicit comments and criticisms. Parents interviewed should include representatives of the diversified ethnic and socio-economic groups prevalent in the community (Berger 1981).
3. Reports on educational issues from parent-teacher groups and other community service groups such as fraternal orders, charitable societies and family service leagues.
4. Professional polls, i.e. the Gallup Poll, an annual survey, which supplies data based on its findings dealing with home and school.
5. Information packets, books, pamphlets and investigative reports developed by organizations dealing with home-school relations and children's rights. National Committee for Citizens in Education (NCCE), Institute for Responsive Education, Chil-

Parent Questionnaire A

If you were principal of the school or director of the child care center, which programs and activities would you have for parents and children? Which of these programs would you use as a parent?

	Schools should offer		I would use	
	Yes	**No**	**Yes**	**No**
1. Parent-teacher conferences				
2. Parent education and preschool programs				
3. Newsletters				
4. PTA or PTO				
5. Parent volunteers				
6. Child care during conferences				
7. After-school programs for children whose parents work				
8. Special support groups for single parents				
9. Parents as resource persons in the room				
10. Parent advisory committee				
11. Parent education and toddler program				
12. Activities and guides for parents to use with children during holidays and spring break				
13. Parents as tutors				

(adapted from Berger 1981)

---

dren's Defense Fund and National Congress of Parents and Teachers are but a few of the national organizations that can assist in supplying information and data analysis for assessing needs.

Survey Mechanisms

A useful tool for conducting a survey of parent concerns is the questionnaire. A questionnaire may be a very specific instrument featuring a check-off procedure as a response to an inquiry. An illustration of this type of diagnostic mechanism is presented in Parent Questionnaire A.

Open-ended questionnaires are still another type of a needs-assessment measuring device. The questions posed on an open-ended questionnaire are broader in scope and more thought provoking. The answers to these inquiries are not easily submitted in written form but may require a seminar format to evoke responses. This type of questionnaire is best illustrated by the following set of questions.

1. What kind of questions are appropriate for parent involvement?

2. What should be the extent of participation in such areas as placement, curriculum planning and evaluation progress?
3. To what extent can parents contribute to the instructional program?
4. What kind of discussion groups should be initiated?
5. What kind of communication links should be established?

(Kroth & Scholl 1978)

Planning Strategies

The use of these devices to determine the concerns and needs of parents should lead to identification of problem areas. A planning initiative then should be undertaken as the next step. In the planning stage specific objectives should be formulated to address the apparent needs of school and home. A committee of administrators, teachers and parents working cooperatively should resolve what those objectives are and how they are best met. For example, parents and teachers may decide that homework is an issue on which both sides have conflicting

Parent Questionnaire B

1. In my job as parent I have the hardest time in:	Very Difficult	Somewhat Difficult	No Problem
a. Being an only parent			
b. Teaching my child to obey			
c. Providing proper nourishment			
d. Making time to listen and play with my child			
e. Disciplining my child			
f. Having patience and understanding			
g. Understanding my child's growth			
h. Other (specify)			

2. To do my job better as a parent I would like training in:	Very Important	Somewhat Important	Not Important
a. Child growth and development			
b. Bilingual-bicultural education			
c. Nutrition			
d. Child behavior and discipline			
e. First Aid			
f. Self-improvement			
g. Home improvement			
h. Techniques in working with the handicapped child			
i. Other (specify)			

(Adapted from Little, John R. and Assoc. 1976)

opinions. Teachers may view homework as an experience carried on outside the school in the form of books, trips and audio-visual materials while parents may consider homework as a written exercise. In the educator's opinion homework is in this instance a supplementary activity used to enrich classroom learning whereas the parent sees homework as a daily written assignment to reinforce classroom instruction. A program designed to focus on the issue of homework would be a way to resolve this conflict. The format might be a series of workshops in which both the parents and teachers participate. Workshop sessions would then presumably consist of value clarification and techniques that could be used to satisfy the requirements of both home and school.

After objectives are stated, considerations should be given to the process of implementing said objectives. A series of meetings, workshops or rap sessions may all be appropriate techniques for outlining the procedures for integration of parents into the educational community.

The following are steps that should be considered when getting started on a program of parent involvement.

1. Define the assignment. Make it simple yet clear, so that teachers and parents understand the nature and limits of their responsibility.
2. Define the role of the participant. Identify the roles that parents and teachers will assume in the assignment. In some areas parents may assume the role of teacher and vice-versa.
3. Give a job description. Clearly describe the specifics involved in any task a parent may perform.
4. Set up training sessions. Parents should be taught the skills and knowledge necessary for the tasks they will be performing. Workshops, information sessions and the use of resource materials are ways of imparting training to parents and teachers alike.
5. Allot time periods for objectives. Some objectives are, by their very nature, short-term in duration

while others are open-ended and on-going. A time limit should be set where it would be counter-productive to conduct the program over a long period of time.

6. Recruit volunteers. All parents are not involved in the planning stages but once the program is underway, the efforts should be made to involve a substantially greater number of parents.

7. Design an evaluation mechanism. Periodically programs of parent involvement should be reviewed to determine whether goals and objectives are being met. Request opinions of those being served as well as those serving.

8. Give parent participants recognition. Assess the efforts that parents have made and apprise them of their contributions. Inform them of how well they have performed and how they might strengthen their skills. Concrete awards such as certificates, ceremonies, and luncheons have special meaning for parent volunteers.

Communication Links

When teachers are convinced of the merits of parental involvement, a partnership program can prove to be mutually beneficial. Parental involvement helps children learn more effectively (Bennett 1968). Invite parents to participate and give them an opportunity to play a significant part in the educational community.

This begins with effective communication between the school and home. Any effort at recruiting more parents and non-parents to serve in a partnership capacity involves good communication links with the community.

The following are sound communication practices established in many schools across the country.

1. Parent conferences
2. Parent newsletters
3. Annual open house
4. Annual curriculum night
5. Annual school calendar
6. Parent-teacher organization or school-community council.
7. Local newspaper
8. Annual grandparents' day
9. Board of Education spokesperson or communication officer
10. Annual Field Day

Activities for Parent Participation

Parent participation programs already in existence in schools today have many elements in common. In fact some activities prevalent in the partnership model can be

found in all schools. The difference is that the thrust here should be for a program of greater involvement and more meaningful participation. Activities included in many programs of parental involvement are summarized below.

Class Mothers/Fathers. Whereas in the past the female parent was assigned to serve as liaison between the classroom teacher and class parents, today more fathers are assuming this responsibility. In this capacity the parent assumes the task of keeping the parents of a particular class informed of various and sundry activities such as class parties, trips and school closings.

Parent Tutors. Parents can be trained to work with individual students or small groups in many areas of the curriculum. Some parent volunteers who are former teachers can assist in training other parents. Students tutoring other students is a valid program which can be included in this category. Parent assistants may be required to supervise in this area.

Resource Personnel. Parents with specialized skills or training could be utilized as resource persons. These volunteers could share their expertise with the entire student body through individual class visits or school assemblies. Parents who have travelled extensively or who have lived abroad can enrich the curriculum by recounting their experiences. Storytelling by parents and especially senior citizens is another activity which can be established.

Classroom Aides. In this category parents can help teachers by taking attendance, monitoring arrivals and departures of students, collecting funds when needed and assisting in the use of hi-tech equipment. Parents can also play informal games with students and supervise periods of free play and recess.

Library Aides. Parents can assist immeasurably in a school library. They can provide an extra pair of hands sorely needed in this facility. Aides can help in filing and typing, maintaining the card catalog and stamping out and returning of books.

Service Aides. As service aides parents assist in field trips, monitor halls and entrances, assist in lunchrooms and participate in fundraisers.

Advisory Boards. Parents who sit on advisory boards are frequently involved in decision-making in such areas as budget, staff selection and general operating procedures.

Student Activity Advisors. Student activities such as student council and school newspaper are areas where parents can provide much needed support. Often these activities are suspended in schools where personnel is unavailable for supervision.

After-School Care. In view of the increasing number of working parents many school districts are now offering after-school care. This is truly an area of school and home partnership. Volunteers can assist recreation workers or teachers in the care and supervision of youngsters whose parents are unable to be at home.

Parent Education Programs. More and more parents, confused about whether they are doing the right thing, are turning to private agencies for skills training in child-rearing. Schools should consider offering courses in parenting and support services to assist families in raising their children. Educate parents to be change agents or educators of their own children (Kroth and Scholl 1978). Schedule workshops when it is convenient for parents to meet such as Saturdays or evenings.

Curriculum Education Programs. Whether it is "new" math or innovative reading programs, parents feel left in the dark regarding teaching practices presently in use. Parents can benefit from refresher sessions with teachers and administrators on the goals and methods employed in the various curriculum areas. Teachers can review with parents what is being covered in class and how to best assist a child with homework and class projects.

Conclusion

While these activities are by no means all-encompassing they do offer opportunities for facilitating programs of parental involvement. There are many ways in which parent services can be rendered more effectively. Much depends on the creativity and willingness of the school personnel.

Educators harried by the pressures and responsibilities of teaching and administration find there are not enough hours in the day to carry out primary programs of responsibility, let alone supplementary ones. An effort to devote time to partnership programs results in benefits to students, to parents and to teachers. Studies have shown that when parents are made part of a comprehensive delivery system, students perform better academically and socially.

It makes sense to encourage parent participation at a time when education is witnessing significant cutbacks in funding. Parents can be utilized to supply that extra pair of hands so that schools may continue to maintain educational standards. Schools wishing to initiate creative and innovative educational programs would need to rely on volunteer assistants to carry out these programs as lack of funds becomes more acute.

As parents become more active in the educational

community, their roles will be more effective in improving school-community relations. Parents who have a voice in decision-making will be a positive influence in public relations. The partnership component will serve to increase a cooperative and constructive relation between home and school.

REFERENCES

Beale, A.V., "Toward More Effective Parent Involvement," *The Clearing House,* January 1985, Vol. 58, 213-215.

Bennet, W.J., *What Works,* U.S. Dept. of Education, Washington, D.C. 1986.

Berger, E.H., *Parents as Partners in Education,* The C.V. Mosby Co., St. Louis, 1981.

Cattermole, J. & Robinson N., "Effective Home/School Communication From the Parents' Perspective," *Phi Delta Kappan,* Sept. 1985, Vol. 67, No. 1, p. 48-50.

Comer, James P., "Parent Participation in the Schools," *Phi Delta Kappan,* Feb. 1986, Vol. 67; 442-6.

Fiske, E.B., "Beyond the Classroom," *The New York Times,* Education Spring Survey, Sec. 12, April 14, 1985, p. 1 & 43.

Johnston, M. & Slotnik, J., "Parent Participation in the Schools: Are the Benefits Worth the Burdens?", *Phi Delta Kappan,* Feb. 1985, p. 430-433.

Kroth, R.L. & Scholl, G.T., *Getting Schools Involved with Parents,* The Council for Exceptional Children, Reston, VA., 1978.

Little John, R. & Associates, *Involving Parents in Head Start; a Guide for Parent Involvement Coordinators,* Washington, D.C., 1976, Office of Human Development, p. 1-1, 1-4.

Parent Associations and the Schools, Policy Statement of the Board of Education, Office of Education Information Services and Public Relations, Brooklyn, N.Y. Oct. 1971.

Trimarco, Teresa A., "Selection Practices of Parents' Organizations in New York City Elementary Schools." Unpublished Doctoral Dissertation, Fordham University, 1965.

Trimarco, Teresa A. and Chapey, Geraldine D. "Participation of Parents in Programs for the Gifted in New York City." *Journal for Education of the Gifted.* Vol. 7, No. 3, pp. 178-191, (1984).

Spodek, B., Saracho, O.N., & Lee, R.C., *Mainstreaming Young Children,* Wadsworth Publishing Co., Belmont, CA., 1984.

Chapter 43
Curricular Change: A Look at the Influences at Work
Louise R. Giddings*

Educational systems in today's society are continually seeking ways to respond to the needs and demands of varied individuals and groups. Many individuals are presently involved in attempts to plan and implement curricular changes. Yet, the task of instituting curricular change requires some analyses of the problems involved in educational change. In 1964, Miles noted that the current interest and involvement of schools in the United States in educational change offered many opportunities to study the problems of change.[1] Miles noted further that this area is one "where our understanding is decidedly less than perfect."[2] Today, interest and involvement in educational change are still apparent, and ample opportunities exist for continued study of phenomena occurring in change processes.

One aspect of the change problem which is salient is that of recognizing and understanding factors which operate to influence the adoption of innovations in schools. Many school and community individuals often cooperate in the implementation of new programs without awareness of the influences which have prevailed to cause such programs to be instituted. Ohme states, however, that in looking for significant change in education, as well as change models, concerned individuals must address themselves to questions such as:

- Who had the idea? A teacher, counselor, a group of students?
- Did it evolve? How?
- What was the process?
- How long did it take?
- What procedures were used?
- What were the problems encountered?[3]

In other words, in the study of curricular change, there is need to analyze the process involved in planning for a new program and to gain some understanding of factors which operate to secure the installation of new projects or programs in schools. Awareness and understanding of influences which operate in the planning stages prior to the adoption and implementation of a curricular innovation can assist responsible individuals in their attempts to plan for and manage change in the schools.

This writer undertook an investigation to provide an explanation of some of the factors that operated in the process leading to the adoption of the Communication Skills Laboratory in a middle school of a northeastern urban community. The conceptualization of the change process as developed by Gordon Mackenzie was used to study the adoption process.[4] The Mackenzie model deals with curricular change as a political process, and Mackenzie asserts that beyond the advocacy of a change or the communication of a proposal to others, the process of exerting influence in favor of a proposed change is based on power.[5]

The Communication Skills Laboratory was an innovation that replaced an English program which some teachers believed stigmatized low achievers and separated them from their peers. The laboratory was designed to help students develop skills in many areas of communication within a setting based on unity with diversity. According to the plan for the program, the innovation was intended to focus on non-verbal communication such as pantomime, body language and photography, as well as on the language arts and literature. Moreover, the program was developed to foster growth in critical thinking, creative thinking, self-instruction, self-evaluation, and a sense of inquiry.

Operationally, adoption was defined as the installation and offering of the Communication Skills Laboratory as a required curricular program in the selected middle school. Considering the relevant aspects of the change process as indicated in the Mackenzie model, the major question which this investigation sought to answer was:

*Dr. Louise R. Giddings is an Assistant Professor, Division of Education, Medgar Evers College, the City University of New York.

Can the Mackenzie conceptualization of the process of curricular change be applied to describe the process leading to the adoption of the Communication Skills Laboratory?

Specifically, the investigation was concerned with the manner in which the curricular change was brought about and with the individuals who facilitated the change. Thus, the inquiry undertook to find answers to the following sub-questions as they related to the nature of the process of curricular change prior to the adoption of the Communication Skills Laboratory:

1.   What curricular determiners facilitated the change?
2.   Who were the participants who helped to effect the curricular change?
3.   What were the sources of power and methods of influence used by the participants in change?
4.   What were the phases in the process of curricular change leading to the adoption of the Communication Skills Laboratory?

This investigation, which stemmed from the work of Mackenzie, was, in essence, an inquiry as to whether the framework provided by Mackenzie could serve as a useful research tool for this investigator. In a preliminary review of the literature on curricular change, the investigator noted one study which utilized the Mackenzie paradigm as a framework of analysis.[6] This study by Dionne described the adoption of the Physical Sciences Study Committee Physics Program by the high schools in one school system. Dionne reported the events in the case chronologically and then employed the Mackenzie framework in analyzing the case. Essentially, the study was based on interviews by Dionne with individuals who had been involved in the change process.

The investigation under review dealt with an innovation which was developed within a school system and based on the perceived needs in the system. Moreover, this investigator was involved in the change process as a participant-observer. Being familiar with the case, the investigator was able to develop procedures which took advantage of her participation in the change.

This investigator became involved in the development of the Communication Skills Laboratory as a research worker engaged in fieldwork related to studies in curriculum and instruction. As a participant-observer involved with the Communication Skills Laboratory, the investigator contributed to the development of the program by:

1.   studying the roles of other participants in designing the curriculum for the Communication Skills Laboratory.

2.   conducting an evaluation and an analysis of the curricular design for the program, and reporting the information to the teachers in order to assist in the improvement of the design.
3.   reviewing and organizing student literature for the Communication Skills Laboratory in terms of reading levels and stated themes of the program.

The procedures used in this study were based on the unique experiences of this writer as a participant-observer. As a result of the investigator's involvement in the change, it was possible to develop a report of the change process based on observations, logs, reports, and data obtained from interviews and questionnaires included in the field component. In addition, interviews were conducted to validate the investigator's understanding of the change process as indicated by the report, and to gain as much additional information as possible concerning the change from other participants and participant-observers.

The general framework of analysis for this investigation was Mackenzie's conceptualization of the process of curricular change. Figure 1 of this report summarizes Mackenzie's effort to "systematize many observations resulting from an analysis of the cases studied."[7] Basically, the rationale points out that participants in curricular change having control of power sources and methods of influence proceed through phases in a process to influence curriculum determiners, namely, teachers, students, subject matter, methods, materials, facilities, and time. Mackenzie points out, however, that the impact of the cultural context is very obvious in his analysis of the change process.[8] In the studies he analyzed, the precise form and emphasis of the reported changes could hardly be understood or accounted for without some knowledge of the setting in which they occurred. An important observation concerning the Mackenzie model is that Mackenzie specifically notes that:

> this analysis is only a beginning step toward a valid description of the process of curricular change under current conditions. More complete and adequate descriptions should be gathered and analyzed to check the validity of this presentation.[9]

As a result of this investigation, it was determined that curricular change occurred at the selected middle school as a result of actions taken by the reading teacher in the school as she perceived a need for change in the English and reading programs. Although the proposed ideas for change were initially received with some reservations on the part of the principal in the school, the reading teacher, supported by the assistant superintendent for instruction in the district, was able to secure approval of the new program by the local school board.

Participants in curriculum change, sources of their power, and phases in the processes of change of the determiners of the curriculum

Cultural Context

Participants in curricular change	Having control of certain sources of power and methods of influence	Proceed through various phases in a process	To influence the determiners of the curriculum
Internal participants	Advocacy and communication	Initiated by internal or external participants	
Students	Prestige	Criticism	Teachers
Teachers	Competence	Proposal of changes	Students
Principals	Money or goods	Development and clarification	Subject matter
Supervisors	Legal authority	of proposals for change	Methods
Superintendents	Policy, precedent, custom	Evaluation, review and refor-	Materials and facilities
Boards of education	Cooperation and collaboration	mulation of proposals	Time
Citizens in local communities		Comparison of proposals	
State legislatures		Initiated by internal participants	
State departments of education		Actions on proposals	
State and federal courts		Implementation of action	
External participants		decisions	
Non-educationists			
Foundations			
Academicians			
Business and industry			
Educationists			
National government			

Figure 1. The Mackenzie Conceptualization of the Process of Curricular Change

Determiners identified as focal points of change when compared with the program which was replaced were: subject matter, teachers, students, methods, materials, and facilities. Much emphasis was placed on the first five curriculum determiners with less emphasis on facilities. Time was not cited by interviewees as a significant focal point in the change.

Internal and external participants were involved in the change process leading to the adoption of the Communication Skills Laboratory, but the faculty itself played the major role in the development of the new programs. Internal participants in the change were identified as: the superintendent, the assistant superintendent for instruction, the administrative assistant for personnel, the assistant superintendent for business, the school principal, the high school English chairman, the school board, and the staff of the Communication Skills Laboratory. Participant-observers were external participants in the change process.

The reading teacher in the middle school and the superintendent for instruction were the influential people in bringing about the curricular change. The reading teacher, who proposed the change, was viewed by persons interviewed as a capable and confident person with a "strong personality" while the assistant superintendent for instruction was able to influence the change because of his administrative position in the school district.

The staff of the Communication Skills Laboratory was influential in planning for the program and implementing it in the school. Varying levels and types of competences and skills were noted in this investigation on the part of staff members as they contributed to the change process. The principal was also influential in facilitating the change, according to the reading teacher, because he presented critical comments to her which caused her to think through more carefully the proposal which she intended to offer.

With regard to the change in general, power bases and methods of influence pointed out in the Mackenzie conceptual model were identifiable. These included: advocacy and communication, prestige, competence, money, legal authority, policy, precedent, and collaboration.

All phases but one in the process of curricular change as conceptualized by Mackenzie were incorporated in the change process at the middle school. The phases were: criticism; proposal for change; action on proposal; development and clarification of the proposal; evaluation, review and reformulation of proposal; and implementation of action decisions. The phase not identified was "comparison of proposals," a phase which is conceptualized to deal with screening or considering various related but alterative change proposals. There was no evidence that competing or alternative change proposals were considered by participants involved in the process leading to the adoption of the Communication Skills Laboratory.

Based on the study by this investigator, the following conclusions were drawn:

1.   The Mackenzie conceptualization of the process of curricular change could be utilized to examine the process leading to the adoption of the Communication Sills Laboratory.

2.   The application of the Mackenzie conceptualization to the process leading to the adoption of the Communication Skills Laboratory revealed that the adoption of the Communication Skills Laboratory was brought about primarily because of the initiative of one dynamic teacher who was supported in her efforts to effect change by the assistant superintendent for instruction.

3.   Accurate and meaningful descriptions of change situations are needed in understanding the process of change and in determining how systems can be managed to bring about desired curricular changes most effectively.

FOOTNOTES

1.   Matthew B. Miles, "Educational Innovation: The Nature of the Problem," in *Innovation in Education,* ed. by Matthew B. Miles (New York: Bureau of Publications, Teachers College, Columbia University, 1964), p. 2.

2.   Ibid.

3.   Herman Ohme, "Needed: Exportable Models of Significant Change in Education," *Phi Delta Kappan,* 53:657, June, 1972.

4.   Gordon N. Mackenzie, "Curricular Change: Participants, Power, and Processes," in *Innovation in Education,* ed. by Matthew B. Miles (New York: Bureau of Publications, Teachers College, Columbia University, 1964).

5.   Ibid., p. 418.

6.   Joseph Dionne, "Curricular Change: A Descriptive Report of the Adoption of Physical Sciences Study Committee Physics by Four High Schools" (Unpublished Ed.D. dissertation, Teachers College, Columbia University, 1965).

7.   Mackenzie, "Curricular Change: Participants, Power, and Processes," p. 400.

8.   Ibid., p. 407.

9.   Ibid., p. 424.

BIBLIOGRAPHY

Cohen, B. and J. Lukinsky. "Evaluator As Change Agent: A Practical Approach In A Limited Time Frame." *Jewish Education.* 49:4-9; Spring 1981.

Dionne, Joseph. "Curricular Change: A Descriptive Report Of The Adoption Of Physical Sciences Study Committee Physics By Four High Schools." (Unpublished Ed.D. dissertation, Teachers College, Columbia University, 1965).

Horn, J.L. "Reading Specialist As An Effective Change Agent." *The Reading Teacher.* 35: 408-11; January 1982.

Jacobson, R.L. "Higher Education Researchers Probe Curriculum Change." *The Chronicle of Higher Education.* 30: 12-13; March 1985.

Mackenzie, D.G. "Moving Toward Education Change— Where Does One Start?" *National Association of Secondary School Principals Bulletin.* 69:12-17; January 1985.

MacKenzie, Gordon N. "Curricular Change: Participants, Power, and Processes," in *Innovation In Education,* Ed. by Matthew B. Miles, New York: Bureau of Publications, Teachers College, Columbia University, 1964.

Miles, Matthew B. "Education Innovation: The Nature Of the Problem," in *Innovation in Education,* Ed. by Matthew B. Miles. New York: Bureau of Publication, Teachers College, Columbia University, 1964.

Ohme, Herman. "Needed: Exportable Models Of Significant Change In Education." *Phi Delta Kappan.* 53: 657; June 1972.

Ornstein, A.C. "Innovation and Change: Yesterday and Today." *The High School Journal.* 65: 279-86; May 1982.

Pipho, Carl. "School Administrators: The Bottom Line Of The Reform Movement," *Phi Delta Kappan.* 66: 165-6; November 1984.

Renfro, W.L. and J.L. Morrison. "Anticipating and Managing Change In Educational Organizations." *Educational Leadership.* 41:50-54; September 1983.

Section VI
Urban Issues
Introduction by James J. Shields, Jr.*

School is the dependent variable in the school-society-family relationship. Schools mirror the societies and the times in which they exist, and pupils mirror the very intense family and peer relationships which are in place long before they enter school and continue throughout their school experiences. In fact, for most children, less than one-third of any given day is actually spent in school.

The current crisis in urban education is symptomatic of a larger crisis in urban life. Creaky public transportation systems, unsafe streets, demoralized police, and overburdened public hospitals all share with the public school an overriding sense that they are besieged with massive problems whose solutions are elusive at best.

Public schools do not appear to have found the means to be much different or much better than the larger society. The articles in this chapter on the new immigrants provide good cases in point. The current wave of immigrants has brought with it new problems of developing a unifying mainstream culture while respecting quite different, often conflicting, and very diverse cultures. The special needs of the ever-growing ranks of children whose disrupted and quirky lives seem to render it all but impossible for many of them to focus on the day to day patterns of discipline required for effective classroom learning.

As the disenchantment with public schools grows, increased attention is being focused on understanding the role of the family in pupil success. As John Dewey has argued, we learn what we do not only in school, but everywhere. Our first schoolroom is the womb, and from there we graduate to the nursery for more advanced education.

Several of the authors in this chapter address the issues of the interrelationship and changing patterns between the family and the school. In particular, the role of family characteristics in intellectual development as measured by such instruments as the SAT is explored. Also, we are told that while the patterns of raising children in families has not changed as broadly as we have thought, there is reason to believe there has been some erosion in the role of deep personal caring in child-parent relationships.

Throughout the chapter the authors reflect an implicit commitment to the belief that the traditional family continues to be the best setting for nurturing self-confident and responsible children. However, there is also the awareness that today many children grow up in families where both parents work, or in single parent families where emotional and financial stress often is severe. Therefore, it becomes clear that any future agenda for school reform has to set as a priority high-quality day care programs.

No exploration of the critical factors which determine pupil success and failure in school is complete without looking at the powerful world of peer relationships. Indeed, chronically poor peer relationships is one of the strongest predictors of a troubled school career. And no problem connected to peers is more fundamental than those related to drugs. Drug prevention programs have become a major vehicle for finding solutions for a whole range of other problems such as high school dropouts, teenage pregnancy, school violence and low achievement levels.

Beyond the challenges of the urban crisis, changing patterns of family relationships, and rampant drug abuse, there are fundamental structural changes in the world of work. One author tells us that by the end of the century approximately two-thirds of all work will be information based. This raises the question of how schools should change their goals and teaching methodologies to prepare those entering first grade today—who will graduate from high school by the end of the century.

*Dr. James J. Shields is Professor, School of Education, City College, The City University of New York.

This change to an information society is primarily an electronic revolution. We face the dissolution of school systems organized around the slow-moving printed word, and the rapid emergence of new educational systems based on the speed-of-light electronic image. A massive reorientation toward learning is now taking place right in the home as a result of the electronic revolution, primarily through the invention of television. The degree to which the urban public school can adapt to this revolution will play an important role in its ultimate success in meeting the troubling challenges embedded in the urban crisis in America today.

Nathan Brenowitz

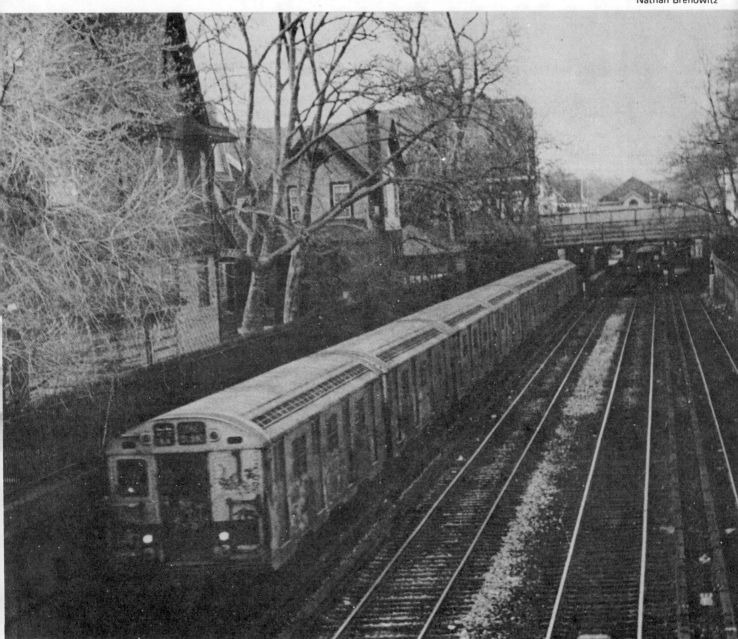

Chapter 44
Urban Population Patterns and Projections
Allan C. Ornstein*

The current crisis in urban education is symptomatic of a general crisis in urban life, particularly the American city. The crisis is in part reflected by the population patterns and projections impacting on urban America; these population patterns and projections have policy implications for educators and especially urban educators. What follows below is an urban population model, along with some future population projections for educators to consider.

City Dwellers Today

There are basically five group of dwellers in the large cities (500,000 or more) in the urban areas of America. First there are the rich and unmarried young who desire the excitement and social opportunities of the city. These people are overwhelmingly white. They do not flee a decaying school system because either they do not have children or they can afford to send them to private school. Instead they want to be close to work, to entertainment, to restaurants, to shopping, and to parks or beaches. As good "liberals" they see a quaintness in urban diversity. Although they tended to be more liberal in the 1960s and early 1970s, and in fact often formed coalitions with minority groups at the expense of other whites, they are becoming less liberal because of the disappearing middle-class buffer against the poor; they are no longer insulated from urban crime, their taxes have increased, and neoconservatism is fashionable now.

Second are the ethnics, deeply traditional, religious, and family oriented. They are firmly rooted to their neighborhoods, to their transplanted cultural institutions—churches, schools, neighborhood clubs, shops and restaurants, to the comfort of speaking the old language with friends and relatives on the street. For these groups, remaining in the city is acceptable so long as their culture and neighborhood can remain intact. They resist neighborhood change and school integration, in part because of racial reasons (partially justified by fears of increased crime and school discipline problems, as well as lowered reading scores and teacher morale) and social and cultural upheaval.

The banks have seen these neighborhoods as "graying" or changing areas and have been reluctant to finance mortgages for young ethnics to live in the old neighborhood. The result is, those who can afford to move, namely second generation ethnics, have moved to the suburbs and have assimilated into the melting pot; those who have been left behind tend to be older and poorer. Although the various ethnics are extremely diverse and different, the media, social scientists, and educators of previous decades often lumped these people into part of the "silent majority," the "hardhat" or the middle American population—fair game for criticism and ridicule. Although most of these ethnics are white and of European descent a recent growing number are Asian. Only recently have social scientists and educators made an attempt to discern between Croations and Serbians, or between Hungarians, Germans, and Poles, or between Chinese, Japanese, and Koreans—corresponding with the growth of ethnic consciousness and cultural pluralism.

Third are a substantial number of economically trapped groups, overwhelmingly white but a growing number of Asians, Hispanics, and blacks, consisting of the following: older folks left behind to endure the city, losing more economic ground each year due to inflation, too poor to retire or if they have already too hard pressed because of a limited pension. Few of the aging poor rely on their children for support, rather on some form of public assistance in terms of housing, social or medical services—living in a fringe area on their own, or in a home for the aged or sickly—facing years of increasing dependency before they die. Since this country was never a traditional society, and having transformed from an inner-directed, industrial society to an other-directed,

*Dr. Allan C. Ornstein is Associate Professor of Education at Loyola University of Chicago.

post industrial society, few of the elderly live with their children. Most of the elderly are independent and live in what are now called "geriatric ghettoes" among the poor and lower middle class, either in the central cities or in areas which are older, have lower housing values, signs of neighborhood deterioration and multi-family dwelling units. To be sure, data suggest that residential age segregation in the cities has increased significantly since the 1950s—corresponding with our aging population and the declining ability of the aged to pay and compete in the free market and high-priced housing.[1]

Part of the economically trapped comprise the lower middle-class, blue collar or white collar workers, who either live in the old neighborhood or in some fringe area which is changing. They are tied to a municipal job— teacher, policeman, fireman, sanitation worker, or park district worker—which requires residence in the city. The requirement is usually a function of the size of the city; the larger the city the more feasible for carrying out a residence requirement due to the increased pool of workers. The requirement may either be a function of the patronage system that exists in the city or a legislated act. They are economically trapped because while many could afford to move to the suburbs, their livelihood would be cut off if they did.

Finally there is a growing number of young and middle aged couples with good education and jobs and earnings in 1980 between $20,000 to $35,000, subjectively, defined as the middle class. They would like to buy a home in the suburbs, but cannot afford the $25,000 down payment and, if they could afford it, the high interest rates for new mortgages prevent them from purchasing even a modest home. Their dream of owning their own home is vanishing. Confronted by a nightmare of sky-rocketing costs that have outstripped their gain in income since the late 1970s, and earning too much to qualify for government programs but too little to take advantage of most tax shelters and investments, they have found it increasingly difficult to get ahead; they too feel trapped economically, even alienated since the good life that was to come after graduation from college has not materialized.

Of course, some of the economically trapped families finally make it to the suburbs; either because their financial situation has improved (largely as a result of both spouses working), or they have changed employment from a municipal job that obligated their city residency.

Fourth are the newcomers to the cities, recent immigrants from Mexico and other parts of Latin America, Southeast Asia, Africa, and Russia. In the minds of many people, the era of immigration to the U.S. ended more than a half century ago. Not so. This land continues to attract to its shores hundreds of thousands of new residents each year. Despite present economic ills, we still

look like the promised land to people looking for a better life. Thus the ebb and flow of legal immigration has surpassed already post World War II rates and is approaching post World War I peak rates.

Legal immigration now accounts for up to one half of the annual growth in U.S. population. Between 1970 and 1980 legal immigration totaled approximately five million, by far the largest influx in more than fifty years, with the highest in order from Mexico, Philippines, South Korea, Taiwan, Vietnam, Jamaica, India, Dominican Republic, Cuba, and Britain. Estimates of illegal immigration, mainly from Mexico, the Caribbean, and Southeast Europe, total 1 to 2.5 million per year, with some 500,000 establishing permanent residence, depending on what report we digest.[2] Legal and illegal immigration rates far surpass the annual mass immigration flow of the early twentieth century. These new immigrants, like their predecessors, tend to huddle in our cities.

Loneliness, language barriers, ethnic prejudice, and the need of finding work fast remain problems, as they did when the European immigrants landed on our shores. The difference is, the newcomers today enter a land that is vastly different from the open, booming America that absorbed the European masses with much ease in prior decades. Moreover, hostilities toward immigrants, especially illegal immigrants, are common—born of economic and population pressures; jobs are scarce and unemployment trends and wages in many sectors of the economy are affected by the immigrants who are willing to work for less money than Americans. Many of the new immigrants, especially the Hispanics who represent the fastest growing ethnic population in the country (15 million represents the legal immigrant population) and possess the least clout for their numbers, have to compete with blacks, urban interests, and other groups scrambling for a share of government dollars, affirmative action progress, jobs, and political representation.

Although some of these refugees have tremendous health problems (especially those from Southeast Asia), and some members of the family are politically or economically trapped in the old country, and some experience acute language and cultural differences, these immigrants will succeed by and large for several reasons. Regardless of family size, most come with a strong family structure supported by traditional values and a culture older than ours which emphasizes the work ethnic, male dominance, and respect for family, school, church and adult authority in general.

Tremendous stress exists among the children to please family elders and teachers, to learn and succeed in school, and learn on the job (which they do, on both accounts according to middle-class standards). Parents and adults come with a desire to work, immediately find it because of their desire to work, and work harder than most Americans; in fact they manage to save money while most of us consume it. Moreover, many of the Asian, Russian, and early Cuban populations come with technological skills and education. The overwhelming majority of the immigrants, legal and illegal, work, pay taxes, and no more than five percent receive welfare—and for a short period of time. Most of them depend on help from friends, family and social service organizations—are driven for a chance to start life again and thus are future oriented; it is this motivation and future perspective which results in benefit for themselves and the nation.

Fifth are the "structural" poor—meaning there are few chances to escape from poverty and this is fast becoming an inherited curse for the children of the poor. We are talking about an inherited poverty, due mainly to unstable and disorganized family conditions, few enriching stimuli at home, little emphasis on learning tasks at home that might facilitate school achievement, and little orientation to the rules and routine of the middle-class school culture and world of technology and bureaucracy.

Although more whites than blacks are structurally poor, a much larger percentage of blacks can be categorized into this group; moreover, the latter are concentrated in cities (50% of the city poor are black). Despite the fact that there is an increasing black middle class escaping the ghetto, there is at the same time an increasing breakdown of the family structure of blacks which perpetuates their poverty class. These families are characterized by large numbers of children, exceedingly high illegitimacy rates and welfare dependency, as well as high delinquency, drugs, arrest rates, dropout rates, and unemployment among youth—largely a reflection of the growing rise of black female-headed households (from 18% in 1949 to 24% in 1963 to 49% in 1979)—which sap the vitality, strength, and money of the cities and schools. While the number of blacks below the poverty line has declined more than 50% in the 1970s for families with male heads, it increased 25% for those with female heads. Similar patterns of increasing breakdown of the Puerto Rican family are evidenced, although not as dramatically; also, their numbers are limited to a few cities.

Future Population Considerations

Whatever our approach to solving our urban problems, certain demographic and economic realistics must be considered. First, the American cities, not only in the frost zone but also in the sunbelt, will be confronted with an increasing structurally poor group functioning outside the system with little prospects for the future. This group is powerless, frustrated, alienated, and envious, and violent urban eruptions should be considered a real possibility in the 1980s. The melting pot theme breaks

down with the structurally poor who are nonwhite. Hence, we have underestimated the difficulty of breaking the cycle of poverty among them. The implications are that the cities and schools, especially in the frost zone, will further deteriorate in terms of quality and financial and social stability.

Absorbing these structurally poor groups into the social and economic system is bound to increase social spending (when the liberal platform returns to Washington) and taxes and decrease productivity rates and the quality of goods and services we produce—in turn increasing our over-all deficits and inflation rates and reducing our economic growth and quality of living—all which are already evident and will probably worsen. This is one reason why the Japanese and Germans are outproducing us in terms of cost and performance (why you and I often buy foreign cars, televisions, cameras, and electronic equipment).

Our standard of living will most likely decline, with or without Reagan economics. Our children and grandchildren will experience this change in living, more than us and more than we may imagine; as a nation our economic downside is just beginning. The problem will be more intense in the cities, especially in the frost zone, because our manufacturing productivity rates are in decline and we are forced to absorb more and more disadvantaged groups into the system. Not only city schools but also many of our public institutions and services face tremendous strain and potential economic collapse (school budgets will be stripped in future years). Indeed, it is easy to spend someone else's money, the public money, but there is only so much we can tax people and only so much money we can print to pay for our social programs and defense needs before the system begins to deteriorate, as it is now, and possibly breaks down.

Of crucial concern is the fact that the manufacturing centers of the frost zone are ailing, and they are expected by some economists to never fully recover from this last recession. The impact on the structurally poor male seeking employment, especially black male, is bleak. These males are looking for work, and given their skills and work history, are losing the very chance to work. The only other option they have, other than unemployment or crime, it so seek jobs in the expanding service industry of janitors, dishwashers, hamburger helpers, and cooks, where salaries are low.

In the meantime, the females of the structurally poor, especially black poor, are being increasingly integrated into the administrative and clerical sectors of the city economics with incomes that would normally bring them out of economically poor categories if their spouses could find viable jobs. The families who are structurally poor, and seeking to out-distance the welfare syndrome, will remain one-income household units, with the woman (not the man) earning that income. Similarly, the single-parent female-headed black (and to a lesser extent Hispanic) family will increase—a tragic trend on black family stability. The message is clear to black teenagers of the inner city, more than half of whom who see little point in learning and drop out of school before graduation.

Second, the large cities of the nation, especially in the first zone where whites are still fleeing, and a few sunbelt cities due to immigration trends, will come to resemble the Third World—with its unemployment and underemployment, poor health and housing conditions, lack of adequate schooling, and squalor. The combined effects of increase in the American black and Hispanic populations, coupled with immigration trends, create this United Nations effect; moreover, as their members grow, they become a larger population of the total city population which in turn fuels middle-class flight.

This population trend has even led to suggestions that the cities try the methods of Third World nations: luring industries into the inner city through tax holidays, duty free zones, low land costs, and free training of workers. While the enterprise zone idea is a hot topic among urban planners and Reaganite supporters, the idea to attract private capital into ghetto areas for tax breaks is untested in the United States; moreover, it misses the point that taxes are seldom the deciding factor where a firm sets up a new branch for investment. The reward-risks and mathematics of the investment have to work out; smart money will not invest in declining areas, much less the inner cities, not for tax advantages if there is a real possibility of losing real money.

As for urban schools, the expansion of bilingual and multicultural programs will be evident in the 1980s. More and more immigrant and/or non-speaking and limited English speaking children will be entering our city schools, and teacher training and school programs should flourish in these areas of concentration.

Third, the cities' middle-class population will become increasingly non-family. Young children striking out for the first time will seek to establish new households in inexpensive neighborhoods near jobs and activities of larger cities. Divorced persons, especially those without children, will likely resettle in cities for the same reason. Middle-aged parents, whose children have grown up and left, will seek the convenience of a smaller residence in middle-income and high rental areas of the city. An expanding number of nonmarried living partners will find the city a viable place to live.

Although the non-family household is increasing and returning to the cities, their numbers are too few to create a statistical impact or to offset the large and continuous increase of structurally poor and immigrant populations characterizing our large cities. Nonetheless, their concentration in neighborhoods create a micro real estate boom

in small, selected parts of the cities, as well as for a concentration of expensive restaurants and boutiques. The result of this boom is the creation of a false impression of urban revitalization and renaissance. To be sure, most of the neighborhoods of the cities, especially in the frost zone, are experiencing decay—adding to the outmigration of middle-class and white households with children.

While our prime goal should be to attract families back to the cities, the statistical facts do not permit this to happen. Fewer children, especially of the middle class, are being born—at least during the last 20 years. A recent survey shows that only 17 percent of the households in the nation fit into the traditional American family format of a husband and wife with more than one child.[3]

Taking note of some vital marriage signs, the marriage rate of women has declined from a high of 109 per 1,000 in 1969–71 to 85 in 1975–77. The remarriage rate has also begun to drop from 166 in 1966–68 to 134 in 1975–77. In the case of young women, the declining marriage rate means not only a delay in marriage but also no marriage at all; we know that the longer young adults postpone marriage, the greater the chance of no marriage. Estimates of the proportion of young women who will not marry (and not have children) have increased from 4–5 percent to 8–9 percent in the last 20 years.[4]

Paralleling the apparent reluctance to enter into marriage is the growing willingness to leave it; divorce rates have doubled from the mid 1960s to the mid 1970s. Moreover, marriage used to mean having children as a matter of course—the only question was just how many children. Since the 1970s, however, there has been a notable increase of young women who plan to have no children; 11 percent among 18–34 year olds in 1978, and 21 percent for 18–34 year olds with a college degree (and the percentage of college educated women is rapidly increasing). Similarly, among currently married women, 18–34, the average number of expected children in 1986 was 3.1; in 1978, it was 2.3; among college educated women, it was 1.5.[5] This means that whatever babies will be born in the near future will be mainly from noncollege women, that is from lower- and working-class households.

Fourth, a baby boom is seen by the mid 1980s—characterized by a small number of two-income upper middle and upper class (with one or no children), a shrinking one-income middle class (representing the traditional family, two or three children), and vast lower class, one headed household (with several children). The later two population groups will be limited in income because of the number of adult persons in the age group crowding the job market, an escalation in inflation, the fact that salaries will not keep up to inflation, and the fact that it will take two salaries to keep ahead of inflation.

Since many of the two-income families will be housed in the cities, demand for luxury goods and services will be high in selected areas of many cities. On the other hand, sales of mass-market durable goods will be much weaker than the size of the baby boom generation would indicate, since the mass of the population will have less real money to spend. In turn, this will detrimentally effect the economy of the frost zone cities—where manufacturing of such goods is focused.

In this connection, the public schools will house fewer middle-class students and more lower-class and financially strapped working-class students. Educators, today, who refer to the coming baby boom (the children of the baby boomers born between the end of World War II and 1960; this makes them between 21 and 36 years old now), are counting heads and not looking at the increasing problems of educating more economically disadvantaged students. The decline of middle-class families, and especially students, will be nationwide but highlighted in the cities where families with children and who are economically mobile will continue to flee.

The typical American household, the one-income family, where income is growing most slowly, will continue to shrink as a portion of the total households in the nation, particularly in the cities, and two income families will continue to grow. By 1990, American society will be divided almost equally among single person households, one-income families, and two-income families; quite different from 1970, when one income families comprised more than half of American households, with two-income families accounting for 26 percent and singles only 22 percent.[6]

Two-income families will grow more rapidly because women will be pushed by slower income growth of their husbands and pulled by more opportunities in the expanding job market. The two-income families will form the bulk of the upper middle class over the next decade or so, and be involved more in conspicuous consuming and leisure than raising a family. Because many of the two-income families are likely to be professional couples, those combined incomes will be substantial. Single professionals will also swell the upper middle class in the cities. The women in these twin groups, however, will change some of their traditional attitudes and behaviors; they will have fewer children.

Fifth, the public schools of the cities have been written off as less than second rate by most knowledgeable parents, and without good schools the cities will not attract nor keep families who can afford to move and pay for better schooling through higher property taxes to the suburbs where education is a relatively superior and physically safe experience for their children. When a middle-class family is economically tied to the city, chances are the children will attend a private or parochial institution, thus avoiding the public schools. The parochial school system alone provides the education of 25 to

40 percent of the elementary and secondary students in Boston, Buffalo, Chicago, Cincinnati, Cleveland, Detroit, Milwaukee, Philadelphia, Pittsburgh, Newark, and St. Louis. More than two thirds of this student population is white, compared to the public schools in these cities which are less than one third white.[7]

Worried educators have already coined a new term to define the trend: bright flight. The private and parochial school boom is skimming off many of the nation's and especially cities' middle-class and able students—and what is even worse, this trend is occurring during one of the biggest baby busts of this century. In the last decade, public school enrollments dropped more than ten percent, and in the 25 largest city school systems it dropped nearly 20 percent; nonetheless, private school enrollments climbed 20 percent nationwide and nearly 30 percent in the cities—and even more in cities like Boston and Los Angeles that have experienced court-ordered busing.[8]

Recent polls by Gallup and Newsweek seem to support the fear that more than 50 percent of parents with children in public school say they have considered the private alternative, and almost 25 percent say they would switch to private schooling if Congress approved a tuition voucher or tax credit of $250 or more. Furthermore, James Coleman's new study argues that private schools are superior in comparison to public schools for both white and minority populations alike, and Andrew Greeley's lesser known study supports this data.[9]

Conclusion

The economically disadvantaged populations of the cities are expanding by natural increase, migration, and immigration, while the middle-class and white populations are producing fewer children and those with children continue to flee the cities. It is indeed a sad note that just when the frost zone cities are desperate to reattract middle-class families, they are witnessing economic decline—adding to the flight of the middle class who are following job opportunities to the suburbs and sunbelt—and the growth of poor families. The irony becomes tragic and potentially explosive because these disadvantaged families find themselves walled in by all the ingredients of the urban crisis—poverty, generation to generation of welfare dependency, discrimination, and political exploitation—compounded today by federal cuts in social and educational programs. As a result, the polarization between the "haves" and "have nots" becomes greater and the crisis point in the cities looms closer—and as the cities' problems snowball they will eventually spill over and affect adjacent suburbs and their respective states, too. This domino trend is only a matter of time, when it will become more obvious to the American people.

FOOTNOTES

1. See Donald O. Coqwill, "Residential Segregation by Age in American Metropolitan areas," *Journal of Gerontology* (May 1978), pp. 446-53; "Housing the Elderly: Challenges for the Future," *Urban Institute Policy and Research Report* (Spring 1981), pp. 14-16; Mark LaGarey et al., "The Age Segregation Process: Explanation for American Cities," *Urban Affairs Quarterly* (September 1980), pp. 59-80.

2. *Chicago Sun Times,* October 26, 1981, p. 4; "Making it in America," *"U.S. News and World Report,* August 17, 1981, pp. 58-61.

3. White House Conference on Families, *Listening to America's Families Action for the 1980s* (Washington, D.C.: U.S. Government Printing Office, 1980).

4. Jessie Bernard, "Facing the Future," *Society* (January 1981), pp. 53-59; Heather Ross and Isabel Sawhill, *Time of Transition: The Growth of Families Headed by Women* (Washington, D.C.: Urban Institute, 1979).

5. Bernard, "Facing the Future"; White House Conference on Families, *Listening to America's Families.*

6. Ross and Sawhill, *Time of Transition.* Also see Bernadette Doran, "Population Experts Say a Surprise Package Might Soon Arrive at Your Schools," *American School Board Journal* (February 1982), pp. 19-21, 24.

7. *Catholic Schools in America, 1981* (Washington, D.C.: Catholic Education Association, 1981).

8. *Ibid; Digest of Educational Statistics, 1980* (Washington, D.C.: U.S. Government Printing Office, 1981); "Why Public Schools Fail," *Newsweek,* April 20, 1981, pp. 62-73; also see Table 1.

9. James S. Coleman, *Achievement in High School: Public and Private Schools Compared* (New York: Basic Books, 1981); Andrew Greeley, *Catholic High Schools and Minority Students* (New Brunswick, N.J.: Transaction Books, 1982).

Van Bucher

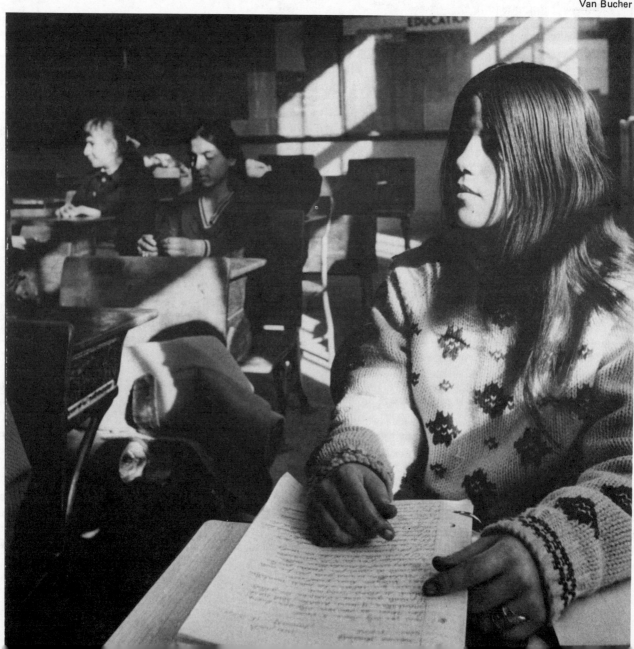

Chapter 45
The New Immigrants
Barry Persky and Leonard H. Golubchick*

As we celebrate the centennial of the Statue of Liberty and the bicentennial of the United States Constitution, immigrants from all over the world beat at our door. The concept of the statue has evolved into a "Mother of Exiles," a sheltering figure holding the beacon of liberty to millions of immigrants. The words of poet Emma Lazarus have become familiar to every school-age child in our country:

Give me your tired, your poor,
Your huddled masses yearning to breathe free,
The wretched refuse of your teeming shore.
Send these, the homeless, the tempest-tossed to me:
I lift my lamp beside the golden door!

Ellis Island, the processing center near the statue, was the point of entry into our shore for more than 70% of the 24 million immigrants who entered the country between 1892 and 1954. It is estimated that 85% of the Americans living today have some family connected with the island.

In the year 1986, the centennial of the Statue of Liberty, which symbolizes the port of entry or door to our shores, the "golden door" is often characterized as being tarnished. The Southwest, Mexican desert borders of our nation, guarded by an understaffed Border Patrol, are involved daily with the smuggling of people and drugs. Men and women pay exorbitant amounts to smugglers to enter the country. In the Caribbean waters off the Florida coast people are crammed into unseaworthy boats seeking refuge in the United States.

Immigration has been a controversial issue before in our history, as it is today. Americans are polarized regarding the needed changes in our immigration laws. Many Americans are concerned that economic, social, and political realities of today may force us to either radically restrict immigration or close our doors altogether. Conversely, many other Americans feel that our immigration policy falls short of what is necessary. They contend that the adoption of a more restrictive immigra-tion policy will severely tarnish our world image as a beacon of light in the darkness of human misery.

Immigrants were welcome with open arms for over a century after our country's founding. The first restrictive laws, the Alien and Sedition Acts of 1798, gave the President broad powers to deport aliens and raised the residence requirement to 14 years. The act was politically motivated in an attempt by the Federalists to restrict the powers of Thomas Jefferson and his followers. The laws were repealed by 1800 when the Republicans gained power. In 1882, Congress enacted our first racist immigration law, the Chinese Exclusion Act. This act resulted from the depression of the 1870s following the completion of the transcontinental railroad. Disgruntled American workers called for the banning of further Chinese workers, who were willing to work long hours at hard labor without complaint. In response to the Chinese workers' thriftiness and willingness to work at any price, the pejorative idiom "coolie labor" was coined. In 1904, Chinese immigration was indefinitely suspended, not to be resumed until 1943. In 1890, the Census Bureau officially declared our western frontier movement closed. This meant the end of our unlimited horizons and need for cheap immigrant labor. As immigrants continued to arrive at our shores, they were accused of draining our natural resources and taxing our social welfare system.

In the 1920s, the United States Congress placed a ceiling on the total number of immigrants allowed to enter our country legally. The proportion of entrants from any foreign country was fixed according to the national origin of the existing United States population. This quota system favored northern and western Europeans. The rise of totalitarianism prevented many people from emi-

*Dr. Barry Persky is Educational Faculty Chair, Walden University, and President of the Doctorate Association of New York. Dr. Leonard Golubchick is Principal of P.S. 20 Manhattan, New York City Board of Education.

grating from Germany, Italy and Russia. The United States itself was so isolationist prior to World War II that in 1939 a proposal to admit 20,000 Jewish refugee children from Nazi Germany failed to pass Congress on the grounds that the German quota would be exceeded. World War II changed the United States from isolationism to internationalism. Congress repealed the ban on Chinese immigration in 1943 and liberalized immigration from India and the Philippines.

The rise in strength and influence of the Communist bloc brought about the passage of the McCarran-Walter Immigration and Nationality Act of 1952, the first major immigration legislation since 1924. President Harry Truman labeled the act as one of the most shameful and discriminatory in our history. In the immigration act of 1965, the national origin quotas were dropped with 120,000 visas being issued to persons living in the Western Hemisphere and 170,000 additional visas being issued to people born elsewhere. Provision was made for spouses and children of United States citizens and political refugees including: Cubans, Vietnamese and Cambodians. In addition to "legal" immigrants, there are the "undocumented aliens," who settle amongst their countrymen where they are virtually undetectable. In 1985 more than 600,000 legal immigrants and refugees entered the country, at the same time that the United States Immigration and Naturalization Service apprehended 1.3 million illegal immigrants. It is estimated that many more slipped into our country undetected. Among the nationalities that immigrated to our shores in 1985 were: Mexicans, Koreans, Vietnamese, Indians, Jamaicans, Chinese, Iranians, English, Dominicans, Salvadoreans, Guatemalans and Filipinos. This does not include the large Cuban population that came to country via Miami.

The statistical data reflect the changing face of two of our largest cities: New York and Los Angeles. New York City's Hispanic population 15 years ago was roughly 950,000 and today it is close to 2 million. Orientals, who numbered 60,000 in 1965, now number over 250,000. In Los Angeles in 1960, one in nine was Hispanic and one in a hundred was Asian. Today one in ten is Asian and a third of Los Angeles County is Hispanic; Hispanics compose over two third of the county's kindergarten enrollment. A good number of the new immigrants are well-educated professionals, who are meeting the American dream of success. Yet for others the adjustment to a new land is traumatic, as they possess little education and few skills. Los Angeles and New York face similar problems in absorbing the new wave of immigrants. Los Angeles has a school enrollment of 550,000 children, of which 117,000 speak one of 104 languages as a first language. Many of these new-comers cling to their own ethnic identity, preserving their language and customs. New neighborhoods, like New York City's Flushing, Queens area,

have become a haven for Koreans. You can walk for blocks without seeing a sign in English.

Many of the new arrivals also cling to their old prejudices, i.e., Japanese look down upon Koreans while Koreans develop new prejudices as they in turn look down upon Chicanos and Blacks. Overall, the new arrivals would like their children to become Americanized, so they can gain status in their new country. The great socializing effects of American television, advertising, and fast food chains, as well as the educational system, contribute to homogenize the children of immigrants. Yet unlike the immigrants of the late nineteenth century and the early twentieth century, today's immigrant population and their children find it possible to maintain their language and avoid becoming fully assimilated. The main factor is the ability to be highly mobile due to easy access to jet transportation and frequent trips back to their homeland. It is relatively simple for Dominicans, Puerto Ricans and Mexicans to travel back and forth to their native lands.

Freda Cheung, Deputy Chief of the Minority Research Resources Branch of the National Institute of Mental Health (NIMH) believes that the way immigrants cope with their new environment may be influenced by how they arrived in this country. For example, immigrants are better prepared mentally than refugees, since refugees feel more uprooted. Ruben Rumbaut, a Cuban refugee and sociologist, has been studying four groups of refugees who have settled in the San Diego area. They are the Hmong from the mountains of Laos, the Khmer from Cambodia, ethnic Chinese from Vietnam and Vietnamese. Rambaut has found that approximately 75% of the refugees live below the poverty line and that 60% of them are on welfare. Due to differing backgrounds there are marked distinctions between the refugees. Those from rural backgrounds have the greatest difficulty. They have the lowest educational level and literacy level; most of them are not able to read or write English. These refugees, the Hmong and the Khmer, are the least skilled, with the highest unemployment rate and lowest income, and are welfare dependent when compared to other refugee groups. The Chinese and Vietnamese, who come from an urban background, are the best educated of all refugee groups and have the least problems of adjusting to their new land. Seventy-five percent of these refugees can read and write English.

Furthermore, today's immigrants from Asia are the most well educated and highly skilled immigrant group that ever came here. This is due to the fact that the Philippines, Taiwan, and India are producing more college graduates, especially in the areas of the sciences, medicine and engineering, than those countries can absorb. As a result many graduates leave their country for a place where they can practice their profession. In addition to these well educated immigrants are those who come from the Middle East: Iranians, Israelis, Egyptians, Lebanese and Russian Jews.

The make-up of the Hispanic populations and their socio-economic status are diverse. In Los Angeles 8 out of 10 Hispanics are of Mexican origin. Approximately 2.1 million are Mexicans, approximately 200,000 are from El Salvador, and approximately 50,000 are Guatemalans, while an additional 100,000 Hispanics came from Colombia, Honduras, Cuba and/or Puerto Rico. These numbers include many illegals, the poorest of whom are the Salvadoreans. New York is composed of an estimated 1 million Puerto Ricans along with a substantial number of Dominicans. The number of Cubans in New York are relatively well educated and occupy high status positions since it was the upper and middle classes that fled Cuba upon Castro's takeover. When we compare Mexicans, Dominicans and those from South and Central America, it is the later groups which hold relatively high levels of education and hold better jobs than their Puerto Rican, Mexican, and Dominican counterparts.

Assimilation to the ways of one's new country is made relatively easier when there are established social networks created by previous immigrant groups. Jewish immigrants of the early twentieth century founded "vereins," Chinese groups continued the "tong" in their new country and Hispanic and Italian groups established social clubs, all of which served as social networks to alleviate anxiety and assist in the new immigrants' assimilation. As time passes, the children of immigrants usually become enmeshed in their new country through education, employment and marriage to non-immigrants. This invariably leads to integration into the mainstream social and economic fabric of the city.

Conversely, the same social and economic forces which assist integration may impede it as well. This is due in large measure to the ease with which immigrants can board planes and return to their homelands in a matter of hours. Thus, when there are extreme stresses in the economic and social spheres one can easily flee. This creates a problem; particularly, with Hispanic and Caribbean groups, in regard to public policy planning. For what has resulted is a great number of families, headed by females, receiving Aid to Dependent Children. Another aspect, which was not common to previous waves of immigrants, is the large number of illegals entering our country. In terms of public policy planning, provisions have to be made for their remaining hidden and falling prey to unscrupulous employers. Their economic and social integration are far more difficult and they create strains upon our institutions such as the educational and health care systems.

The impact of the recent wave of immigrants will become increasingly significant in the future. Harold Hodgkinson projects that shortly after the turn of the century one of every three Americans will be nonwhite. Currently the majority of students in our 25 largest city school systems are minorities. Demographers predict that as a result of low white birth rates and immigration that California will become the first mainland state to have a population whose majority is made up of minorities by the year 2010. In the coming years the pluralistic society in America will be even more diverse. For educators that translates into working with a far greater range of ethnically diverse children than ever before. The schools' present record of working with lower class Black and Hispanic children is dismal. By all indications, the growing number of America's future young people will be poor, nonwhite, limited-English proficient and from broken homes headed by uneducated adults. Can our schools as they are presently functioning prepare these generations for higher education, active citizenship, and tomorrow's advanced workforce?

BIBLIOGRAPHY

Cafferty, P. *The Dilemma of American Immigration: Beyond the Golden Door.* San Francisco: Transaction Books, 1983.

Ehrlich, Paul R. *The Golden Door: International Migration, Mexico and the U.S.* New York: Ballantine, 1979.

Kennedy, John F. *A Nation of Immigrants.* New York: Harper and Row, 1971.

Haskins, James. *The New Americans, Cuban Boat People.* Hillside, New Jersey: Enslow Publishers, 1982.

Hodgkinson, Harold L., et al. "A Population in Motion," *Education Week,* May 14, 1986, pp. 13-37.

Philipson, Loren and Llerena, Rafael. *Freedom Flights.* New York: Random House, 1980.

Chapter 46
Educating for the Information Society
Harlan Cleveland*

Shortly after the attempted assassination of President Reagan in 1981, Secretary of State Alexander Haig announced on television from the White House that "I am in control here. . . . " That statement produced neither reassurance nor anger from the American people: rather, the response was nervous laughter, as in watching theater of the absurd. We, the people, know by instinct that in our pluralistic democracy no one is, can be, nor is even supposed to be "in control." By constitutional design, reinforced by the information-rich conditions of work, we live in a nobody-in-charge society.

In a nobody-in-charge society, where decisions are made by consensus and committee, policy is made by an upside-down version of the traditional pyramid of power. Russell Baker, probably the best satirist currently practicing, captured the essence of this anomaly in an ironic dialogue with himself several years ago:

"What does this country need today?"

"Leadership. . . . The country yearns for new leadership for a new era."

"If led, will the country follow?"

"If given the right kind of leadership, the country will surely follow."

"But what kind of leadership is the right kind?"

"The leadership that leads the country in the direction it wants to take."

"And what specific direction does the country want to take?"

"Who knows? That's for the leader to figure out. If he is the right kind of leader, he will guess correctly."

" . . . Am I wrong (Baker asks) in concluding that it isn't leadership the country wants in a president, but followership?"

Russell Baker was not wrong. High policy—that is major changes in society's sense of direction—is first shaped by an inchoate consensus reached by the people at large.

If you find this upside-down pyramid hard to visualize, you are in distinguished company. The classic expression of this wearied cynicism is still Walter Lippmann's brooding book *The Phantom Public,* in which he announced his conclusion that "we must abandon the notion that the people govern. Instead," he continued, "we must adopt the theory that, by their occasional mobilization as a majority, people support or oppose individuals who actually govern. We must say that the popular will does not direct continuously but that it intervenes occasionally." The task, Lippmann thought, was "to find ways for people to act intelligently but in ignorance."

Walter Lippmann was the most brilliant pundit of his time—but he never ran for office or even ran an organization. No political leader or corporate executive could operate on his premise and survive.

Tick off in your mind some major shifts in U.S. policy these past twenty years:

- The federal government was the last to learn that the war in Vietnam was over.
- Richard Nixon and his immediate staff were the last to tumble to the fact that the president had fumbled his way out of office.
- The tidal waves of social change in our time—environmental sensitivity, civil rights for all races, the enhanced status of women, recognition of the rights of consumers and small investors—were not generated by the established leaders in government, business, labor, religion, or high education. They boiled up from people (and new leaders) who had not previously been heard from.
- The nuclear power industry was derailed by the very large numbers of plain people who concluded that the experts had not done their homework on nuclear

*Dr. Harlan Cleveland is Dean of the Hubert H. Humphrey Institute of Public Affairs, University of Minnesota. Reprinted with permission of the author from *Change* magazine, July, 1985.

safety, on nuclear proliferation, and on the disposal of radioactive waste—yet were, nevertheless, pushing this new source of energy down their throats.

- American women had stopped having so many babies long before school boards and government planners adjusted to no-growth or slow-growth assumptions.
- People were opting for smaller cars well before Detroit caught on.
- There was a grassroots movement toward an ethic of qualitative growth while government and business leaders were still measuring "progress" by quantitative aggregates.
- Americans became interested in energy conservation and solar energy while the ranking alarmists on energy policy in and out of government were still pooh-poohing sun-based alternatives to imported oil, driving around in gas-guzzling limousines, and failing to practice conservation in their own organizations.

Sprinkle on your own illustrations, to taste.

What seems to happen is that if the question is important enough, people-in-general get to the answer first. Then the experts and pundits and pollsters and labor leaders and lawyers and doctors and business executives and foundation officers and judges and professors and public executives—many of them chronically afflicted with hardening of the categories—catch up in jerky arthritic moves with all deliberate speed.

Journalists and educators serve as gatekeepers, moving all this information from its specialized sources to the general public, where it is then circulated through powerful but informal interpersonal networks. Only then, when the policy decision is long since made and the experts have finally done the programming, written the editorials, raised the money, painted the directional signposts, and staged the appropriate media event, the publicity heroes and heroines come forth, the people that *People* magazine thinks are our leaders. They climb aboard the train as it gathers momentum and announce for all to hear the new direction of march—speaking by television from the safety of the caboose.

It's more and more obvious: those with visible responsibility for leadership are nearly always too visible to take the responsibility for change—until it becomes more dangerous to stand there than to move. It is not a new idea: "I am a leader," Voltaire wrote, "therefore, I must follow."

The Informatization of Society

This state of affairs has been brought about by the two interdependent macro-trends of out time: the sudden emergence of new information technologies, and the sudden emergence of a new *attitude* toward new technologies.

It is still shocking, forty years later, to remember that the Manhattan Project, the huge secret program that produced the atomic bomb during World War II, did not employ on its staff a single person whose full-time assignment was to think hard about the policy implications of the project if it should succeed. Thus, no one was working on nuclear arms control—though I.I. Rabi says he and Robert Oppenheimer used to discuss it earnestly over lunch. We have been playing catch-up, not too successfully, ever since.

The Manhattan Project was not, however, an exception; it was the rule. For three hundred years, until the 1970s, science and technology were quite generally regarded as having lives of their own, each with an "inner logic," and an autonomous sense of direction. Their self-justifying ethic was change and growth. But in the 1970s, society started to take charge—not of scientific discovery, but of its technological fallout. The decision not to build the SST or deploy an ABM system even though we knew how to make them, the dramatic change in national environmental policy, and the souring of the nuclear power industry, bear witness.

The most prominent and pervasive consequence of the people's concern about the impacts and implications of new technologies is characterized by a French coinage, "l'informatisation de la societe," which we will Americanize to "informatization." It will serve as well as any to describe what is happening to some of our key concepts and conceptions as information becomes the dominant resource in "post-industrial society." (The new word is certainly better than "post-industrial," which describes the future by saying it comes after the past.)

The revolutions that began with Charles Babbage's "analytical engine" (fewer than 150 years ago) and Guglielmo Marconi's wireless telegraphy (not yet a century old) started on quite different tracks. But a quarter of a century ago, computers and telecommunications began to converge to produce a combined complexity, one interlocked industry that is transforming our personal lives, our national politics and our international relations.

The industrial era was characterized by the influence of humankind over things, including nature as well as the artifacts of humankind. The information era features a sudden increase in humanity's power to think and therefore to organize.

The "information society" does not replace, it overlaps, the growing and extracting and processing and manufacturing and recycling and distribution and consumption of tangible things. Agriculture and industry continue to progress by doing more with less through better knowledge, leaving plenty of room for a knowledge economy that, in statistics now widely accepted, accounts for more than half of our workforce, our national productivity, and our global reach. (*The Econo-*

mist recently estimated the information sector at 56 percent of the U.S. economy.)

The actual growing, production, and extraction of things now soaks up a good deal less than a quarter of our human resources. Of all the rest, which used to be lumped together as "services," more than two-thirds are information workers. By the end of the century, something like two-thirds of all work will be information work.

If information (organized data, refined into knowledge and combined into wisdom) is now our "crucial resource"—that's how Peter Drucker describes it—what does that portend for citizenship, and for the education of citizens? The answer has to start with a close look at the inherent characteristics of information considered as a resource. These provide some clues to the vigorous rethinking that lies ahead for all of us:

Information Is Expandable.   In 1972, the same year *The Limits to Growth* was published, John McHale came out with a book called *The Changing Information Environment*. It didn't sell three million copies in sixteen languages, but it may prove to have been the more prescient of the two studies. McHale argued that information expands as it is used. Whole industries have grown up to exploit this characteristics of information: scientific research, technology transfer, computer software (which already makes a contribution to the U.S. economy that is several times the contribution of computer hardware), and agencies for publishing, advertising, public relations, and government propaganda to spread the word (and thus to enhance the word's value).

Information Is Not Resource-Hungry.   Compared to the steel-and-automobile economy, the production and distribution of information are remarkably sparing in their requirements for energy and other physical and biological resources. Investments, pricing policies, and power relationships that assume the more developed countries will goble up disproportionate shares of real resources are overdue for wholesale revision.

Information Is Substitutable.   Information can, and increasingly does, replace capital, labor, and physical materials. Robotics and automation in factories and offices are displacing workers and thus requiring a transformation of the labor force. Any machine that can be accessed by computerized telecommunications doesn't have to be in your own inventory. And Dieter Altenpohl, an executive of Alusuisse, has calculations and charts to prove that, as he says, "The smarter the metal, the less it weighs."

Information Is Transportable.   Words and numbers can be transmitted at close to the speed of light. As a result, remoteness is now more a matter of choice than geography. You can sit in Auckland, New Zealand, and play the New York stock markets in real time—if you don't mind keeping slightly peculiar hours. And the same is true, without the big gap in time zones, of people in any rural hamlet in the United States. In the world of information-richness, you will be able to be remote if you want to, but you'll have to work at it.

Information Is Diffusive.   Information tends to leak—and the more it leaks the more we have. It is not the inherent tendency of natural resources to leak. Jewels may be stolen; a lump or two of coal may fall off the railroad car on its way from Montana; there is an occasional spillage of oil in the ocean. The leakage of information, however, is wholesale, pervasive, and continuous. In the era of the institutionalized leak, monopolizing information is very nearly a contradiction in terms; that can be done only in more and more specialized fields, for shorter and shorter periods of time.

Information Is Shareable.   Shortly before his death, the great British communications theorist Colin Cherry wrote that information by nature cannot give rise to exchange transactions, only to sharing transactions. Things are exchanged: if I give you a flower or sell you my automobile, you have it an I don't. But if I sell you an *idea* or give you a *fact,* we both have it.

An information-rich environment is thus a sharing environment. That needn't mean an environment without standards, rules, conventions, and ethical codes. It does mean the standards, rules, conventions, and codes are going to be different from those created to manage the zero-sum bargains of market trading and traditional international relations.

The Erosion of Hierarchies

The historically sudden dominance of information resources has, it seems to me, produced a kind of theory crisis—a sudden sense of having run out of basic assumptions. And somewhere near the center of the confusion are the difficulties caused by thinking about information (which is to say symbols) using concepts developed for the management of things—concepts such as property, depletion, depreciation, monopoly, "inevitable" unfairnesses, geopolitics, the class struggle, and top-down leadership.

The assumptions we have inherited are not producing satisfactory growth with acceptable equity either in the capitalist West or in the socialist East. As Simon Nora and Alain Minc wrote in their landmark report to the president of France: "The liberal and Marxist approaches, contemporaries of the production-based society, are rendered questionable by its demise."

The most troublesome concepts are those which were created to deal with the main problems presented by the management of things—problems such as their scarcity, their bulk, their limited substitutability for each other, the expense and trouble in transporting them, the paucity of information about them (which makes them comparatively easy to hide), and the fact that, being tangible, they could be hoarded. It was "the nature of things" that the few had access to them and the many did not.

Thus, the inherent characteristics of physical resources (natural and manmade) hastened the development of hierarchies of *power based on control* (of new weapons, of energy sources, of trade routes, of markets, and especially of knowledge), hierarchies of *influence based on secrecy,* hierarchies of *class based on ownership,* hierarchies of *privilege based on early access* to valuable resources, and hierarchies of *politics based on geography.*

Each of these five bases for discrimination and unfairness is crumbling today—because the old means of control are of dwindling efficacy, secrets are harder and harder to keep, and ownership, early arrival, and geography are of dwindling significance in getting access to the knowledge and wisdom which are the really valuable legal tender of our time.

Suppose you and I were living in a large wooden structure, without noticing that termites have eaten away its supporting pillars from the inside. Any day now, we may lean against a pillar and it will turn out to be a hollow shell. Something like that is happening to the hierarchies we have grown accustomed to in a civilization based on industrial production.

Let's examine more closely, as a "for instance," just one of these five eroding hierarchies: the familiar pyramid of power based on control, which has been the building block of bureaucratic, corporate, and military organizations.

Power and Participation

Knowledge is power, as Francis Bacon wrote in 1597. Therefore, the wider the spread of knowledge, the more power gets diffused. For the most part, individuals, corporations, and governments don't have a choice about this; it is the ineluctable consequence of creating—through education—societies with millions of knowledgeable people.

We see the results all around us, and around the world. More and more work gets done by horizontal process—or it doesn't get done. More and more decisions are made with wider and wider consultation—or they don't

"stick." If the Census Bureau counted each year the number of committees per thousand population, we would have a rough quantitative measure of the bundle of changes called "the information society." A revolution in the technology of organization—the twilight of hierarchy—is already well under way.

Information was always the basis of human organization, of course. Those with better or more recent information (Moses with his tablets, generals with their fast couriers, kings with their spies and ambassadors, speculators with their quick access to markets for gold, diamonds, or ownership shares, security forces with their sources of rumor and gossip) held sway over the rest of humankind.

But, once information was capable of being spread fast and wide—rapidly collected and analyzed, instantly communicated, readily understood by millions—the power monopolies that closely-held knowledge used to make possible were subject to accelerating erosion.

In the old days when only a few people were well educated and "in the know," leadership of the uninformed was likely to be organized in vertical structures of command and control. Leadership of the informed is different: it results in the necessary action only if it is exercised mainly through persuasion and by consulting those who are going to have to do something to make the decision a decision. When people are educated and are not treated this way, they either balk at the decisions made or have to be dragooned by organized misinformation backed by brute force. (Examples of both results have been on recent display in Poland.)

In an information-rich policy, the very definition of control changes. Very large numbers of people empowered by knowledge—coming together in parties, unions, factions, lobbies, interest groups, neighborhoods, families, and hundreds of other structures—assert the right or feel the obligation to make policy.

Decision making proceeds not by "recommendations up, orders down," but by the development of a shared sense of direction among those who must form the parade if there is going to be a parade.

Collegial, not command, structures become the more natural basis for organization. Conferring and "networking," not "command and control," become the mandatory modes for getting things done.

Planning cannot be done by a few leaders, or even the brightest whiz-kids immured in a systems analysis unit or a planning staff. Real-life planning is the dynamic improvisation by the many on a general sense of direction—anounced by the few, but only after genuine consultation with those who will have to improvise on it.

More participatory decision making implies a need for much information, widely spread, and much feedback, seriously attended—as in biological processes. Participation and public feedback become conditions precedent to decisions that stick. That means more openness, less secrecy—not as an ideological preference but as a technological imperative. (Secrecy goes out of fashion anyway, because secrets are so hard to keep.)

Education for Citizenship

Lets consider now the implications of "informatization" for the education of a society. In the upside-down pyramid, where the people really do make the policy, leadership is continuous dialogue–not an act, but an interaction between leaders and followers. The preparation of self-selected leaders is an important piece of the puzzle. But the whole puzzle is much larger: it is how citizens at large learn to make policy on issues that affect their destiny.

Education is the drivewheel of citizenship in the informatized society. With information now America's dominant resource, the quality of life in our communities and our leadership in the world depend on how many of us get educated for the new knowledge environment—and how demanding, relevant, continuous, broad, and wise (not merely knowledgeable) that learning is. Our task as educators is to make sure that during the half-century or more that our average student will live, he and she will also be *alive*. How are we doing?

We now have a national system of post-secondary education to which more than two-thirds of our high school students aspire. Such a system will obviously serve multiple purposes: education as an investment (for the poor), education as a consumer good (for the affluent), education as a device for avoiding decisions about what to do next (for the unattached, the uncertain, and the unemployed). But whatever the individual purpose of "going to college," the social contract in American higher education is clear enough: colleges and universities, and especially the public colleges and universities, are the egalitarian means for making an aristocracy of achievement acceptable in a democratic society. It is now part of our democratic ethos that if you apply the merit principle to a large enough body of students with a fair enough representation of previously disadvantaged kinds of people, the resulting discrimination is permissible. This double ethic suits the students fine: they want an equal chance to go to college, but they also want a job when they get out.

Of course, no one is much good at forecasting the job market: the science of what people will be doing for a living is still the most primitive part of a still adolescent discipline.

The critics of higher education are judging by a simpler standard: if a job isn't awaiting the student as soon as he or she acquires credentials, then the system of higher education is not working the way it should. Most educators, by contrast, think their most important task is not to train for a meal ticket the week after graduation, but to educate for fifty years of self-fulfillment: to help students develop a capacity for learning that will be a continuing asset, and a joy, for decades to come. Our egalitarian target is not an equal crack at a first job, but an equal chance at a full life.

In this longer time perspective, the attempt to quantify human resource requirements is bound to produce nonsense. In a society of increasing information-richness, the content of many, perhaps most, jobs a generation hence is unknowable today—just as the children of yesteryear were unable, through the ignorance of their parents and guidance counselors, to dream of being astronauts, nuclear physicists, ecologists, computer programmers, television repairmen, or managers of retrieval systems. (It was not until quite recently that the category of "guidance counselor" was added to the roster of our school systems.) Already a decade ago, the U.S. Department of Labor was guessing that by the year 2000, two-thirds of 1974's kindergarten students would be filling jobs which did not yet exist.

I have set down elsewhere my skepticism of the forecasting racket. Do not suspend your own skepticism as I now try, with an impressionist's broad brush, to project the kinds of work that are bound to be especially valued in a knowledge-rich society.

There will be more "information" and "services" work, and proportionately fewer "production" jobs, to be had. Machines will keep on eating up routine and repetitive tasks; the jobs left for people to do will require more and more brainwork, and more skill in the people-to-people relations, which machines are no good at.

"Computer literacy" will be part of knowing how to read, write, compute, and communicate. (That doesn't mean more than a rudimentary understanding of the architecture and electronics of microprocessing; it does mean understanding what computers, linked to telecommunications, can do for us—just as most of us understand an automobile's functions without being able to repair it.)

Despite tenure systems and retirement benefits, people will move around even more than they do now—from place to place, from function to function, from career to career.

Work, and therefore education for work, will become less competitive and more organized around cooperation.

There will be a growing market for education as a non-polluting leisure-time "consumer good." Already some union contracts entitle workers to time off for education; Italian metal workers, for example, are entitled by contract to 150 hours of education a year.

A growing proportion of the demand for higher education will be for "recurring education"—the 1980's international in-word for what used to be called "adult" or "continuing" education.

Education for leadership in varying forms will be a growth industry, because the proportion of the population that performs some leadership functions will keep growing.

More and more people will work at the management of international interdependence—in the federal government, multinational corporations, private voluntary agencies, and international organizations both public and private (if you can tell the difference). International travel, for work and for leisure, and the expansion of global telecommunications will also keep spreading, therefore swelling the demand for people with training in cross-cultural communication.

This is a vision of full and fulfilling employment. Will there be enough jobs to go around? No one knows. What Howard Bowen said in the 1970s still seems a good guess in the 1980s: that "two centuries of history have revealed no secular trend toward greater unemployment as technology advances." There is no finite amount of "work" to be divided up among a given number of "workers." Work, along with capital, expands with our capacity to use what is new in new ways for new purposes. The United States did not get to be a great nation by redoing in each generation what it used to do well in the one before—like making propeller aircraft or mechanical adding machines or oversized automobiles. It got there by constantly thinking up new things to do—like linking computers to telecommunications—before others did.

Education for Integrative Thinking

How are we doing in teaching wisdom—the get-it-all-together way of integrative thinking?

The academy's students, and its outside critics too, notice that the vertical academic disciplines, built around clusters of related research methods, are not in themselves very helpful in solving problems. No real-world problem can be fitted into the jurisdiction of any single academic department. As every urban resident realizes, we know every specialized thing about the modern city—but we seldom "get it all together" to make the city livable, efficient, safe, and clean.

As they awaken to problem solving, students therefore gravitate to those of the academy's offerings that seem to promise an interdisciplinary approach. These offering are sometimes disappointing. A course on environmental issues may be taught by an evangelist less eager to train analysts than to recruit zealots. A workshop on a "problem" may mask a research contract for a client (the government, a corporation, a wealthy donor) who knows the answer and is looking for ammunition

and an academic seal of approval for a predetermined course of action.

We all know that the only truly interdisciplinary instrument is not a committee of experts, but the synoptic view from a single integrative mind. In university education, what is too often lacking is an interdisciplinary role model up front by the blackboard.

Even so, many students prefer offerings that promise to cut across the vertical structures of method and help them construct homemade ways of thinking about the situation as a whole.

The revolt against methodology is also powered by the quickening interest in ethics—which started even before Watergate. A growing number of students come to college after some life experience—in the army or on a job or in a commune. They are groping for purpose, for effective ways of asking "Why?" and "Where are we supposed to be going, anyway?" Disciplines that seem neutral about purpose, modes of analysis that are equally applicable to killing people or building low-cost housing, make these students uncomfortable.

The students' intuition may not be wrong. Yet, they face an impressive phalanx of opposition to their instinct that the vertical disciplines should be stirred together in problem-solving, purpose-related combinations. Access to academic journals, collegial admiration, and promotion and tenure are not achieved by having lunch with colleagues in other departments. In addition, the external critics are for once on the professors' side: the division of knowledge into manageable compartments enabled the alumni to develop self-esteem and earn a decent living, so they don't understand why the curriculum has to be controversial.

But doesn't the new knowledge environment place a much greater premium on integrative thought? Won't we have to take a new look at higher educational systems that award the highest credentials for wisdom to those who master the narrowest slices of knowledge?

We are born, aren't we, with naturally integrative minds. I suspect that a newborn baby knows from the start, by instinct, that everything is related to everything else. Before a child is exposed to formal education, its curiosity is all-embracing. The child hasn't yet been told about the parts, so it is interested in the whole.

The more we learn, ironically, the less tied together is our learning. It's not situation-as-a-whole thinking, it's the separation of the specialized kinds of knowledge that (like racial prejudice) "has to be carefully taught."

Holistic learning comes especially in grades K to 4; the fourth-grade teacher is perhaps the premier generalist in our society. (Think of the variety of subjects on which she—it usually is "she"—has to be able to answer the question "Why?") Farther up the ladder of formal schooling, we do manage to persuade most children that the really important questions start with "When?" and "Where?" and "How?" and especially "How much?" Fortunately for the nation and the world, some young citizens persist in asking "Why?"

Jasmina Wellinghoff, a Twin Cities scientist and writer, writes about her first-grader:

> When my six-year-old learns that we heat the house with forced air, she immediately wants to know who is forcing the air, where natural gas comes from, and how it got stuck underground. After I have done my best to explain all this, comes the next question: "If we didn't have natural gas, would we die in the winter?" There you have it. Geology, engineering, physics and biology, all together in a hierarchy of concepts and facts.
>
> However, a few years from now my daughter will be studying the structure of the earth's crust, combustion, hydraulics and the classification of living beings—all in different years and quarters, neatly separated, tested and graded.

It is a well known scandal that our whole educational system is geared more to categorizing and analyzing patches of knowledge than to threading them together. Yet the experts obviously don't have the answers, and we are exposed to daily and dramatic demonstrations of experts in the service of expertise rather than in the service of values. What we've been neglecting is education for breadth.

Now the good news. Just in time, new instruments that can be used for thinking in breadth are at hand.

The computer, the complex simulations it makes possible, and its hookup to a worldwide network of electronic communications, now make it possible for individuals and small groups to analyze enormously complex natural systems (global weather), economic markets (the international monetary system), technologies not yet deployed, decision "trees," models of voting behavior, crisis management, and conflict resolution. Tools such as these empower those who learn to use them to make complex judgments in the more mindful knowledge of alternative futures. Systems thinking has created new ways to help encompass in a single mind some approximation of "the situation as a whole," as it relates to the problem being studied.

Don't get me wrong. There are dangers in excessive dedication to systems analysis. Part of the body count in Vietnam is certainly traceable to quantifying the tactics of war while neglecting the impressionistic strategies of peace. Still, it is useful for decision makers to be able to count what can be counted—as long as they remember that if it can't be counted, that doesn't mean it doesn't count.

The machines that are so useful in processing information are, of course, stupid beyond belief. Despite the attribution to them of "intelligence" (in the much misunderstood phrase "artificial intelligence"), they can still only count (very fast) from zero to one and back again, and transmit the results (at nearly the speed of light, in large and increasing volume) from place to place around the world. People have to do all the rest—define the human needs and purposes, select and analyze the relevant data, fix the assumptions to be made, stir in the inferences and insights and imagination, form the organizations, make the decisions, issue or implement the instructions, and above all, deal with other people.

Time for a New "Core"

The people who will perform these functions will be mostly college men and women. What should they be learning, for this purpose, during the years they are students?

It would be nice if the dilemma were simple. but the ancient clashes between "training" and "education," between "vocational" and "general," between honing the mind and nourishing the soul, divide the outside critics, the professional educators, and the students, too.

Just now our favorite way to resolve the dilemma is to delegate it to the individual student. We "maximize the student's options" by creating a bewildering proliferation of courses and programs of study, a cafeteria of the intellect using what the food service people call the "scramble system."

For the limited numbers of students who know just what they want and why, the new freedom doesn't work badly. But most students expect and need some guidance in creating an intellectually nutritious trayful of reading, discussion, writing, computing, and work experience.

My guess is that if U.S. colleges and universities continue to proliferate courses, external pressure groups and the state and federal governments will sooner or later impose social, economic, and even political criteria, on curriculum-building in higher education. At the graduate level such coercion is already felt to some extent, as governments bribe the universities with research funds to teach what political leaders think is important—and know is safe. At the undergraduate level, if our ultimate curricular principle is the cop-out called "maximum options," the outsiders will, in the end, tell the academics what to teach and the students what they can learn at the public's expense.

The answer, as usual, is not to settle the argument by choosing one of the dilemma's horns or the other. Honing the mind and nourishing the soul are both functional in the new knowledge environment. What we need now is a theory of general education that is clearly relevant to life and work in a context of the information age—a rapidly changing scene in which uncertainty is the main planning factor. Perhaps, in the alternating current of general and job-oriented education, it is time for a new synthesis, a new "core curriculum"—something very different from Columbia's World Civilization, Syracuse's Responsible Citizenship, or Chicago's Great Books, yet still a central idea about what every educated person would know, and have, and try to be.

I had a chance, not long before his untimely death in 1982, to consider with Stephen K. Bailey the make-up of a new "core." Bailey had been vice president of the American Council on Education and president of the National Institute of Education, and had thought long and hard about curricular reform in higher education. We concluded that such a core would not have much to do with learning "facts." It is said that each half-hour produces enough new knowledge to fill a twenty-four-volume edition of the *Encyclopedia Britannica*. Our world of indiscriminate erudition turns out millions of new books and articles and pamphlets in a year's time. Most of the facts we learn in school are unlikely to be true for as long as we can remember them.

(The last time I took physics, in the mid-1930s, my instructor told me the atom couldn't be split. When I studied Keynesian economics with a young Oxford tutor named Harold Wilson, I learned that inflation and recession were periodic, but occurred at opposite ends of the business cycle; the idea that they might be glued together in persistent stagflation was not mentioned. This remembered learning has not been very useful to me, of late; it didn't seem to work very well for Prime Minister Wilson, either.)

If, however, we think hard about the requirements of the new knowledge environment, and consult the instincts and perceptions of our own future-oriented students, I think we could construct a new "core curriculum" from such elements as these:

- Education in integrative brainwork—developing the capacity to synthesize, for the solution of real-world problems, the analytical methods and insights of conventional academic disciplines. (Exposure to basic science and mathematics, to elementary systems analysis, and to what a computer can and cannot do, are part, but only a part, of this education.)
- Education about the social goals, public purposes, costs, benefits, and ethics of citizenship—to enable each educated person to answer for himself or herself two questions: "Apart from the fact that I am expected to do this, is this what I would expect *myself* to do?" and "Does the validity of this action depend on its secrecy?"
- A capacity for self-analysis—through the study of ethnic heritage, religion and philosophy, and art and literature, leading to the achievement of some fluency in answering the question, "Who am I?"
- Some practice in real-world negotiation, in the psychology of consultation, and the nature of leadership in the knowledge environment.
- A global perspective, and an attitude of personal responsibility for the general outcome of public life—passports to citizenship in the interdependent world.

The fusion of computers and telecommunications, and developments in bio-technology, are the basis for a legion of new activities, new things to do, new "jobs," on Earth, in the oceans, in the atmosphere and outer space. The number and quality of "jobs" will be a function not of physical constraints but of the human imagination. Will we use our imagination to create full employment at fulfilling work? In the words of Barbara Ward: "We do not know. We have the duty to hope."

There are two predictions to which I would assign a high probability value. The first is that people who do not educate themselves—and keep reeducating themselves—to participate in the new knowledge environment will be the peasants of the information society. The second is that societies that do not give *all* their people an opportunity for relevant education, as well as periodic opportunities to fine-tune their knowledge and their insights, will be left in the jetstream of history by those that do.

Chapter 47
Family Configuration, Intelligence, and the SAT

Eric L. Lang*

During the last ten years educators, parents, politicians, and psychologists have debated the influences underlying the changing pattern of Scholastic Aptitude Test (SAT) scores of American students. Of particular interest was the sudden upswing in SAT performance which began in 1980, after 17 years of steadily decreasing scores. Causal responsibility for changes in the national SAT averages has typically been attributed to two institutional agencies: the school system and the family. While it is relatively easy to come up with conjectures about how each of these agencies could influence trends in test scores, none of these conjectures meet strict scientific standards. However, a scientific theory has been developed which is able to explain these trends in a rigorous and testable way. The theory, known as the Confluence Theory, accounts for children's intellectual growth by estimating the influence of family configuration factors, like size and sibling spacing. The purpose of this paper is to review briefly some of the relevant research on how family configuration influences intelligence, illustrate the descriptive and predictive power of the confluence theory—highlighting its application to SAT trends, and discuss several practical considerations of this research.

Before discussing the impact of family configuration on intelligence it is important to clarify some relevant terms and limitations. In this paper, three aspects of family configuration will be considered: number of children in a family, children's birth order, and the temporal spacing among children in a family.

Unfortunately, the concept of intelligence is not so easy to define. At present educators and research psychologists are searching for a theoretically sound conceptualization of intelligence. Because the theoretical roots of intelligence are uncertain, it has become common practice to define a individual's intelligence as his score on one or more standardized IQ tests. Testing and defining intelligence in this way is like defining a bird as "an animal which lives in a bird-cage." This circular definition of intelligence has not lent itself to productive in-

quiry, and it remains to be seen whether current efforts at untangling this problem will be successful. Although several issues about intelligence will be discussed later, it is not the purpose of this paper to resolve the conceptual ambiguities surrounding intelligence testing, or to examine the differences between IQ and aptitude tests. Standard IQ tests generally correlate well with each other, and with different tests of intellectual performance, like the SAT. Therefore, because the correlations between different IQ tests are usually substantial, no distinction will be made among the various IQ measures reviewed in this paper.

Much of the interest in the effects of family configuration on intelligence was sparked by survey research reported in the 1950s which demonstrated a negative association between an individual's IQ score and the total number of siblings reported by the individual at the test time (Anastasi, 1956; Gille et al, 1954; Scottish Council for Research in Education, 1953). This negative association means that as the number of children in a family increases, the average intellectual performance of the children decreases. The average correlation evidenced in these studies was about -.30. When this negative correlation is expressed in terms of percentage of children scoring below average, we see that of the 70,805 children tested in the Scottish Council investigation, 37% of the only children scored below the average, compared to 60% of the children with four siblings, and 71% of the children with seven or more siblings. Since then, a number of studies have shown support for the finding that children with many siblings tend to perform worse on IQ tests (see Heer, 1985 for a review), and aptitude tests (Zajonc, 1983) than children with few siblings.

Although one interpretation of this finding is that family factors influence intellectual outcomes, an alternative explanation suggests that some other factor influ-

*Dr. Eric L. Lang is Research Associate, Institute for Social Research, University of Michigan. The author thanks Robert Zajonc for his comments on a draft of this article.

ences family factors and intelligence in separate but similar fashions. If this were so, the negative correlation between family size and intelligence would be coincidental, not causal. To illustrate a coincidental association of this kind, consider the fact that every year in New York as more ice cream cones are sold, less ski equipment is rented. Although these two events are correlated, changes in ice cream sales *do not cause* changes in ski equipment rentals. Instead, both types of sales are influenced by warm weather. Thus, ice cream sales and ski equipment rentals are related to each other by coincidence because both are influenced by a common factor, which is seasonal weather. In the case of intellectual performance, a similar argument asserts that the socio-economic status (SES) of a family is responsible for the relatedness of family size with intelligence. This argument contends that, on the average, low SES families are larger than high SES families, and that children from low SES families score lower on intelligence tests than children from high SES families. Thus, both family size and intelligence are influenced by SES, rather than by each other. According to this logic it is a statistical coincidence that large family size is related to low intelligence scores.

There are simple statistical tests which can distinguish between coincidental and causal relationships. If the relationship between family size and intelligence is coincidental because of an SES influence, then the correlation between them should disappear when the influence of SES is statistically controlled for. Zajonc (1983) tested this idea and found that the relationship between number of siblings and their intellectual performance tends to remains significant, albeit reduced, when SES is controlled for. Thus, the SES influence does not account for the relationship between family size and intelligence. To date, no factors have been found which indicate that the relationship between family configuration and intelligence is merely a coincidence. By testing and eliminating alternative explanations in this way, the idea that family configuration factors influence intellectual performance is supported.

It is difficult to assess the effect of birth order on intelligence because the birth order influence is confounded somewhat with the number of children in a family. For example, a fifth born child (i.e., a large birth order) will normally grow up in a family composed of five or more children. In this case, knowing the child's birth order is nearly equivalent to knowing how many children there are in the family. However, a first born child (i.e. a low birth order) may come from either a small or large family, depending on whether he is an only child or the eldest of many. Therefore, to adequately test for an independent birth order effect on intelligence, comparisons among individuals of different birth orders should be made for several different family sizes. For example,

to understand the intellectual effects of being born second rather than first, a researcher should compare second-born children from small, medium, and large families to first-born children from small, medium, and large families. Unfortunately, because very few studies like this have been done, researchers are not certain about the intellectual effects associated with each birth order.

The discussion presented earlier in this paper indicated that children with many siblings perform worse on intelligence tests than children with fewer siblings. However, sometimes a researcher will not have information regarding how many siblings each test-taker has. In the event that a researcher knows only the birth order of each test-taker, then birth order can be used as an approximation of the number of children in a family. Here is why. Let us refer to the number of children in a family as a "sib-group." If Anne is the fifth-born child in her family then she has always had four older siblings in her home environment. Thus, Anne's large birth order is a good indication that she may suffer the intellectual disadvantages of growing up in a large sib-group. Because having a large birth order is nearly always equivalent to having a large sib-group, researchers can use birth order information in place of sib-group information, when the latter is not available. But what about low birth order? As discussed above, a first-born child (birth order = 1) may be an only child or the first born child of a large sib-group. Thus, the question is, does knowing that an individual has a low birth order tell us anything important about the sibling environment that the individual grew up in? The answer is yes. Because we are interested in how many siblings a child is exposed to while growing up, even a low birth order can be used to approximate sib-group size information. This is because the first born child of five grows up in a different sibling environment than the last born child—and this difference is of the same form as a sib-group size influence. For example, in a family with five sons born at two year intervals, the eldest son lives two years as an only child, four years in a sib-group of two, six years in a sib group of three, and so forth. In contrast, the last born son grown up entirely in a sib-group of five. Consequently, the first born child of five grows up with a smaller *average* sib-group than the last born child of five. Therefore, when sib-group size information is not available, birth order information can be used in correlations and other calculations to approximate the influence of sib-group size on children' intelligence.

In addition to the studies of children's IQ and aptitude scores, other research on family configuration effects has shown that having fewer siblings is related to higher educational attainment, even when parental IQ, age, and several different SES factors are statistically controlled for (Olneck & Bills, 1979; Sewell et al, 1980). Similarly, first born individuals are found in greater than chance proportions among candidates for the National Merit Scholarship, University Professorships, and the Presidency of the United States. In short, the bulk of relevant research indicates that family configuration factors assert a significant and independent influence on children's intellectual development. The following section attempts to explain this link.

The Confluence Theory

The confluence theory (Zajonc, 1976, 1983; Zajonc & Markus, 1975) asserts that family configuration factors help determine a child's cognitive development by way of intellectual stimulation provided by the family environment. For example, the last-born child of five closely-spaced children will spend much of her time exposed to her siblings' limited vocabularies, undeveloped logic, and immature approaches to life's uncertainties. In contrast, an only child will spend relatively more time exposed to parents' well-developed vocabularies and mature intellects. Thus, on the average, the presence of many closely-spaced siblings "dilutes" the intellectual environment relative to a small sib-group environment.

The confluence model is a mathematical equation designed to assess the impact of birth order, sib-group size, and sibling spacing on intellectual development. A major strength of the model is that it accounts for dynamic change in the intellectual milieu encountered by a child as old siblings mature and new siblings arrive. Mathematically,

> The confluence model is written in the form of a first-order difference equation whose terms are yearly increments in the intellectual growth of a child. Its principal element represents the child's intellectual environment at every year of his life until the time the child is tested. As an approximation, the quality of the family's intellectual environment is estimated on the basis of an average of the *absolute* intellectual levels of all the family members. We are not averaging IQ's, which is a score *relative* to chronological age, but in our calculations, we use absolute levels, more akin to mental ages. (Zajonc, 1986, p. 862)

By employing a calculus equation in this way, the confluence model takes into account the familial history of annual changes in the intellectual environment surrounding each child.

The confluence model also accounts for a birth order effect related to the *positive* intellectual contribution of having a younger sibling. Although the presence of additional siblings generally depresses the intellectual environment, there is a temporary but definite intellectual

benefit for having a younger sibling to teach and help. This is not surprising, given that teaching a concept or skill usually requires the teacher to think about the relevant information and to manage its communication. "Teaching benefits" regarding child-to-child tutoring of this kind have been well documented by research (cf Levine, 1986). Unfortunately, in many cases, the intellectual benefit acquired through teaching a younger sibling is eclipsed ultimately by the deficit to the overall intellectual environment resulting from the younger sibling's low intellectual contribution. Furthermore, not every child is in a position to be a teacher. Because only children and last-born children have no younger siblings, they have little or no opportunity to benefit from the intellectual rewards of being a teacher. Consequently, as several large studies have shown, only-children demonstrate a relatively small intellectual advantage over children from two-child families, and in some studies, the two-child environment is superior (Zajonc, 1983). Similarly, unusually poor intellectual performance by last-born children may result from sib-group size effects are not alleviated by the benefits of having a younger sibling to teach.

However, the last-born child's "non-teacher deficit" can be overcome. As the confluence model illustrates, several different factors work in concert to influence the intellectual environment of each child. For example, the confluence model shows that a group of siblings who are very close in age to each other will grow up in a poorer intellectual environment than a similar group of siblings spaced farther apart in age. In the case of the last-born's non-teacher deficit, much of the detrimental effects of that birth position can be attenuated by a longer spacing between the last-born child and his or her older sibling(s). The longer spacing results in a more mature intellectual environment for the last-born's development; a benefit which may counteract completely the non-teacher deficit (Zajonc, 1976).

Although the confluence model is expressed in terms of the changing intellectual conditions that occur in an individual family's development, it can readily be applied to large populations. For example, in the confluence model calculations, instead of using a value to represent the number of children in one family, a researcher could represent the *average number of children per family* in some population of interest. Extending this idea then, changes in the average family configuration of a population should parallel later changes in the average intellectual performance of children from that population. In the United States, for example, the average sib-group size increased from 1.5 in 1945 until its peak in 1963 when the average newborn was a family's third child. Thereafter, the average sib-group size decreased until 1979 to a sib-group size of 2. Did the intellectual performance of American students over the last 35 years correspond to this dramatic change in American family patterns? The answer is "yes"—at every grade level.

Zajonc (1986) compared annual changes in the average sib-group size of Iowa families (which were representative of sib-group changes in the nation at large) to annual changes in the average scores of children on the Iowa Basic Skills Test (IBST). He found that the trend of IBST scores for cohorts born between 1950–1975 described a U-shaped curve that corresponded well[2] with the trend in Iowa sib-group sizes. At the bottom of the curve (low test scores) were children born in 1962, the year of large sib-groups. This pattern held true for Iowa elementary school students, junior high school students, and high school students as well, thus supporting the confluence hypothesis that changes in family configuration correspond to subsequent changes in intellectual performance.

As high school students approach graduation many of them take the Scholastic Aptitude Test, which is an admission requirement for most colleges. In 1986, over one million students in this nation took the SAT. The test is designed to assess students' intellectual ability to handle college study. It is, therefore, not surprising that Americans have been interested and concerned about annual changes in the national SAT scores. Of particular concern was the decline of SAT scores between 1963 and 1980 from a national average of 490 to 445.[3] Since 1980, the national scores have been rising steadily, such that a chart of their pattern over the last 15 years illustrates a U-shaped curve. At the bottom of the curve are students born around 1962, as predicted by the confluence model (see Figure 1). Thus, the SAT trend parallels the primary and secondary school test trend, all of which correspond to annual changes in average family configuration. Statistically, Zajonc (1986) has shown that two thirds of the variation in national SAT performance can be attributed to family factors described by the confluence model. In other words, most of the changes in national SAT scores from year to year illustrate a pattern which is explainable in terms of the average family configuration pattern that was evident seventeen years earlier, when the test-takers were born.

Although the confluence model has demonstrated empirical power to assess family configuration influences on intellectual performance, what support has been found for theoretical assertions regarding the intellectual environment as the medium of change? In a recent review of longitudinal research on the family environment and early cognitive development, Gottfried (1984) concluded:

> The relationship of birth order to home environment also showed a generalizable finding. In the studies investigat-

Figure 1. The Relationship Between Birth Order and SAT.

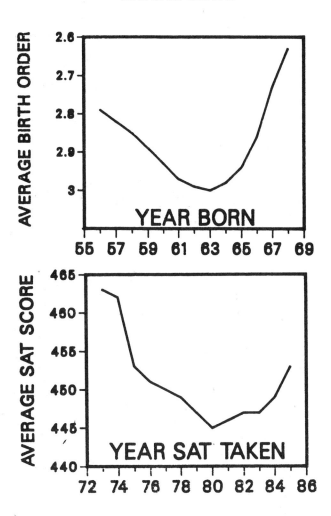

The upper panel shows the national average birth orders of children born between 1956—1968. The lower panel shows the national average SAT scores achieved by each of these cohorts seventeen years later. (Adapted from Zajonc, 1986; with permission of the author)

ing this relationship, the data indicated that firstborns, compared to later-borns, received a more intellectually stimulating environment. . . . Thus, the evidence is reliable that during infancy and the preschool years, firstborns compared to later-borns have environments that are advantaged for enhancing intellectual skills. This holds for children differing in race and SES. (p.332)

In the same review, Gottfried (1984) cites evidence for similar effects related to sib-group size and crowding (room: person ratio).[4] In sum, there is substantial support for the psychological aspects of the confluence theory.

Practical Considerations

Understanding the role that family configuration factors play in the course of intellectual development leads to several important considerations regarding family planning, the educational system in this country, and the SAT.

With respect to the SAT, one of the most important considerations for the future derives directly from results of confluence research. Because national SAT scores are predictable on the basis of national family patterns observed 17 years prior to the testing year of interest, then average SAT performances for the next 17 years should be equally predictable based on recent family patterns that have already begun to influence American children. According to Zajonc (1986), SAT scores in this nation will increase to between 510-515 at the turn of the century. At that point, average scores can be expected to decrease slightly because of the slowly rising birth rate of the 1980s. As citizens, it is important that we understand this trend and the role of family configuration factors so that we can be informed appraisers of national news and intelligent decision-makers on educational and related issues.

Although the confluence model accounts for a substantial part of the intellectual performance of large populations, how relevant is the model for the development of a single family? In general, the confluence model is a poor predictor of the total intellectual development within one family. For example, the SAT score of any particular individual may be influenced by a host of factors including the caliber of school curriculum taken and exposure to SAT preparation materials. SAT performance is also enhanced if one has chosen parents with sound genetic contributions. Moreover, it is important to remember that the confluence model is not designed to account *for all* factors contributing to intellectual development. Rather, the confluence model assesses only the contribution of family configuration factors to intellectual performance. Because non-confluence factors may easily obscure family configuration effects in a particular family, confluence predictions are less reliable for individuals than for large populations. This is an important point. Because nearly everyone knows one or many large families with intellectually gifted children, the confluence model would seem to be wrong. However, we should expect some large families to have gifted children, just as we should expect some wives to be taller than their husbands. The point is that the more families included in a study, the more likely we are to find that, *on the average,* husbands are taller than their wives, and children with many siblings perform worse on intelligence tests than children with few siblings. Thus, confluence model predictions are most reliable when applied to large populations.

Nevertheless, confluence research has practical implications regarding individual families. Although the development of children depends on many factors, the intellectual environment of the home is more likely to be inhibited by many children born at short intervals than by fewer children born farther apart. Furthermore, this handicap may be quite resilient to change. In a recent study concerning the effects of an early educational intervention program on children from disadvantaged families, Boat, Campbell, and Ramey (1986) found that children provided with a five-year (five days per week) preschool program demonstrated higher average IQ than children in a control group who did not participate in the program. Although these researchers also expected that the educational program would reduce the intellectual gap between first-born children and later-born children, they found instead that "provision of intensive programming did not override the effect of birth order" (p.32). Interestingly, their study indicates that the birth order difference *increased* as a result of the educational intervention. This suggests that first-born children may be more receptive to the benefits of educational intervention than later-born children, and that later-borns may have an enduring educational disadvantage.

Another practical consideration regarding the research presented thus far involves the conceptualization of intelligence. Although IQ and aptitude test scores reflect some form of mental ability, such tests are limited in their focus and sensitivity. Recent research on this topic (Frederiksen, 1986; Walters, 1985; Wagner and Sternberg, 1984) suggests that commonly used tests of intellectual performance measure a narrow range of logical-mathematical and linguistic ability, and overlook other forms of intelligence including pragmatic, kinesthetic, interpersonal, and artistic intelligence. Broadening the conceptualization of intelligence is necessary to reflect the diversity of problem solving and creative abilities that occur in real world situations. The best scientist, for example, is not simply a logical methodologist juggling equipment and data; he or she must possess an aptitude for creative insight as well as the ability to make practical research decisions which maximize resources and minimize disabilities. Tests of such abilities and alternative forms of intelligence are currently in the experimental phase of development. Thus, although family configuration effects have been demonstrated in a variety of intellectual domains including mathematics, English, reading comprehension, general information, and abstract reasoning (Claudy, 1976), it is important to remember that these forms of intellectual expression do not account for the total spectrum of human intelligence.

As mentioned earlier, the decline of national SAT scores through the 1970s caused much concern among parents and education administrators. This concern instigated President Carter, the College Board, the Educational Testing Service, and several other groups to establish committees to investigate and resolve the issue. Several reports and many hypotheses later, no clear interpretation of the decline had emerged. Little or no attention was given to results of confluence research.

After the SAT scores began increasing in 1980 there was no shortage of groups willing to take credit for the turnaround. By the mid 1980s President Reagan had pronounced that the SAT turnaround was due to "the American people who, in reaching for excellence, knew to reach back to basics."[5] This is an interesting conclusion given that there is no research which demonstrates how the decline and rise of national SAT scores depends on "back to basics" factors. The only line of research that reliably explains and predicts the national SAT pattern is the confluence theory, which says nothing about a back to basics influence. It is possible that such an influence may account for some of the 33% of the SAT trend not accounted for by the confluence model. However, valid support for this argument is lacking.

What is most interesting, given the current focus on the SAT trend, is that the confluence theory including supporting evidence and *a prediction of the 1980 SAT turnaround was published in 1976* (Zajonc, 1976). Since then, Zajonc and his colleagues have published several papers that expand and further validate the confluence model. Despite this, in his latest state-by-state review of public education the Secretary of Education, William J. Bennett, reported that the rising SAT scores indicated that "the movement to raise academic achievement standards and restore discipline is showing results."[6] Statements like this are simply not supported by relevant scientific research. Consequently, until education officials acknowledge and comprehend the contribution of confluence theory toward understanding intelligence and educational outcomes, the quality of educational policy development in this country may be at risk.

In summary, a substantial amount of research concerning the effects of family configuration factors on intellectual performance indicates that such factors can be important determinants of the intellectual environment in the home. Specifically, research on the confluence model was used to articulate the agents of influence and illustrate how the national SAT trend is affected by family configuration patterns. Several educational and familial implications of this research were discussed briefly as well as the issue of political attention. Although more research will certainly be needed to understand the subtleties inherent in family configuration effects, no amount of research may be enough until parents, teachers, and education officials comprehend available information and consider its implications.

FOOTNOTES

1. Research Associate, Institute for Social Research, University of Michigan. The author thanks Robert Zajonc for his comments on a draft of this paper.
2. Average correlation = -.73, very high statistical significance.
3. These figures represent the average of both halves (math and verbal sections) of the SAT. Possible scores on each half of the SAT range between 200 and 800, with a standard deviation of approximately 100.
4. The research on crowding aspects of the family environment is interesting because it suggests that some of the intellectual deficits of a large sib-group environment may be ameliorated by increasing the personal space available to each child in the home.
5. State of the Union Address delivered February 5, 1986. Mr. Reagan made a similar statement in his 1985 State of the Union Address of February 11, 1985.
6. Speech delivered February 20, 1986.

REFERENCES

Anastasi, A. (1956). Intelligence and family size. *Psychological Bulletin, 53,* 187-209.

Boat, B.W., Campbell, F.A., & Ramey, C.T. (1986). Preventive education and birth order as co-determinants of IQ in disadvantaged 5-year olds. *Child: care, health and development, 12,* 25-36.

Claudy, J.G. (1976). Cognitive characteristics, family size, and birth order. Paper presented at the meeting of the American Psychological Association. Washington, D.C.

Frederiksen, N. (1986). Toward a broader conception of human intelligence. *American Psychologist, 41,* 445-452.

Gille, R., Henry, L., Tabah, L. et al. (1954). Le niveau intellectuel des infants d'age scolaire: la determination des aptitudes; l'influence des facteures constitutionnels, familiaux, et sociaux. *Inst. Natl. Etudes Demographiques: Trav. Doc.,* Cahier 23.

Gottfried, A.W. (1984). *Home environment and early cognitive development: Longitudinal research.* New York, Academic Press.

Heer, D.M. (1985). Effects of sibling number on child outcome. *Annual Review of Sociology, 11,* 27-47.

Levine, M. (1986). Docemur Docendo (He who teaches, learns). *American Educator,* Fall, 22-25.

Olneck, M.B., Bills, D.B. (1979). Family configuration and achievement: Effects of birth order and family size in a sample of brothers. *Social Psychology Quarterly, 42,* 135-148.

Sewell, W.H., Hauser, R.M., Wolf, W.C. (1980). Sex, schooling, and occupational status. *American Journal of Sociology, 86,* 551-583.

Scottish Council for Research in Education. (1953). *Social Implications of the 1947 Scottish Mental Survey.* London, University London Press.

Walters, J.M. (1985). The theory of multiple intelligences: Some issues and answers, in R. Sternberg and R. Wagner (eds.) *Practical intelligence: Origins of competence.* Cambridge: University Press.

Wagner, R.K. & Sternberg, R.J. (1984). Alternative conceptions of intelligence and their implications for education. *Review of Educational Research, 54,* 2, 179-223.

Zajonc, R.B. (1976). Family configuration and intelligence. *Science, 192,* 227-236.

Zajonc, R.B. (1983). Validating the confluence model. *Psychological Bulletin, 93,* 457-480.

Zajonc, R.B. (1986). The decline and rise of scholastic aptitude scores: A prediction derived from the confluence model. *American Psychologist, 41,* 8, 862-867.

Zajonc, R.B., Markus, G.B. (1975). Birth order and intellectual development. *Psychological Review, 82,1,* 74-88.

American Federation of Teachers

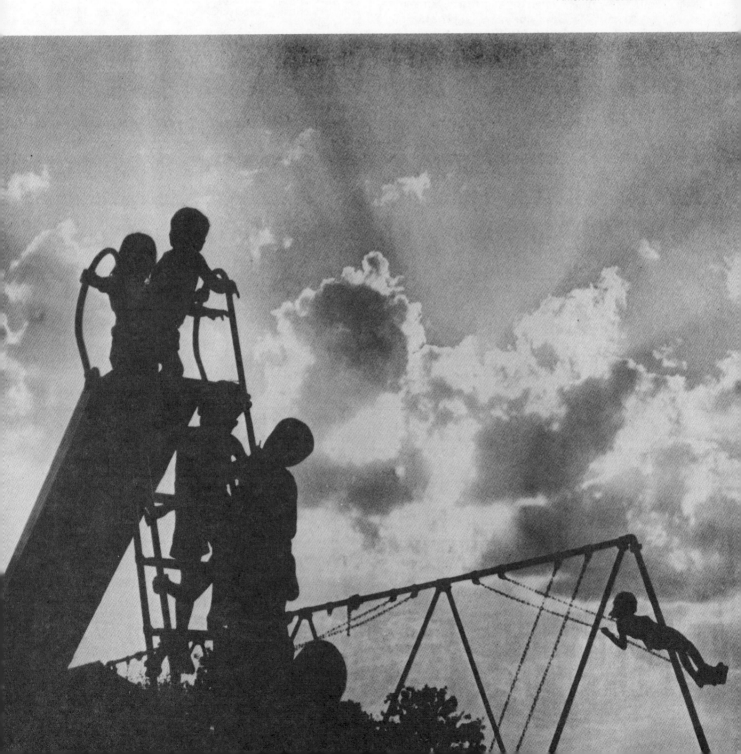

Chapter 48
Day Care for Young Children: A Vital Resource for Children and Parents
Paula L. Zajan*

Introduction

Group care for young children has existed whenever mothers have had to leave their children with others for varying periods of time. Such care may range from the informal minding of a child by a relative or neighbor to highly organized educational facilities for larger groups. The term "day care" usually denotes programs that provide services to children for the entire day and the youngsters who attend may be infants, toddlers, pre-schoolers or school-age children.

Day care facilities can be found throughout the world and their availability, quality and variety of programs are influenced by cultural, economic, social and political considerations. In the United States, day care has been available on a limited basis, usually serving low income families and funded by Federal and local government. In recent years, day care centers sponsored by a variety of organizations, agencies and businesses have been established and are expanding rapidly to meet the needs of families at all income levels. Clearly there is a trend toward making day care facilities available to all those who demand and need them but there are questions as well: Should all children attend day care centers from an early age? Is it desirable to separate young children from their home environment? Is the value of the experience consistent with the very considerable cost of providing day care services? Are day care programs able to meet the needs of children and their families?

The Needs of Children

Research studies have emphasized that the first five years of a child's life are generally thought to be the period of most rapid growth (Bloom 1964). It is during these years that the child's physical and intellectual capacities develop most quickly and personality traits and attitudes toward self and others most firmly established.

There is no question that many families are able to provide their children with all the physical, social, emo-

tional and intellectual support and stimulation needed for them to realize their full potential. Indeed, research studies conducted by Burton White conclude that it is the family that makes the greatest impact on the child's total educational development and that the crucial time is during the child's first three years of life (White 1975). Even under optimum conditions, raising children in today's world is difficult; but there are countless numbers of children who do not have the benefit of families that can give them the time, care and guidance that is required.

Child Rearing in a Rapidly Changing, Complex Society

A report by the Labor Department (*New York Times,* March 16, 1986) describes the changing composition of the American family and rapid rise in the number of mothers who work outside the home. The study shows that nearly 50 percent of American women with children under one year worked, as compared to 25 percent in 1970. For some mothers, working outside the home is a matter of choice, but for many it is an economic necessity. The rise in separation, divorce and single parenthood has resulted in the single mothers of these households often becoming the sole support of themselves and their children. The Department of Labor report notes that the proportion of single mothers who were employed full-time ranged from 38 percent of those with children under a year old, to 79 percent of those with children under three years old, to 84 percent of those whose children were from six to seventeen years old. In all, the report goes on to say, 25 million children—over half of them with married parents—are in families where the mother is regularly at work for at least part of the day.

In addition to economic and social conditions, children, particularly those in urban settings, are confronted with additional handicaps. How often are city children able to run, climb, jump, shout, roll in the grass, skate

*Dr. Paula L. Zajan is Professor, Early Childhood Education, Hostos Community College, The City University of New York.

and do all of the wonderful, physical things young children love and need to do? Apartment living does not encourage such activities. How often are young children able to make friends and enjoy social contacts on their own? Fears for children's safety may limit these activities. Far too often the cramped apartment and television set determine what the young child will do all day.

Day Care Services Vary

It is for these and many other reasons that families have sought day care services for their young. There are, however, wide variations in the centers and day care can mean different things to different people.

For some, it is a place where children from infancy to school age can be taken care of during the day in safe, healthy surroundings. Others demand that the center provide an educational program in addition to custodial care. Still others look for a program that concerns itself with the developmental needs of the child—physical, social, emotional and intellectual. Some would include the needs of the child's family, be they parent education, health care or social services. Some see the day care center as a focus of community involvement, with parents and members of the community entirely responsible for the on-going program. Others again look to governmental or individually controlled facilities where a minimum of responsibility is required.

Essential Features of Quality Day Care

Day care, as the name implies, generally means all-day care from early morning until evening. When children spend up to ten hours each day for five days each week, it is incumbent upon the center to provide the maximum quality environment for children who spend the largest percent of their waking hours away from home.

Perhaps the most essential feature of a good day care center, and the one most difficult to define, is the quality of life that exists within it. In such a center, the child's well-being, physical, social, emotional and intellectual, takes top priority. All facets of the program focus on the child as an individual and as a member of the group. The staff: director, teachers, assistants, social worker, secretary, cook and custodian all play important roles in determining whether the climate within that center is supportive and stimulating or whether it is passive, custodial or even destructive. The feelings, attitudes and communication among the staff members, among the staff members and children and among the children themselves, give many clues to the quality of life within the center.

There is no question that a knowledgeable, harmonious staff deeply concerned with the needs of children, makes the difference between an adequate program and a

good one. One of the main responsibilities of the center director is to hire competent staff and to continually upgrade their performance through on-the-job staff development. The director should have firsthand knowledge and experience in working with young children and their parents in addition to administrative and supervisory skills. The teachers and assistants must have, at the very minimum, the physical and emotional health as well as the skills necessary to work with young children in an all-day setting.

Although the emotional climate takes top priority, the physical environment cannot be overlooked. A good day care center should be a place that is safe, clean and spacious. Classrooms should be bright and well-ventilated with sufficient storage and work space. Rooms should not be overcrowded. State or city health codes frequently determine the number of children in a classroom according to their age, the number of adults in the room and the size of the facility. The three-year old group usually has 8-10 children; the four-year-old group from 10-12; and the five-year-old group from 15-20. In infant and toddler programs, the ratio of children to adults is smaller. In addition to the classrooms, there may be a large free activity room for children to use when inclement weather prohibits outdoor play.

Large muscle activity in an outdoor yard or on a roof top is a "must" for young children. Whatever the arrangement, there should be sufficient protected space for children to move freely and to use outdoor equipment such as climbing apparatus, wheel toys, sandboxes, large hollow blocks, balls and the like. In addition to "child space," there must be "adult space": offices for the director, secretary, nurse and social worker as well as room for staff and parents' activities, a basically equipped kitchen and storage space.

Programs in day care centers vary and they are generally influenced by the educational beliefs of the center director and teachers. In centers where there are advisory boards consisting of parents, community members and professionals, input as to the educational content as well as operating procedures may be made by the advisory body.

Some centers' programs are very unstructured and free with little direction from the adults. Children in these programs are encouraged to choose their own activities within a flexible time schedule and great emphasis is placed on activities and experiences initiated by the children. Creativity and self-expression are highly valued in these centers and one would not be likely to see adult directed art projects or large groups during story time or music. Children work at their own pace individually and in small groups and the adults take their cues from the spontaneous activities of the children.

At the other end of the spectrum, there are highly

structured, adult-dominated programs. In these centers, children follow a tightly organized schedule and there may be little opportunity for flexibility and spontaneous activity. There are many adult-initiated group activities such as in art, science and language. Emphasis is placed on preparing children for subsequent schooling and in such centers, formal reading and mathematics readiness programs may be observed.

Falling in between, there is a broad range of programs that follow a middle road, taking those facets which are compatable with the philosophy and beliefs of the staff and parents within that center. Although most center directors and teachers might say that they are concerned with the development of the whole child, physically, socially, emotionally and intellectually, it is the underlying attitudes and beliefs of the adults and the pressures that are brought to bear that ultimately determine the type of program.

A developmental child care center is not only concerned with the environmental and educational aspects of the program but also with the additional comprehensive services that are offered to the children and their families. These would include health services, counselling and guidance, social services and the like. In many centers, men and women from the immediate community are hired to assist the professionals in providing these services. These assistants may lack the formal educational credentials, but they are knowledgeable about their communities and can speak to the families as neighbor to neighbor. When appropriate, these workers may be bilingual and this brings an added dimension to the program.

In a comprehensive child development center, parents are encouraged to be active participants in the life of the center. They are urged to voice their opinions in the running of the center; to volunteer their time or skills whenever possible; and join in the parents' activities be they educational, social or recreational. Staff members establish good relationships with the parents and work actively to keep them informed of their children's progress through individual and group meetings.

A Typical Day in the Center

Those who have not had the opportunity to observe a day care center in operation, may wonder what goes on during a typical day. Usually the children start arriving at about 8:00 a.m. but many will not appear until 9:00 a.m. The first hour is a flexible one filled with greetings, good-byes, brief parent-teacher conversations, short visits, the putting away of outer wraps, informal health inspections, and perhaps a first or second breakfast. Once everyone has settled down, the daily program begins.

Let us assume that we are visiting the four-year-olds today. There will be about 12 children in the group. Usually the first hour and a half is devoted to a work and play period in which children are free to choose from among countless activities and materials.

The room will most probably be divided into areas of interest such as the doll house, block corner, workbench, easels, fingerpainting table, science area, library, sandbox, clay corner, mathematics table and music area. There will be low storage shelves holding a variety of manipulative materials which the children will bring to their tables to work with. These would include puzzles, pegs and peg-boards, small construction and block materials, crayons and games. Children may have access to a tape-recorder, primer typewriter, or even a computer. The children are free to move from one activity to another providing the activity does not become overcrowded. The adults in the meantime are actively involved with the children. They may be helping some, talking with others, preparing materials or working with a small group on a special project.

A good deal of learning goes on at this time and the children are deeply involved in what they are doing. It is interesting to observe the relationships among the children: Who are the ones who always play alone? Who are the ones who are the leaders in group play? Who are the ones who are able to concentrate on an activity for some length of time?

This is also a time for verbal expression and interaction as small groups gather around the sandbox, plan a structure in the block corner, or enact a family scene in the house area. This may also be a time for release of tension as we observe children hammering nails, pounding clay or spanking the doll. Children develop small-muscle coordination and hand-eye coordination as they build block towers, put puzzle pieces in their trays, or place pegs in their peg-boards. Creative expression is encouraged by easel painting, finger painting, clay work, and cutting and pasting. There is mathematics going on as children estimate the amount of sand needed to pour into a cup or measure the piece of wood that must be sawed to complete a boat. Science is not forgotten as children care for the class pet, water plants, use the magnet or other science materials.

When it is time to clean up, the room becomes a beehive of activity as children put away the materials, tidy the shelves, sweep the floor, clean the sink and do all the things necessary to put the room back together again. After the routine of washing up, there may be a brief group activity such as a discussion of the weather, which children are absent, a finger play or song followed by the midmorning snack of juice and crackers. Afterwards the group may go to the outside play area or take a walk in the neighborhood to visit a local store or observe something within the immediate area such as the post office, a construction site, or a tree whose leaves are changing. Then it's back to the room to prepare for lunch. As the room is being readied for the noon meal, the children may listen to a story, sing songs, play the rhythm instruments or have a discussion.

Lunch is a highlight of the day and in most day care centers it is a full, nutritious hot meal prepared in the kitchen by an experienced cook. For many children, this may be the only full meal in the day. The food is brought to each room and is usually served family-style. Children are encouraged to help in setting the tables, passing the food and finally in the cleaning up. Less emphasis is placed on formal table manners or coercing the children to eat than on a relaxed meal in which children and adults converse freely and enjoy each other's company.

As the children finish their lunch and clean up after themselves, they may take a library book or quiet table toy while the room is prepared for nap time. In all-day programs, children sleep on cots in a darkened room. Although four-year-olds may resist naps, they usually settle down after the long active morning and sleep for an hour or more.

When the children wake up, they may play quietly for a while until the entire group is ready for the afternoon activities. These may include another work-play time, outdoor play, some special activity such as a film or another snack of fruit or milk; then gradually the parents or older siblings arrive to take the children home and the day is at an end.

Variations in Day Care Programs

The day care program described above is one that is commonly found in group day care centers throughout the country. These centers may be sponsored through local government agencies and supported by Federal and local funds. This pattern of subsidized day care cannot begin to meet the needs of those who wish to place their children in all day programs and, given the concern over Federal deficits, there is little likelihood of increased funding in the near future. Day care centers sponsored by religious groups, public schools, colleges, and social service agencies have also played an important role in providing needed services, and while they, too, have been growing in number and variety there is still an insufficient number to meet the demand.

A more recent development has been day care underwritten by private corporations with the support and encouragement of Federal and local government. Work-related day care centers are not a new idea and in countries such as Russia (Bronfenbrenner, 1973) and China (Sidel, 1973) child care facilities are provided from in-

fancy through pre-school. In the United States during World War II, centers such as those established by the Kaiser shipyards in Oregon could be found in factories and defense plants but they eventually disappeared once the war was over. Today, however, there is a growing trend toward centers that are sponsored and fully or partially funded by hospitals and large businesses. Over 2,000 corporations such as Procter and Gamble, American Telephone and Telegraph and International Business Machines provide some form of child care assistance and have found that it pays off with higher productivity and less employee turnover (*New York Times,* August 4, 1985). Many companies that are located in depressed urban areas use the day care program to attract employees to work in their factories and offices. They often open these centers to residents of the community as well. The Stride Rite Shoe Corporation of Boston is a case in point, having established its first center in 1971 in Roxbury, Massachusetts and a second when the corporate offices moved to Cambridge in 1981 (Working Parents, Volume 2, #6).

The sponsorship, funding and location of work-related day care centers vary widely. Decker and Decker have categorized these programs into on-site day care; off-site work-related day care; the consortium model in which several companies work together to sponsor a center; and work-related day care centers that are supported indirectly by companies which subsidize the centers financially or provide other kinds of support services.

In some states, local government agencies have assisted companies and community groups in developing day care centers within their communities. An example of such a center is the Merrimack River Community Child Care Center in Lawrence, Massachusetts. This program is sponsored by the Greico Brothers, a manufacturer of men's clothing, and supported through union contributions and private donations. The initial funding of this program was made by the Massachusetts Industrial Finance Agency and was an outgrowth of the Day Care Partnership Initiative, a two-year program begun by Governor Michael S. Dukakis in January 1985. The purpose of this program was to develop a model day care system in cooperation with schools, businesses and local government (New York Times, February 23, 1986).

Another variation of day care is the Family Day Care Program. In this type of program, a mother within her home will take care of approximately five children, ranging from infants through school-age children. The mother is hired by the sponsoring agency and her health, character and home conditions are checked. She receives training in a nearby resource center and on-the-job training by supervisors who visit her in the home. This program has many positive aspects such as a more intimate home environment and is especially good for younger children or those who might have difficulty adjusting to a large group.

There are still other variations of day care such as infant day care centers and programs that operate under private franchise systems.

Clearly there is no one pattern of day care service but all programs, regardless of sponsorship and funding, should provide quality care. Major problems include setting minimum standards and providing on-going supervision.

Careers in Early Childhood Education

For the student who has not yet decided upon a career, working with young children can offer many interesting possibilities in addition to providing service to the community and opportunity for deep personal satisfaction.

High school graduates can frequently obtain part or full-time employment as teacher aides or can volunteer their services. These jobs give the student experience in working with young children in a group setting under the direction of a more experienced person. The aide is not expected to assume overall responsibility but will be given tasks that supplement the activities of the teacher and the assistant. Aides should not only be limited to the housekeeping tasks such as setting up the room or distributing materials although these are important, but should also work with the children on a one-to-one basis providing individual attention and support as needed.

Educational Issues

Most day care center directors encourage their personnel to seek advanced training. Students who have graduated from a two-year program in early childhood education such as those offered by many community colleges, are able to secure positions as assistant teachers. With an additional two years of college and a bachelor's degree, the student is then eligible for certification as a teacher.

What was once strictly a woman's job is no longer such. Many men are seeking to work with young children and are being encouraged to do so. The realization that young children should have many male adult models with whom they can identify is one important reason for this trend. This is especially true in one-parent homes or when the male influence is limited or weak. There is also the awareness that young children are influenced by stereotyped sex roles and activities. This can be alleviated by

observing males and females in interchangeable roles such as those related to the physical care of children, housekeeping activities and the like.

Regardless of vocational interest, learning about children, how they grow and develop and the skills needed to work with them can help young people become better parents themselves. Preparation for parenthood should not be left to chance, good luck or some of the child-rearing customs that are part of the folk culture.

Conclusion

For those who question the concept of all-day care for young children, there are countless others for whom day care centers fulfill a tremendous need. Young children, growing up in families when both parents work or brought up by parents who may be struggling with the emotional and financial demands of single parenthood, need the nuturance and care that good day care programs can provide. Whether these programs are funded publicly, privately or by a combination of the two, they must assure quality care for the families they serve. If we truly believe that children are our most precious natural resource, then providing the best facilities for their optimum growth and development should be high on the list of national priorities.

BIBLIOGRAPHY

Bloom, Benjamin S. *Stability and Change in Human Characteristics.* New York: John Wiley and Sons, Inc., 1964.

Bronfenbrenner, Urie. *Two Worlds of Childhood. U.S. and U.S.S.R.* New York: Pocket Books, 1973 (Paperback Edition).

Decker, Celia A. and Decker, John R. *Planning and Administering Early Childhood Programs.* Columbus, Ohio: Charles E. Merril Publishing Company, 1984.

Article in the "New York Times," August 4, 1985.

Article in the "New York Times," February 23, 1986.

Article in the "New York Times," March 16, 1986.

Editors, "A Step Ahead in Corporate Care" *Working Parents.* Year-End Issue 1985. Volume 2, Number 6: 10-13.

Sidel, Ruth. *Women and Child Care in China.* Baltimore, Maryland: Penguin Books, Inc., 1973 (Paperback Edition).

White, Burton L. *The First Three Years of Life.* New Jersey: Prentice Hall, 1975.

Chapter 49
Who's Minding Our Kids? A Defense of the Traditional Family
Rita Kramer*

Some hundred and fifty years ago a visitor to this country, observing "the rude indifference which is so remarkably prevalent in the manners of American children," added, "I have conversed with many American ladies on the total want of discipline and subjection which I observed universally among children of all ages, and I never found any who did not both acknowledge and deplore the truth of the remark. In the state of Ohio they have a law that if a father strike his son, he shall pay a fine of ten dollars for every such offense. I was told by a gentleman of Cincinnati that he had seen this fine inflicted there at the requisition of a boy of twelve years of age, whose father, he proved, had struck him for lying. Such a law, they say, generates a spirit of freedom. What else may it generate?"

It is no wonder that Frances Trollope, or as Mark Twain called her, "poor, candid Mrs. Trollope," was, as he put it, "so handsomely cursed and reviled by this nation." Even then feelings ran high on the question of how we, as individuals and as a society, should raise our children. We are a self conscious nation, free to ask such questions, and for two hundred years we have been listening to those, from Cotton Mather to Dr. Spock, who are ready to give us the answers. Beyond Dr. Spock we now have the feminists, the egalitarians, and various other kinds of reformers in government, the media, and the academic world, all seemingly agreed on at least one aspect of social policy—the need to bring about greater equality; to facilitate it and—if that doesn't work fast enough—to require it.

Now what does this have to do with how we bring up our children—as individual parents and as a nation?

I think something has gone wrong in the way we interpret equality and that this misunderstanding is affecting the lives children live in their families and in their schools and eventually, by determining what kinds of adults they become, must have an effect on the nature of our society.

The equality on which the idea of this country was based was intended to mean two things: equality before the law—the same protection granted to all citizens—and equality for each to go as far in any direction as his own capacities would take him.

However imperfectly realized, this was the ideal that defined this nation. Is it still so? I think not, and ironically it is from efforts to do good—perhaps of a kind that cannot really be done at a price we want to pay—that many of our troubles come.

The questionable "good" I refer to is the guaranteeing of the results, not just the chance to compete for them, and the price of that is a degree of social control that can change the nature of the free society we are talking about preserving.

The belief that everyone is owed something more than freedom from restraint, something more than an opportunity to make the most he can of himself, is only one aspect of the distortion of the ideal of equality. It is embedded in a context of values that threatens to replace the traditional ones of effort, accomplishment, and self-control, of competing to achieve some goal for the sake of which one has to work hard and even make sacrifices, and of the idea that to live a full life one must care for others—not "humanity," just a few real people—more than for one's self and that this kind of commitment is most appropriately realized in marriage and family life, which means raising children together with all its pains as well as pleasures. Disappearing, too, is the idea that there are certain moral imperatives—rights and wrongs for everyone—and certain loyalties, certain values worth dying for.

These traditional values—middle-class values if you will—are threatened today by a contempt for the pursuit of excellence and for loyalty, by the belief that rewards

*Rita Kramer is the author of *In Defense of the Family: Raising Children in America Today* (Basic Books). This article is based on a speech she gave at a symposium on "Raising Children for a Free Society: Parents, Schools, and Public Policy" sponsored by the Manhattan Institute for Policy Research at the Harvard Club in New York City on February 3, 1983. Reprinted with permission from the Summer 1983 issue of *American Educator,* the quarterly journal of the American Federation of Teachers.

should be distributed regardless of effort, by the encouragement of self-expression and self-gratification rather than self-restraint, and by the definition of sexual activity as a kind of sport unrelated to lasting commitment and unrelated to childbearing and, therefore, acceptable in any form.

If we go back to the question with which we began—what kind of children do we need for a free society?—surely the answer is to be found in those traditional aspects of character like conscience and loyalty, the capacity to defer gratification of one's impulses, to work toward the accomplishment of a long-range goal, to empathize with others, and to nurture the young, even at some cost to one's self. A free society is one that can do without too many restraints because it is made up of individuals able and willing to exercise a degree of self-restraint. We need children with character—what psychoanalysts call ego strengths—the interconnected abilities to love and to work; to form early, long-lasting attachments to others, and to learn from them about the outside world and later invest one's energy in mastering some aspect of its varied possibilities to produce something as well as one can. That something can be some good or service, it can be knowledge, and it can be children.

The best means we have of producing such children is through the traditional family. Weaken it, and we're in trouble.

What are the crucial factors that influence individual development and what do they have to do with the agency of the family?

We all go from helpless infancy to mature independence through a series of stages as different in particulars as they are universal in sequence.

What happens in infancy that in some way determines everything that comes after is the formation of a strong, mutually satisfying attachment between the infant and one consistent care giver—optimally its own mother. The baby learns as they get to know each other that his needs will be met, that a recognizable *other* outside himself meets them. What is being learned in the context of a mutually engaging dialogue is a sense of the world as a basically good place, of others as givers of pleasure whom it is worthwhile pleasing, even by sometimes giving up some of one's *own* pleasures. This process takes place in the context of the hundreds of little transactions over bed and bath, table and toilet, that make up the small child's daily life. His home is his school, his mother is his teacher (his father, too, in his own way), and the lessons he learns—or doesn't—are the basis for what comes later when he goes to another kind of school away from home. Unless he has become attached to someone special enough and important enough to be worth giving up some of his infantile pleasures for, accepting the first

restraints of civilization, he won't develop the capacity for self-restraint he'll need in order to learn later on.

Through a process of identification with his parents' clearly expressed but not violently imposed rules he will internalize those rules and make them his own. It's a subtle and complicated process by which a child comes to recognize someone as of such unique importance that when that person makes demands, those demands must be accepted as part of himself rather than as external structures to be followed only when someone is looking.

This internal structure is conscience, and it begins only when the givers of love and the setters of limits are the same figures. It is in the resolution of the child's ambivalence toward parental figures of authority that character is born.

This process requires only the care that most normal people give their own children as a matter of course and without too much thought. But it is too important to leave to strangers and cannot be done very well by professionals in institutions, by groups of people who come and go in the child's life, or by anyone who isn't familiar with the subtle, individual ways that the child expresses his needs. For that reason, mothers who *have the option* do themselves and their children a disservice if they don't care for them themselves during the earliest years of life—the first three years, certainly, and until they go to school if possible. And those who would deny that it makes any difference who takes care of a child all day, that a little carefully scheduled "quality" time is enough to establish a parental relationship, do those who are listening to them a disservice.

The demand for day care for infants and young children to enable mothers to add to the family's discretionary income, or "realize" themselves in the job market, is one of the things that threatens to weaken the family. It weakens the connections between its members and robs children of what they need most to meet the outside world: a sense of belonging to a family with well-defined roles and recognizable rules, a sense of being a competent boy like one's father or girl like one's mother and the desire to grow up like the one and be loved by someone like the other and do all the mysterious and rewarding things they do together and out in the world with other grownups.

Restoring the prestige of mothering and of the intact two-parent family is only the beginning. Parents remain crucial to their children's lives, but their influence lessens somewhat when it comes to be shared with authorities outside the home.

And what the all-pervasive media have not done to deemphasize the importance of mothering the very young by telling women almost anything they can find to do is more important to the world and more fulfilling to themselves, they get another crack at during the school years.

The latency years, from about the time a child gets his second set of teeth until reaching puberty, are crucial in their own way. They are years in which the community has traditionally protected the child from the distractions of sexual arousal in order to master the skills and become acquainted with the ideas he'll need if he's to take his place as an adult in an increasingly complex, demanding, sometimes bewildering world. Those long, slow hours of childhood are for the reading and thinking, the puzzling and fantasies that give definition to the developing self. Books—the ones that have stood the test of time—open the world of the past without which no one understands the present, the world of heroes and quests in which the child sees reflections of himself and his desires.

The same questions, the same conflicts, have been around for generations. Some answers have proved better than others, and they, along with a measure of delight and the ambiguity that enlarges the mind and resonates in later life, are in the books kids don't have time for when they watch TV after school, don't even know about when they aren't even assigned anymore. We offer instead the latest "Young People's Books" dealing with up-to-date matters like drugs, divorce, menstruation, contraception, and race relations—in language purposely limited to the sixth-grade level.

If we do not teach the skills to understand and transmit our culture, which is a literary one, how will it be carried on? Through television? Through Family Life and Sex Education?

This is the name of a curriculum that no longer concerns itself primarily with what its planners scornfully refer to as "the plumbing" but with a store of information and a set of beliefs about sexual behavior that makes it a casual matter, equally acceptable in whatever form it takes. (For a look at the attitudes and values implicit in these courses, see "The New Sex Education" by Diane Ravitch in *The New Leader,* December 13, 1982, and "Teaching the Young About Sex" by William J. Bennett in *American Educator,* Winter 1980.) In Family Life and Sex Education the only thing that's wrong is feeling guilty. So we teach our children every attitude about sexual behavior except thoughtfulness and responsibility, remove from it all meaning except the gratification of the moment, tell them it's all right to do whatever feels good; in fact the only thing they're never told is *not* to do it. Not *yet.* We take care of that with contraceptives for kiddies.

All this, of course, is said to bring about greater freedom. We might ask, with Mrs. Trollope, what else it may generate.

The lessons not learned in sex education are taught in Values Clarification, a course of study that makes it clear

that all values are equally meaningful—or meaningless—since they are all subjective. Values Clarification teaches one thing: to be sure of your own feelings, of what it is you want. Clarified values stop short with gratification of a rather primitive and immediate nature and never consider that an individual might be gratified by doing right, even at some cost to his appetites. (William J. Bennett and Edwin J. Delattre evaluated the values curriculum in "Moral Education in the Schools" in *The Public Interest,* Winter 1978, and "Where the Values Movement Goes Wrong" in *Change Magazine,* February 1979.)

When parents find out what actually goes on in these cources, they sometimes make a fuss, feeling that their privacy has been invaded and their prerogatives taken over, but their confidence has been weakened along with their authority. Who wants to be called a reactionary?

Parents who are strong and sure individuals will take a stand against the cheapening and debasement of language, literature, and human experience where they can, but what they deserve from the schools and the media is, if not support, at least less undermining. What they deserve from government policymakers is more understanding of the real needs of children and less readiness to use publicly funded programs to subvert the authority of the family and weaken the ties that bind the generations in their effort to bring about social change, to effect an equality that denies distinctions between the sexes and the generations, as well as between degrees of merit and accomplishment.

But even strong parents will find they have their work cut out for them far beyond childhood: Adolescence begins at puberty, probably lasts too long, and ends presumably when the young adult has consolidated a sense of identity—sexual and vocational—sufficient to result in a commitment. By a vocation I mean a life lived in accordance with a self-chosen plan directed toward some achievement over time. Law and medicine are vocations, as are journalism, teaching, commerce, government . . . and mothering.

When I say of adolescence that it goes on too long, I'm not referring to its reputation for discomfort. Puberty is a biological event, but adolescence is a social construct designed to do many things, from keeping the young out of the labor force to providing a necessarily extended period for learning about the world and one's self. Neither of these tasks of the teenager is made any easier by the attitude taken by the social scientists, who encourage, and the media, which exploit, the notion that it is the phase-related business of the adolescent to rebel—against himself, his parents, and his society. Since the adolescent often finds rebellion an easy way out of the harder tasks that face him, he is all too ready to comply and live out the fantasies of the very parents and teachers he is presumably rebelling against. But many careful studies in recent years have shown that the tribulations of highly visible but small numbers of over- and under-privileged youngsters do not represent the average expectable experience of youth in this country, most of whom are more interested in joining the adult world than changing it—at least until they can learn more about how it actually works.

We owe them a chance to develop in a family with a mother and a father committed to their nurture, schools that transmit the rich culture that is their heritage together with the skills to extend it, and a public policy that doesn't do away with too much of their freedom, too many distinctions, in its zeal for equality.

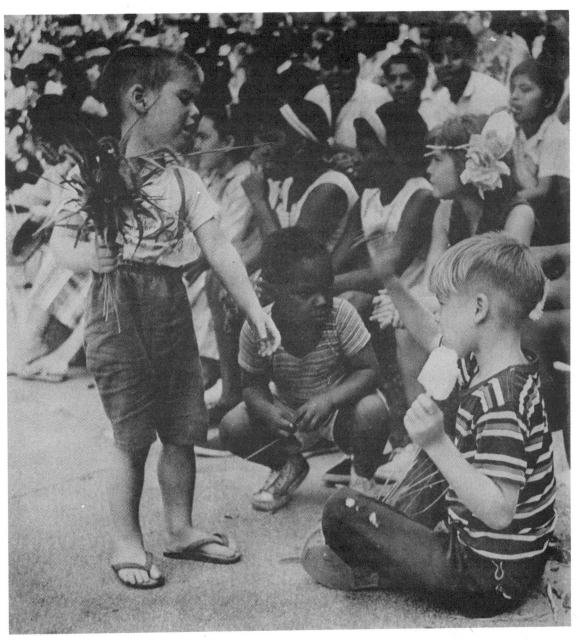

NYC Board of Education, Office of Continuing Education

Chapter 50
Children and the Welfare State: The Changing Role of Families

Mary Jo Bane*

The United States, like the other industrialized countries, is experiencing quite dramatic changes in the structure of its families and households. We see low fertility rates, low marriage rates, increasing numbers of one-person households, smaller household size on average, high and increasing labor force participation rates among women, and increasing numbers of single-parent families. These changes have generated considerable speculation about the "decline of the family" and the quality of contemporary private life. Most sharply, they raise the question of whether the state is being forced to take on responsibilities that families assumed in the past, or conversely (and more insidiously) whether the expansion of the welfare state itself has undermined the family and reduced its role.

Changes in the American family reflect three underlying trends, all of which are tied to long-term economic and social developments, and none of which, therefore, seems likely to be reversed in the next decade or so. The first trend is toward low or zero population growth leading to a population with a relatively small number of children and a large number of elderly. This stable, older population is due to a combination of low fertility rates and low mortality rates and now characterizes most industrialized countries. The second trend, which is probably both a cause and an effect of the first, is toward greater equality and independence for women. Women have gained political suffrage, birth control, and some measure of economic equality in most countries. Women continue to move from the exclusive devotion of their time and energy to home and family toward greater and more equal participation in economic and political activity. The third trend, a more general manifestation of the second, is toward greater autonomy and independence in individual living arrangements. People today feel less bound to spouses, parents, and children and more free to live and support themselves independently.

These three trends lie beneath the changes in family and household structure that most countries are experiencing. I believe they are also shaping a new set of attitudes toward, and social structures for, the care of dependents.

Our society includes a large proportion of dependents who require care and support from the able-bodied adult population: children, frail elderly, sick, disabled, handicapped, and retarded. Historically, these groups have been cared for mostly at home, in families, by women. Women generally assumed the responsibility for care and performed those tasks as part of their domestic roles. This continues to be the case. Most of the care of the old, the young, the sick, and the handicapped is still provided informally by women in their roles as wife, mother, daughter, and neighbor.

Nonetheless, there have been recent changes in the pattern of caring for dependents. Although the vast majority of children still live at home and are cared for by parents, out-of-home paid or public care of children is increasing almost everywhere. The elderly typically no longer live with their children, even when they are frail and in need of care; increasing proportions live alone or in congregate settings. Adult dependents have become more independent, living away from family and asking that care be provided in their own homes. Women are also becoming independent, asking that their husbands, and indeed society at large, share the responsibility for care so that women can participate more fully in other activities. These trends occur within a general demographic shift that has produced fewer young but more older dependents. Thus we see more households that include no workers, and more public and private resources being spent to provide support and care to dependents.

Are the changes in the characteristics and living arrangements of the dependent and in patterns of provid-

*Dr. Mary Jo Bane is Associate Professor of Public Policy at Harvard University's Kennedy School of Government. Reprinted with permission from the Summer 1983 issue of *American Educator,* the quarterly journal of the American Federation of Teachers.

ing for their financial support and physical care cause for alarm? They may be, but that depends on the answers to two other questions: Do these changes unacceptably reduce the quality of care for dependent groups? Will these changes reduce social integration and the sense of responsibility that people in the society feel for each other?

Discussions of the care of dependents usually focus on the changes that have been taking place within the family itself. But we can also look at changes in that sector of the economy that provides care and service to dependent groups. Like changes in family structure, changes over the last two decades in the social welfare sector of the economy have indeed been dramatic.

The Social Security Administration estimates the amount and proportion of total national spending on social welfare each year, primarily the care of dependents. These estimates show that public and private spending in the United States on income maintenance, health, education, welfare, and other services increased from about 16 percent of GNP in 1960 to about 27 percent of GNP in 1978, with most of the growth taking place in the public sector. This dramatic growth in social welfare spending could have come about in two different ways: from the transfer of services that would otherwise have been provided in families by unpaid workers (and thus would not have been calculated in the GNP) to the public and private monetized sectors of the economy, or from the provision of new services or higher quality services that supplement the care provided by families.

The substantial movement of women, especially mothers, into the paid work force suggests that we may simply be moving care from the family into the wage-and-salary sector. In the United States, the labor force participation rate of women aged sixteen and over went from 36 percent in 1960 to 50 percent in 1980; the labor force participation rate of married women with children at home went from 28 percent in 1960 to 54 percent in 1980.

This makes it appear that a massive transfer of caretaking responsibilities from families to paid caretakers in public or private institutions must have taken place over the last few decades. But the segments of the work force that logically ought to be absorbing this displacement do not seem to have grown in nearly the same proportion as the number of unpaid family workers has declined. Women not in the labor force, most of whom describe themselves as "keeping house," went from 51 percent of the 15-to 64-year-old female population in 1960 down to 40 percent in 1979. But over the same period private household workers and out-of-home childcare workers declined from 2.5 percent of the work force in 1960 to about 1.6 percent in 1979. Nonprofessional health workers (aides, etc.) increased from about 1 percent to about 2

percent of the work force. Thus the proportion of the work force engaged in caring for dependents stayed roughly constant from 1960 to 1978—and very small.

Other evidence that the entry of women into the paid work force has had less effect on the care of dependents than might have been expected comes from recent surveys on how children, the sick, and the elderly are indeed cared for. In the United States in 1975 only about 23 percent of children under two years and 25 percent of three- to five-year-old children were cared for by someone other than their parents more than ten hours a week. Only 4 percent of children under two years and 11 percent of three-to-five-year-olds were in formal day care or nursery school more than ten hours a week. These numbers are no doubt higher than in 1960 but they are still not very high. In the late 1970s only about 5 percent of the elderly were in institutions. Of those needing help, surveys show that most received it from family members.

At least in the United States, the movement of women into the work force does not seem to have been accompanied by a massive displacement of family care by the paid economy. Instead, it appears that women have taken on paid jobs *in addition* to their caretaking within the family. This has been partly assisted by other family members taking on additional responsibilities and by a decrease in the amount of housework that gets done by anyone. To some extent, this is because women are filling with paid work what was perhaps relatively unproductive time—while older children were in school, for example. (In the United States in 1980, only about 40 percent of the married mothers in the labor force were year-round full-time workers.) Or perhaps men and women are simply working harder and longer.

Whatever the explanations, not much of the dramatic growth in social welfare can be attributed to the displacement of family care. Rather, the evidence suggests that what we are seeing is mainly the provision of new and higher quality services by the social welfare sector. We see this in health, education, social services, and income security.

Health. About 34 percent of United States social welfare spending in 1978, or 10.2 percent of GNP, was devoted to health, the fastest-growing component. The vast bulk of health spending goes for hospitalization, physicians' services, drugs, and other goods and services that have never been, and indeed cannot be, provided by families. A portion of health spending, however, does go for nursing homes and other forms of long-term care—care that might otherwise have been provided by families. To some extent, nursing home care provided by professionals probably represents an improvement in the quality of care that the frail elderly and chronically ill receive. Nonetheless, the growth in spending on nursing home and long-term care might be one measure of the amount of displacement of families. Spending on nursing home care increased from 2 percent of health spending and 0.1 percent of GNP in 1960 to 8 percent of health spending and 0.8 percent of GNP in 1979. Despite this increase, the vast bulk of health spending can mainly be attributed to new or higher quality services, not changes in family care.

Education. About 23 percent of U.S. social welfare spending in 1978, or 6 percent of GNP, was for education, up from 4.4 percent of GNP in 1960. Most of this represented an expansion of educational services, especially for higher education. Preschool education also grew rapidly. In 1976, 20 percent of three-year-olds and 42 percent of four-year-olds were enrolled in nursery school or kindergarten, up from 7 to 21 percent in 1960. To the extent that nursery school is used by parents as a type of day care, increased spending on nursery school could be considered a displacement of the family, but most parents see nursery school as an educational and developmental institution and, thus, as supplementary to families. Even if all the spending on nursery school and after-school programs is considered displacement, however, it remains a trivial proportion of the growth in spending on education.

Social services. About 3.5 percent of U.S. social welfare spending in 1978, or 1 percent of GNP, went for social services such as day care, child welfare services, homemaker services, school breakfasts and lunches, and so on. Most of these services probably could have been provided by families, although perhaps not at the same level of quality provided by professionals. These services cause the most displacement, but are a very small proportion of total social welfare spending.

Income security. About 36 percent of U.S. social welfare spending in 1978, or 10 percent of GNP, was spending for income maintenance—social insurance and cash transfers. This was a very rapidly growing component of spending, up from 6 percent of GNP in 1960. About 85 percent of this spending was public, with the rest private pensions and private insurance.

Social Security, pensions, and public assistance might be thought of as pure social transfer payments whose sole purpose is to relieve families of the financial burden of supporting the retired, disabled, unemployed, and otherwise poor. There is another way of looking at income security programs that suggests that a large portion of this spending growth is new services.

Both private pension plans and social insurance involve substantial "intra-personal transfers"—that is, savings during working life for later spending during retirement, or insurance payments for unemployment or disability. The intra-personal component of these programs should probably be subtracted from estimates of social welfare spending. Truly intrapersonal transfers seem irrelevant to the general question of displacement of family care, although forced intra-personal transfers may result in some new spending on goods and services that would not otherwise have been purchased.

But social insurance (and other pension funds that do not operate strictly as annuities) still involves some transfers between people, since most beneficiaries now receive much more in benefits than would be expected on the basis of a normal market rate of return on their contributions. (This is likely to be true for most beneficiaries in the United States at least until the second or third decade of the 21st century.) Other income maintenance programs, for example Aid to Families of Dependent Children, AFDC, and general assistance, can be thought of entirely as inter-personal transfers.

In one sense, all these programs do represent replacement of family support. Money once changed hands privately; now it changes hands through taxes and transfers. The public transfer system is also used to purchase goods and services that might otherwise have been provided by families. Elderly men and women may now purchase food and help with household tasks without relying on their sons and daughters. But in another sense even the transfer system embodies a substantial component of spending on new and higher quality services. Most notably, the transfer system purchases the ability to live independently and maintain separate households for many elderly people and many single mothers. The privacy and autonomy that most elderly, disabled, and single people seem to prefer is probably the most expensive new service now purchased by the social welfare system.

One set of questions to be raised about the "new services" component of social welfare spending concerns how much should be spent relative to other government activities and whether this spending represents an efficient use of resources. Another set of questions, more directly relevant to families and the future, comes from the "displacement" component and from the fact that almost all the new services are being provided through monetized, and in many cases, public systems rather than through families. Indeed, part of the concern about the "decline of the family" comes from a sense that the quality of care provided outside the family is inferior to that provided by family members. Although this is no doubt correct in some cases, it is clearly not true across the board. But this view is so widely shared that it may be worth examining in detail with regard to children and the elderly.

Children. As was noted earlier, the increased labor force participation of mothers in the United States does not seem to have been accompanied by a corresponding increase in paid, out-of-home care of preschool children.

Relatively few parents use full-time nonparental care, especially for infants. Most seem to adjust the work schedule of family members to minimize the need for paid care. Parents mostly supplement their own time with informal arrangements, particularly babysitters who are relatives. For three- to five-year-olds, parental and informal care is increasingly supplemented by nursery school.

So the modal family in the United States still relies substantially on parental care, supplemented by nursery school and other arrangements. Much of the concern about the quality of care is therefore misplaced. The trend toward out-of-home care is much slower and has gone much less far than most people imagine. The biggest change—nursery school attendance—is one that most people consider a desirable improvement in the quality of care. I expect that the trend toward out-of-home care will continue at a very slow pace, with most parents choosing to adjust their own work lives to have time to care for their young children themselves.

Nonetheless, it is possible that the trend toward nonparental care will accelerate. We could conceivably see larger proportions of children spending more time in out-of-home care. The social-science evidence of what the effects would be for preschool children is by no means clear. The relative costs and benefits seem to depend on, among other things, the talents and motivations of the parents, the age and personality of the children, and the characteristics of the care facility.

The biggest concern seems to be that as children spend less time in the home they might not establish psychological bonds with their parents sufficiently strong to develop trusting and loving relationships. Psychologists do not know how much time, in what kinds of settings, jeopardizes these bonds. The normal pattern of child care in the United States does not seem to jeopardize them, but the trends are worth watching and one hopes that research into the question continues.

Elderly and disabled. Independent living for the elderly is strongly preferred both by the elderly and the families with whom they would otherwise live. The benefits of privacy and independence seem to outweigh those of companionship and shared labor, especially among most of those who can afford to live alone. Although loneliness can be a problem, it can be reduced through social contacts with family and friends. No doubt some elderly people live alone by necessity rather than choice, and the quality of their lives is no doubt lower than it would have been had they lived with family, but in general the living situations of most of the elderly have not deteriorated due to independent living.

Nursing home and other institutional care for the impaired and handicapped raises more difficult questions. One probable effect of paid care is that it provides a minimal standard of care. For many, this may represent an improvement over what they would have received at home. For others, the availability of institutional care may mean that they are placed in institutions rather than cared for in homes that would have been both adequate and humane, and would have provided more genuine personal concern, social contact, and individual dignity. In general, social research suggests that nursing homes and institutions are last resorts for families who can simply no longer care for an elderly or handicapped person at home. It could be that forcing certain families to provide care at home would result in higher quality, more personal care, but not in general.

So the new patterns of care for children, the elderly, and other dependents in the United States do not represent a decline in quality; indeed, they may mean an improvement over what would have been provided in the absence of changes in families and the social welfare system. This is partly because families continue to provide the vast bulk of care for children, and a substantial amount of the care of the elderly and chronically ill. Social welfare institutions and services supplement what families have always done and continue to do.

This new balance of family care and paid care is likely to continue, particularly for children; if it did not, that would be disturbing. If a larger and larger proportion of care for dependents occurred in the market and public sectors, and if family care came close to disappearing (which it conceivably could for the sick and the old, though I think not for children), this could be tragic. The tragedy would be that professionally provided care in segregated settings might not be provided by someone who genuinely loves and respects the dependent person. Caring could become a job, done by people who are paid for it and who have no personal investment in the well-being of those for whom they care. Interactions become routine and impersonal; although sustenance is provided, love, empathy, and companionship are not. A second effect might be that with less direct contact between the dependent and the working populations, the able-bodied adults who pay for the care might not know them as people, understand their situations, and be concerned about their well-being. This could easily lead to lower levels of financial support and quality of care, especially in hard times.

The changing role of women, which underlies all these transformations, raises another danger. Compassion and responsibility, expressed through personal concern and care, historically have been the virtues expected of women in their role as wives, mothers, daughters, and friends. The responsibilities of men have been in the public arena, to make the money to support dependents. Men have not been expected to personally care for children, the elderly, and the sick. As women enter the paid labor force, the division of labor and moral responsibility has become less clear. This seems an entirely appropriate move toward greater equality for women; the danger, of course, is that personal compassion and responsibility will be lost, rather than shared, as women spend more of their time in paid labor and caretaking is turned over to professionals.

In fact, this may not be happening. One reading of recent history sees the expansion of social welfare services along with substantial caretaking by families as an indication of *more* compassion for the responsibility toward the needy. Nevertheless, personal concern and care must remain. No one has paid much attention to nourishing these virtues in and through public institutions and policies; this may be the most profound challenge the welfare state now faces.

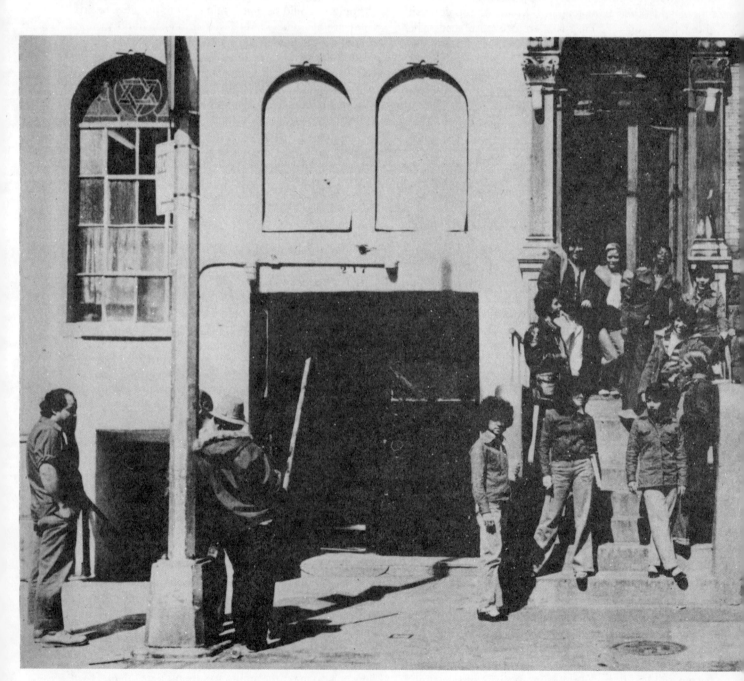

Ellen Meltzer

Chapter 51

The Powerful World of Peer Relationships

Julius Segal and Zelda Segal*

The Biblical scene is the Palestinian desert. Abraham and Sarah have been miraculously blessed in their latter years with a son, Isaac. Living in their household is the bondwoman Hagar, and her son, Ishmael, fathered earlier by the same Abraham.

In what may be the earliest recorded recognition by a parent of the power of peers, Sarah orders her husband to "cast out this bondwoman and her son." Ishmael, she fears, is an unwholesome influence, and despite Abraham's protestations, Sarah insists that he be removed from the environment of young Isaac.

The episode reflects an attitude characteristic of most adults concerned about the future of the young. Countless parents and teachers have similarly observed either with satisfaction or alarm the influence of friends on the lives of children. In the last quarter century, these convictions have been validated by numerous child development researchers. Their data are convincing. Sarah was right. Peers do, indeed, exert considerable force—positive as well as negative—on the destiny of a child.

The process begins in early childhood. At first, as two-year-olds, children typically engage only in "parallel play"—that is, alongside rather than with other children. While they enjoy the company of others, they do not yet fully recognize that friends have something unique to offer. Gradually, however, usually sometime between the age of three and four, children are likely to find themselves interacting in a purposeful way with a friend or two who are now part of their everyday lives—in the yard, in the nursery, in the park. Now it is only a short psychological step to group play, group friendships, and a selection process by which the young relate especially to those peers who are most meaningful to them. From this point onward, the child's destiny will be determined in part by the power of peers.

Indeed, in certain aspects of development, peer relationships emerge as a predominant force. As University of Minnesota psychologist Willard W. Hartup, a leading researcher on the subject of children's friendships, puts

it: "In some very critical areas, relations with co-equals is the key." Here are four of them:

Finding out how to deal with aggression. Parents can hardly provide a natural environment for the testing and modulation of aggressive behavior. The sometimes rough, give-and-take play experiences necessary for learning how to handle anger and hostility are incompatible with the nature of the child's bond with the mother. Children cannot easily experiment with "letting it all hang out" toward someone on whom they are still dependent and to whom they are still securely attached. Fathers, because their play with children is often more intense, may be in a position to contribute more to the child's learning about aggression, but it is doubtful whether they alone can effectively socialize even their male children' aggressive impulses. How can children effectively learn everything to be known about handling aggression, asks Hartup, in a relationship where somebody is always bigger and more capable than they?

Nature, it seems, has dictated that the child's relations with other children ultimately contribute more than adult-child relations in learning how to deal appropriately with aggressive instincts. Among their peers, children can feel safe in revealing their frustrations and rebellion in a way that is impossible at home. And in the rough and tumble of play, they can learn to act out these feelings in an acceptable fashion—discovering along the way the consequences of going too far.

*Julius Segal is a psychologist and writer who served for nearly thirty years on the staff of the National Institute of Mental Health. His latest book, *Winning Life's Toughest Battles: Roots of Human Resilience,* is published by McGraw-Hill. Zelda Segal is a school psychologist specializing in problems of early intellectual development. The Segals are authors of *Growing Up Smart and Happy,* also published by McGraw-Hill, and are contributing editors to *Parents* magazine. Reprinted with permission from the Summer 1983 issue of *American Educator,* the quarterly journal of the American Federation of Teachers.

Learning about sex. When we were children, our parents viewed the task of teaching us "the facts of life" as a sacred responsibility. It was inevitably one of the most awkward and poignant moments of family life when father or mother took a deep breath and attempted to discuss the "unmentionable." Today, of course, some of the responsibility for sex education is being shared by the schools. Our parents could hardly have known that in the matter of their children's sexual development, adults do not typically play the lead role.

"If parents were given the sole responsibility for the socialization of sexuality," says Hartup, *"homo sapiens* would not survive." No one, of course, would discount the well-intentioned efforts at sex education by adults, but as in the case of aggression, the often intense and emotional adult-child relationship is hardly well suited to serve as a conduit to the bewildering world of sex. Parental modesty, discomfort, lack of information, and lack of explanatory ability are additional impediments.

Even when parents make a deliberate effort to educate their young in sexual matters, most children continue to get their information from one another. Playmates can be free with each other in a manner not easily accomplished in the family setting. They can describe feelings and exchange questions without the inhibitions that usually exist even in the most modern and liberated households. To be sure, peers offer each other a great deal of misinformation, too, but ultimately, their free interactions help educate them and provide an important basis for their sexual attitudes.

Developing moral standards from within. Very young children typically behave as if they believe that society's rules are eternal and unchanging and that the power of parents and teachers to dictate standards of behavior is inviolate and total. In order to grow into maturity and independence, however, each child must eventually turn to living by standards of behavior that arise from within rather than from outside.

For an internalized moral sense to develop, the child needs opportunities to see the rules of society not only as dictates from figures of authority but also as products that emerge from group agreement. Such opportunities are richly provided through the social give and take among friends. A peer group inherently contains the dynamic interpersonal checks and balances that significantly nurture the development of a moral sense. Children are constantly arriving at value judgments about each other—accepting, rejecting, and criticizing each other's behavior, responding to each other's actions, helping each other arrive at decisions about what types of behavior are wrong and what are right.

Learning to behave with empathy—to put yourself in another person's position and to share responsibility for another's well-being—also requires experience with friends as much as directives from the child's elders. While it is true, of course, that altruism is often learned by modeling the altruistic behavior of adults, it is in their peer relationships that children find important opportunities to practice kindness and concern for others. Indeed, such interactions are often the key to helping transform the egocentric child into a human being with the kind of social consciousness and moral sensitivity that spring from the heart.

Finding emotional security. Many parents, deeply committed to the emotional well-being of their children, are frustrated at times over their inability to provide the emotional support, encouragement, or healing that a child appears to need at moments of stress. Once again, it is important to acknowledge that often it is peers rather than adults who are best able to fulfill this role. It is in the peer group that children find others functioning at their own level of emotional development. Only with them can they interact as equals, comparing their perceptions of life and sharing their stresses and conflicts.

As a result of their interactions with friends, children come to know that, psychologically, they are not alone—that their strange feelings of isolation or fear or guilt are shared by others. It helps when you are five, for example, to discover that you are not the only little person who feels anxious about school or sad about a pet that died. Like the rest of us, children need their own "social support system."

It is from their peers, moreover, that many children find ego-boosting strength through unqualified acceptance. Good friends typically permit each other to behave inappropriately on occasion without enduring severe criticism or losing face. Of course, children need the applause and approval of their elders, but those who are admired without reservation by their friends as well are likely to develop a special pride and self-confidence in dealing with the outside world.

Despite their demonstrable value to the child, peer relationships continue to pose a distinct threat for many adults. It is not unusual for teachers as well as parents to view friendship networks with suspicion and concern. They are fearful that friends will exert an unwholesome influence, causing behavior, motivation, and school performance to deteriorate. It is as if all our careful child-rearing and educational strategies will come to naught because of those "bad apples" in the yard, the playground, or the classroom. The result can become a contest: Who will control the destiny of our children? We who gave them life, support, and training, or friends who are likely to tarnish or even destroy their future?

Such conflict is almost always unwarranted. Studies show that friends do not typically work at cross purposes with the positive influences of parents and teachers. Indeed, the relationship between the child's standards of behavior and those of the significant adults in their lives is surprisingly high. The peer culture just does not disturb the child's sense of identification with committed parents and teachers as much as is popularly assumed. Rather than erasing the positive values taught in the home, the friends our children make in the world outside can actually extend and expand them.

It cannot be denied, of course, that the young, especially adolescents, can be led astray by a deviant peer group—into drugs, drink, sexual promiscuity, or delinquency. But unwholesome peer influences are likely to be significant mainly for children who grow up in environments lacking sufficient stability, direction, and warmth. Youngsters who feel insecure and without moorings carry out into the world a consuming need for acceptance by others. They have few misgivings about letting their parents or teachers down since they have little to lose in the first place. Acceptance by the peer group—*any* peer group—is all the acceptance they feel they are going to get, so they are willing to adopt its values, including distinctly antisocial values, at any cost. In effect, what children indiscriminately grasp for in their friends is what they have failed to find at home. Those who grow up enjoying solid family bonds are less likely than many parents fear to align themselves with peers who do not share parental values and standards.

Happily, that continues to be the case for most children today, even as family ties appear to be weakening. In satisfying the needs of their friends, and in seeking to have their own needs met, children come to appreciate a good deal about the reciprocal quality of human interaction. In learning to be generous with their peers, supportive of them, angry with them, and forgiving of them, they learn critical lessons about the nature of human comradeship. It is through their friends that they discover how to accept others as well as themselves—to give love and to find love.

Experience with peers is not a superficial luxury to be enjoyed by some children and not by others but a necessity in childhood socialization. Unlike Sarah in the biblical desert, we cannot today so easily manipulate the peer relationships of our children or pick their friends for them. We may help guide children in the selection of their companions, but having done so, we must leave friendships to ripen in their own way. Given what psychology teaches us about the power of peers, a critical task for adults—both teachers and parents—is to act as enthusiastic matchmakers between children and rewarding friends. We will serve the next generation best if we accept the power of our children's peers, recognize their presence, and work with rather than against them.

Anyone who has interacted for a time with children soon recognizes, of course, that not all of them enjoy satisfying interaction with friends.

"He just doesn't seem to get along with his friends."

"She just won't interact with other children." Such comments are frequently made about children who have trouble forming satisfying peer relationships. The reasons vary, of course, from one child to another, but certain patterns seem to stand out.

To begin with, some children are, by temperament, simply unable to make friends easily. A group of investigators, after studying more than a hundred children from birth through elementary school, concluded that one distinct group of them can be described from the very beginning as "slow to warm up." They are typically less upbeat than others, their responses are bland, they tend to withdraw from their first exposure to any new experience, and they take a long time to adjust to change. "A child who stands at the periphery of the group in nursery school may be anxious and insecure," say the researchers, "but he may also be expressing his normal temperamental tendency to warm up slowly." Even more extreme are children who are downright fearful and timid—a trait, according to Harvard developmental psychologist Jerome Kagan, that seems to be more enduring than others with which children come into the world.

Some children have trouble forming friendships because their insecurities result in displays of hostility, driving others away. Others, in contrast, manage somehow to become the scapegoat in a group. They seem to emit signals that they can be taunted or have jokes played on them. Eventually, they may give up trying to make friends, withdraw, and begin playing the role of "loner."

Still others seem to crave the companionship and attention of adults rather than peers—as if they wish to avoid the competition of their own kind. Such children often depend on teachers for emotional support. They become the "teacher's pet," and thus may further alienate their friends.

Keep in mind, too, that some children may be outgoing enough under normal circumstances but are passing through a stressful time that causes them to withdraw. A child who is anxious or depressed is no more likely to be gregarious than you or I when weighted down by feelings of fear and hopelessness.

Because the dynamics of poor peer relations vary, there is, of course, no one-for-all rule to help overcome the problem. Sensitivity to individual differences is the key.

Slow-to-warm-up or timid children require considerable patience. They seem to do best when encouraged to try new experiences—including experiences in a group—but allowed to adapt at their own pace. Too much pressure heightens their natural inclination to withdraw.

As Stanford psychologist Philip Zimbardo points out, teachers can help draw out shy students by arranging for them to participate in studies or classroom tasks with peers who are especially understanding and accepting and by encouraging other children to include them in their activities. Grouping children together who have common interests can also prove useful.

It helps also to find opportunities to build up the withdrawn or hostile child's self-esteem—for example, by encouraging areas of expertise and offering praise for the child's accomplishments. And when reluctant children do interact with their classmates, they should be reinforced for their efforts.

In encouraging children to overcome roadblocks in their peer relations, it is important for teachers and parents to work as a team, sharing observations and ideas. The world of friendships extends far beyond the classroom, and efforts to encourage its development should be coordinated and consistent.

There are cases, of course, when no interventions seem helpful, and these deserve special attention. Indeed a growing body of evidence—from both clinical observations and systematic research—suggests that chronically poor peer interactions may be one of the most potent early indices of later psychological difficulties. Put another way, if you were to survey all of the facets of a child's life, the one that might be the clearest "tip off" to the quality of the child's adjustment is the ability to enjoy rewarding friendships.

The evidence stems, in part, from a series of follow-up studies completed decades ago by psychologist Merrill Roff, in which children with problems in adjusting to peers were found many years later to suffer more than the usual range of mental health difficulties. Roff's results are now buttressed by more recent studies that also portray problematic later adaptation among such children. The prognostic power of peer interactions has been highlighted, for example, in the research of University of Rochester psychologist Emery L. Cowen and his colleagues. From their poor peer relations, a number of first-grade children had been flagged as being at greater risk for mental health problems later on. After thirteen years, these very children did, in fact, appear with a disproportionately high frequency as clients for mental health services.

To be sure, the pattern is hardly inviolate. Studies show, for example, that some creative and contented people were "lone wolves" as kids. But whether they were at odds with their peers or just wanted to spend time alone, they seemed likely also to be blessed with a number of very positive traits: flexibility, assertiveness, self-assurance, a sense of humor, curiosity, venturesomeness, resilience to stress, and constructive ways of reacting to problems.

On the other hand, when consistently poor peer relations are the dominant theme in a child's life and when the pattern is accompanied by other disturbing signs, such as rebelliousness, anxiety, depression, and acting-out behavior, teachers should consider helping to direct parents to sources of early professional intervention.

Chapter 52
The Drug Dilemma: Monster on the Loose
Leonard H. Golubchick*

When the former Soviet Premier Nikita Khrushchev visited the United Nations and pounded on the desk with his shoe while exclaiming, ''We'll bury you'' in reference to the United States, he must have had one eye on the expanding heroin epidemic in the United States at that time.

In order to understand the drug problem we must look inward and to our environment which produces a certain life-style and value system which creates the atmosphere which pushes the child to the brink of death in the form of drug abuse. Many times it is the upwardly mobile middle class parent who doesn't take the time to solve his own problems. Financial problems, familial problems which may lead to divorce, extremely active social lives, etc., all blind parents to their child's cry for help or their child's need to have someone to listen to them. So who's to blame if their child falls prey to peer pressure or rebels and takes drugs just to get a parent's attention? Likewise, in impoverished neighborhoods, parents are too busy trying to survive and to conquer bureaucratic mazes to attain basic services, or might have joined the throngs of homeless, to pay heed to warning signs that their child is headed on the path toward drug abuse.

Regardless of socioeconomic background, ethnic origin, or religious or political persuasion, drugs affect all alike. We cannot say who will be an addict or an abuser of drugs, but we can point to certain areas in which noticeable changes from the norms can help identify a preuser, an experimenter, or an abuser. The indices include: school attendance, grades, discipline, character of homework turned in, physical appearance, compulsive lying, being withdrawn, radical changes in behavior, wearing of sunglasses at inappropriate times to hide dilated or constricted pupils, stealing, association with known drug users (including drinking), lack of interest in school activities, appearing disoriented, drowsy, and even falling asleep in class. One must note that you cannot accuse a child of drug abuse without having a thorough investigation.

In recognizing the danger signs which may cause drug abuse, it is incumbent upon us to seek preventative measures. We must provide positive alternatives to drug use, positive peer groups, as well as intervention services. A massive commitment must be made so that necessary funding is provided. It seems that we always expend massive resources in the treatment of an ailment rather than in the prevention of it.

My work in drug prevention programs and as a principal has taught me that one turns toward drugs as a result of an unmet psychological need. The most influential factor in meeting one's needs in the environment is the one provided by the parents. A person could come from a financially poor home but could be richer than a wealthy person in terms of the presence of stable family life and consistent role models; both of these provide the impetus for the formation of a realistic value system and positive self-concept, while providing love and acceptance—all of which are necessary for good mental health and the development of a strong enough psyche to withstand peer pressure and say no to drugs.

A person who has a good self-concept isn't about to ''dope'' himself up with crack or pills or stick a needle in his arm because he can't cope with reality or certain life situations. A person who is not loved or accepted may take drugs just to be noticed. Thus, just as a child in school may be disruptive in order to get attention which is translated into love by the child; so too, drug taking becomes an attention getting device. Here the individual is trying to say: ''Listen to me . . . look at me . . . I am a person too.'' Furthermore, one who is socialized with a value system which would enable him to ''make it'' in this world will not turn to drugs. Moreover, a person who might succumb to drugs as a method of escaping from reality is one who becomes easily frustrated as a result of school life, job pressures, peer pressures, culture con-

*Dr. Leonard H. Golubchick is Principal of P.S. 20 Manhattan, New York City Board of Education.

flict, poverty, and alienation from the mainstream of the dominant society.

Overall, a person who has tendency to drug abuse is one who feels alienated from society and loved ones, and who has failed to cope with stress and reality, as well as failing to cope with anxiety, conflict, and emotional tension. Such a person, as a result of failing in school, perceiving that he's failing in his job or marriage, or unable to find a job might conclude, "I'm feeling low. I need something to make me feel good." He may "run into" an acquaintance who might offer him something that will make him "feel good." Although he knows that drugs are bad and illegal, his confused value system may rationalize: "Well, I could pick myself up. I'm no addict; what harm will it do?"

Thus, if a person has not developed the psychological processes to meet the strains and stresses of daily life and has not internalized a socially acceptable value system, then all the information, statistics, and first-hand knowledge about the dangers of drug abuse will be of no avail.

The Extent of Drug Use and Abuse

Drug abuse is one of the major social problems which erodes one's potential in our society. According to statistics gathered by the Alcohol, Drug Abuse and Mental Health Administration (1986), drug addiction clearly surfaces as our nation's number one health problem. It is estimated that close to 50 million Americans are addicted to nicotine. Some 13 million are abusing and are addicted to alcohol. Some 600,000 Americans are addicted to hard-core narcotics (heroin and methadone), with 250,000 of these addicts residing in New York City (New York State Division of Substance Abuse, 1986). One million Americans abuse tranquilizers and barbiturates. Between 4 and 5 million Americans use cocaine at least once a month—with 21.6 million having tried it at least once. An estimated 53 million Americans have used marijuana.

The price of drug abuse and addiction to our society is frightening. Drugs cost our society several hundred million dollars per year. Drug addiction is also our number one crime problem. Inevitably all addicts must lead a life of crime in order to support the monkey on their backs. The average addict's habit costs $30 a day. This means that an addict's habit for seven days a week—52 weeks a year—costs $10,950 for the year. Many habits range up to $100 a day. The average crack habit runs $300 per week. It takes $8 in stolen property to retrieve $1 in cash. So to support a $30 a day habit, the addict has to steal $240 a day or $87,360 a year (U.S. Justice Dept.). Police commissioners in New York City and New Orleans have estimated that drug addicts commit 50% of all property crime in their cities. Of all arrests, 85% were addicts. Alcohol is involved in more than 66% of our nation's

homicides, 50% of its rapes, and 70% of assaults, not to mention the staggering figures related to alcohol-connected automobile accidents and fatalities.

In a survey, the United States Justice Department found that heroin addicts and crack addicts committed 100,000 burglaries, robberies, and car thefts every day. This represents about 20% of all property crime committed in the United States. In Baltimore, Maryland a study over an 11 year period demonstrated that only 231 heroin addicts were responsible for 500,000 crimes.

The problem of the drug epidemic has also affected productivity in the workplace. Estimates range from 10% to 32% as to the number of workers using drugs on the job. Not only are these workers less productive, they are more prone to injury.

The highest rate of drug abuse has been among the 12-17 group and the highest rate of narcotic abuse has been among the 18-34 age group. This does not portend well for our society. The statistics also reveal that most first time drug abuse occurs before high school and that 61% of all high school seniors have tried one or more illegal drugs (National Institute on Drug Abuse).

Crack, a form of cocaine that has been processed for smoking, has been spreading in epidemic proportions. Of new admissions to drug treatment, 80% have been cocaine related (New York State Division of Substance Abuse, 1986). It is feared that the crack epidemic will be worse than the heroin epidemic of the 60s. Crack's attractiveness as a drug is due to the fact that it is relatively inexpensive, readily available, and can be smoked at the flick of a cigarette lighter. Crack gives an immediate high, and the stigma of taking a drug with needles (with their inherent dangers) and the dangers of free-basing cocaine are not there. Crack comes in small vials ranging from .3 cc. to .85 cc., and when filled with crack the vials sell for $5 to $450 (NYS Division of Drug Abuse).

Crack—crystallized cocaine that is smoked rather than snorted—stimulates the central nervous system and the brain. After long term use crack can induce severe depression, hallucinations, and paranoia; and after short term use it becomes highly addicting. An addict with a $300 a week habit (a senior in high school) stated, "Once you start smoking crack you can't put it down—it's very addictive—it's a monster." Crack's immediate gratification and strong high is followed by a crash where the user reaches emotional rock bottom; feels anxious, drained, and severely depressed. This may lead to taking amphetamines or tranquilizers. A crack user was quoted as saying, "When you come down, you're a million times worse . . . you feel horrible. Your next worry is when you're going to get more and how." (The Citizen Register, June 1, 1986).

The American Journal of of Drug and Alcohol Abuse (1985) has found that much drug use is accompanied by alcohol abuse. Evidence indicates that alcohol abuse often accompanies cocaine abuse. The effects of alcohol are supposed to calm the negative side effects of cocaine. Historically, there has been joint abuse in the sequential and combinational use of opiates and alcohol. In fact, during the 19th and early 20th centuries, narcotics were taken to reduce or cure alcoholism. There has been recent evidence demonstrating the abuse of alcohol with methadone use.

Additional risks with drug taking have been the incidence of AIDS among intravenous drug users. In New York State, 30% of the reported AIDS cases have been among intravenous drug users. Due to this fact, AIDS has been spreading to the heterosexual population. Deaths due to AIDS among intravenous drug users have increased significantly over the past few years.

Basically, there is one drug problem in the United States that goes practically unnoticed, and that is pill taking. Mainly through television and other commercial media we have become accustomed to the notion that a pill is the best way of dealing with the daily ''Blahs,'' the upset stomach, the hammer pounding on the head, and lightning bolts shooting through your sore muscles. In the United States today 35,000,000 Americans use sedatives, stimulants, or tranquilizers obtained by legal prescriptions. Approximately one million of these persons have become drug abusers. In 1970, five-billion doses of tranquilizers, three-billion doses of amphetamines, and five-billion doses of barbiturates were produced by drug manufacturers. These drugs have found their way into the American black market. The House Select Committee on Crime found that one firm was shipping drugs to a golf hole in Tijuana, Mexico, from which it found its way back into the American black market (Berstein and Lennard, 1973).

Valium and Librium are taken by more then twenty-million people in the country. Valium is the most prescribed drug in the Western World (Librium is #3) and has been prescribed for ailments ranging from insomnia, alcoholism, to painful sexual intercourse. These two anxiety reducing drugs are used whenever the users feel anxious or tense. Fifty-seven million prescriptions for Valium were prescribed in 1975 and some 15% of the adult population of Western Europe use the drug regularly. Valium and Librium act like alcohol or barbiturates in that they depress the central nervous system and produce the following effects: drowsiness, lack of coordination, mental confusion, and slurred speech. A person under the influence of Valium or Librium, when driving, is as dangerous as a person under the influence of alcohol.

As in the case of taking other drugs, persons taking Valium and Librium to reduce anxiety and tension develop a psychological dependence (the person thinks he cannot function or face difficulties without the drugs). A tolerance level is built up, that is, a tendency to take larger doses just to achieve the same result. Thus, after constant use, a physical dependence develops. If the person abruptly stops using the drug after long use, the person will experience painful withdrawal symptoms.

High school and college students have mixed Valium and alcohol at parties to ''get high.'' Valium's and Librium's side effects have been: drowsiness, headaches, nausea, fatigue, skin rash, anxiety, insomnia, and hallucinations. In some cases, instead of reducing anxiety and producing calm, the drug leads to rage and hostility. Librium has also been linked, as well as the tranquilizer Meprobamate (Miltown and Equanil), to the frequency of serious birth defects. And there has been a link between tranquilizer use and learning disabilities. The evidence at this point has not been conclusive and further research is needed.

Valium and Librium have many medical uses. They are mostly used as muscle relaxers and to ease the pain of muscle spasms, arthritis, backaches, multiple sclerosis, cerebral palsy, and heart seizures and strokes. Valium is also given to women at childbirth, since it relaxes the uterine muscles.

Another problem drug that is prescribed to thousands of school children is Ritalin. Ritalin is a behavior changing drug and is related to the amphetamines or pep pills. Although when taken by adults the drug acts as a stimulant, it has the opposite effect when taken by children. Ritalin is advertised as a treatment for children who have ''minimal brain damage'' or who are ''hyperactive.'' Schools often refer children who cannot sit still or pay attention or who are hyperactive. For short term use Ritalin might have the desired results in the classroom. Ritalin's side effects are loss of appetite, sleeplessness, instability, and stomach pains. Long term use can interfere with normal growth. With the emphasis on special education in increased funding for special problems, the use of Ritalin for hyperactive children might become an anachronism for some children.

It must be noted that drug abuse is a worldwide problem. In Britain, it is estimated that heroin addiction is increasing by approximately 5,000 individuals per year. Britain has tried to solve its problem through a program known as Heroin Maintenance. This is a program where the addict registers with a government sponsored clinic and receives a free daily dose of heroin. Considering that 15 years ago there was no heroin problem, heroin maintenance is not the answer.

Sweden's drug problem began after World War II. The major problem is amphetamine abuse or speed addiction.

Alcoholism, marijuana, heroin, barbiturate and amphetamine abuse is prevalent throughout Europe; and this includes the Communist bloc countries as well as Russia. In many instances, illicit drugs have been introduced to European students by Americans. In France, where wine drinking is the national pastime, a serious teenage drinking problem has evolved where Monday in school is a day spent mollifying the effects of the weekend hangover. In Moslem countries, Greece, and India, hash is the drug of abuse. Moreover, besides wide-spread growth in Turkey, Indochina, Thailand, Communist China, and Mexico have become areas where opium is grown and eventually reaches the streets of our cities.

In retrospect, I believe that the emphasis in our society should be placed on prevention; thinking in terms of the benefit to human life and society if we can prevent a person from becoming an addict.

In a drug prevention program, it is incumbent upon the workers to utilize the group in a positive manner. My emphasis in such a program is to provide positive alternatives to drug abuse through organizing a peer group with positive goals. In this group, peer pressures would enforce conformity to life goals which help one to "make it." Such a group would also help to decrease anxiety; to enable one to develop coping mechanisms to deal with life problems and situations; to give a feeling of success and power via involvement in decision-making processes; and to create friendship ties with group members. The activities of the group would consist of rap sessions, recreational and cultural activities, and trips.

In order to interest the group and to keep group solidarity, I utilized athletics. Team sports were organized. Pride in self evolved as a result. In a sport such as basketball, dependence upon one another in the form of teamwork is a necessity. Leadership and self-discipline can be developed. Through sports, I have found that one's personality shows through. For example, if an adolescent becomes easily frustrated in his life's activities, this can be viewed on the basketball court. As such, the sport, if positively directed, can become therapeutic in alleviating anxieties which cause frustrations. Thus, it helps the adolescent to cope with his feelings. In rap sessions, the way one behaves on the court (i.e., throwing the ball in anger or cursing and berating a teammate) can be discussed and evaluated in relation to the goals of the group and the activity.

Thus, through certain positively directed team activities one can learn how to cope with certain life situations.

Moreover, the life space of the individual can be so arranged through peer pressure and carefully directed activities so as to effect positive change and to create a new sense of awareness and power. Also, through group support and one's successful functioning in the group, one's self-concept can become more positive.

Another specific prevention technique is the utilization of peer leadership activities. These activities are to enable youngsters to learn how to make decisions, and they assist in developing leadership skills. Also, there is the utilization of classroom cycles where students are taught listening and communicating skills.

Moreover, no drug prevention program can succeed unless there is a balance between teachers, counselors, paraprofessionals, and student aides (older students who can provide a positive role model) who are workers in it. Such a program must have the support of the school's staff, administration, parents' association, and community in which it functions. For once a program stops serving the children and becomes a political tool, as it has in many New York City school districts, then it not only is failing in its purpose, but above all, it is failing the youngsters it purports to serve.

BIBLIOGRAPHY

Alcohol, Drug Abuse and Mental Health Administration Report, 1986.

The American Journal of Drug and Alcohol Abuse, 1985.

Bernstein, A., and Lennard, Henry, "Drugs, Doctors and Junkies." *Society* 10,4 (May/June 1973), pp. 14–26.

Cohen, Sidney, The Drug Dilemma. N.Y.: McGraw-Hill (1969).

Cuskey, W., and Krasner, W. "The Needle and the Boot: Heroin Maintenance." *Society,* 10,4 (May/June 1973), pp. 45–53.

Helm, Stanley, "Predisposition to Alcoholism." Resource Book for Drug Abuse Education, U.S. Dept. of Health, Education and Welfare (1971), pp. 87–89.

Fact Sheets, U.S. Dept. of Justice, Washington 1986.

National Institute on Drug Abuse, Report, 1986.

New York State Division of Substance Abuse, Report, 1986.

Yolles, Stanley. "Managing the Mood Changers." *NYC Educational Quarterly* (Spring, 1971), pp. 2–8.